Born to Talk

Born to Talk

An Introduction to Speech and Language Development

FOURTH EDITION

Lloyd M. Hulit
Illinois State University

Merle R. Howard
Illinois State University

Boston • New York • San Francisco
Mexico City • Montreal • Toronto • London • Madrid • Munich • Paris
Hong Kong • Singapore • Tokyo • Cape Town • Sydney

Executive Editor and Publisher: Stephen D. Dragin
Series Editorial Assistant: Meaghan Minnick
Marketing Manager: Kris Ellis-Levy
Production Editor: Janet Domingo
Editorial Production Service: Omegatype Typography, Inc.
Composition and Manufacturing Buyer: Andrew Turso
Electronic Composition: Omegatype Typography, Inc.
Photo Researcher: Omegatype Typography, Inc.
Cover Administrator: Linda Knowles

For related titles and support materials, visit our online catalog at www.ablongman.com.

Between the time website information is gathered and then published, it is not unusual for some sites to have closed. Also, the transcription of URLs can result in typographical errors. The publisher would appreciate notification where these errors occur so that they may be corrected in subsequent editions.

Library of Congress Cataloging-in-Publication Data

Hulit, Lloyd M.
    Born to talk : an introduction to speech and language development / Lloyd M. Hulit,
Merle R. Howard. — 4th ed.
        p.   cm.
    Includes bibliographical references and indexes.
    ISBN 0-205-45331-7
    1. Language acquisition.   2. Speech.   3. Language and languages.   I. Howard, Merle R.
II. Title.

P118.H85   2006
401'.93—dc22

                                                                                2005047553

Printed in the United States of America

10 9 8 7 6 5 4 3 2 1   HAM   09 08 07 06 05

To the most important people in our lives,
with immeasurable love and gratitude

Pamela, Yvonne, Carmen, Scot, John, Christopher,
Lance, Benjamin, Peyton, and Brianna
Bonita and Lane

Contents

Chapter 7

The Building Blocks of Speech   307

Chapter 8

Language Diversity: Regional, Social/Cultural, and Gender Differences   334

Chapter 9

One Tongue—Two or More Languages   376

Chapter 10
Speech and Language Disorders   404

Appendix
The Anatomical and Physiological Bases of Speech, Language, and Hearing   431

Name Index   465
Subject Index   473

Preface

It has been observed that during a child's first year of life, her parents cannot wait for her to talk and walk. These same parents spend the next seventeen years telling her to sit down and shut up! Why do children talk? Why do children walk? The simple and correct answer to both questions is—because they can. This book is devoted to helping readers understand that children talk because they are born to talk, because they can talk, because they have a biological urge to talk, and because that biological urge is supported by social pressures and needs that demand talking. Even though we authors have studied speech and language development and disorders for many years and have taught a wide range of courses on these topics to thousands of students, we retain the same curiosity and awe about speech and language that we had when we began to study and teach. In fact, the more we learn about speech and language, the more convinced we are that the whole process is probably impossible. In the pages that follow, we want to share our enthusiasm for this subject. We hope to stimulate in our readers the same passion that has driven us to appreciate the complexity, power, and enormous creative potential of language in all its expressive forms.

Although this book is grounded in relevant research literature, we did not intend to write a scholarly treatise. Although all university professors must serve in many roles, we view ourselves first and foremost as teachers. The purpose of this book is to teach, and the style clearly represents the manner in which we each approach teaching in the classroom. When we teach, we do not merely present information: We explain and provide examples. We ask questions and try to anticipate questions that will or should be asked by our students. When we introduce new concepts, we thoroughly explain the terminology. We review information already discussed to provide a foundation for new information. We reach forward to help students understand where we are headed and to sense what the final outcome will be. We prefer to err on the side of providing too much information rather than on the side of assuming too much knowledge. Above all, we believe that learning should be stimulating and enjoyable, and we have tried to write a book that is stimulating and enjoyable to read. Many books written by professors are heavy on jargon. This book is not. It was impossible to avoid the jargon entirely, of course, because jargon is the language of the discipline, but when we used these terms, we did not assume familiarity.

One of the difficulties involved in writing a textbook is that one must write the book to meet the needs of instructors who teach certain targeted courses, but if the book is to be an effective teaching tool, it must be addressed to the student. We have tried to walk the line between the instructor's needs and student's needs carefully. We will gladly admit, however, that when these needs appeared to collide, we chose to communicate as clearly and directly as possible to the students who will read the book. In doing so, we have created what we hope is a reader-friendly introduction to speech and language development.

The first edition of this book was used in courses representing a number of disciplines and was read by students with widely varying academic backgrounds. We have kept this wide audience in mind as we prepared each new edition. Some readers, for example, will be less familiar than others with information pertaining to the anatomy and physiology of speech, language, and hearing. We have included this information in the appendix (*The Anatomical and Physiological Bases of Speech, Language, and Hearing*). Majors in speech–language pathology and audiology may want to consult this material for purposes of review, but it is strictly introductory and is not intended to include all one needs to know about the structural and functional bases of human communication.

Several chapters of the book have been written as independent units: Chapter 8 (*Language Diversity: Regional, Social/Cultural, and Gender Differences*), Chapter 9 (*One Tongue—Two or More Languages*), and Chapter 10 (*Speech and Language Disorders*). These chapters can be included or deleted without affecting the book's integrity.

In the fourth edition, Chapter 10 has been significantly reduced. We believe that a chapter on disorders is relevant in a book devoted to the development of speech and language, but readily acknowledge that this chapter must be included with an appropriate degree of perspective. For that reason, the sections on speech disorders—phonological/articulation, voice, and fluency difficulties—have been reduced to very basic introductions. Because this book is concerned with language, however, the section on language disorders in Chapter 10 has been fully retained.

The most noticeable change to the fourth edition is the addition of Chapter 9 (*One Tongue—Two or More Languages*). This chapter is, in some ways, an extension of Chapter 8 (*Language Diversity: Regional, Social/Cultural, and Gender Differences*). Since the first edition of *Born to Talk* was written, the demographics of the United States have changed dramatically. As the nation has become more culturally diverse, leaders have been challenged to face the issue of bilingualism among the populace, particularly among those who have immigrated to the United States. The issue, as we address it in Chapter 9, is about more than language. It is about culture and about the choices people have to make when they embrace the United States as their new home.

Chapter 7 (*The Building Blocks of Speech*) is not an independent chapter, but the subject matter does pose a unique problem for those who write about speech and language development. The topic—the development of the speech sound system—must be addressed because it is absolutely fundamental to speech as an oral expression of language, but how and where should it be addressed? We chose to keep the language chapters together, make references to phonological issues in these chapters as necessary, and insert a separate, more comprehensive chapter on phonology following our discussion of speech and language development. Note, however, that Chapter 7 has been written so that it can be moved to the beginning or the end without affecting understanding of the material in any other part of the book.

The primary focus of this book is on language. Chapters 1 through 6 are devoted to language development. Whereas other books divide language development according to the various components of language (i.e., syntax, morphology, semantics, pragmatics, etc.), ours is a *real-time* presentation of development, divided by stages. We have integrated our discussion of the components within each stage. This will allow the reader to sense what the child is receiving and producing at each developmental level and will facilitate an understanding of how one aspect of language affects all other aspects.

It is important that instructors and students alike clearly understand the purpose of Chapter 1 (*A Connection of Brains*). This chapter is not designed as much to present information as it is to pique the reader's interest. We understand that some students who read this book will already have some background in speech and language, but others will not. Students with little or no background in speech–language pathology or linguistics have probably not given much thought to the process of human communication. The sole but important purpose of Chapter 1 is to prod the reader into thinking about language as a unique human experience and to appreciate speech as an incredible means by which messages encoded in language forms can be transmitted from one human brain to another human brain. This purpose is met by considering a classic linguistic essay written in 1960 and an equally classic view of brain-to-brain connection originally written in 1973 and updated in 1993. We believe that students cannot truly appreciate what is now understood and believed about language and language development without understanding the historical context from which the present knowledge originated. Chapter 1 provides that context.

Before we get to our acknowledgments, we want to address the gender strategy used in writing this book. As husbands and as members of a profession that is more than 80 percent female, we are sensitive to the gender problem in communication. We are also frustrated by the limitations of American English pronouns. For this reason, we decided to alternate the use of feminine and masculine pronouns, with the understanding that these pronouns are intended to be gender-neutral in all contexts. We also decided that referring usually to the child in the singular (versus the plural *children*) would be consistent with our intention to create an image of *one* child whose speech and language development we study through the pages of this book.

There are occasional personal references in this book, indicated by first-person pronouns and by phrases such as *my sister, my daughter, my grandchildren,* and *my father.* All of these references are reflections of the life experiences of the senior author.

We want to acknowledge the invaluable contributions of several people. Howard Davis created the anatomical figures in the appendix. Pamela Hulit provided computer assistance in creating a number of tables included in the book. We appreciate the special talents of these people and are grateful for their efforts on our behalf.

We want to acknowledge Dr. David L. Tucker for his contributions to Chapter 6. Dr. Tucker, whose primary scholarly and teaching focus is reading, is a professor in Illinois State University's Department of Specialized Educational Development. The material in the section of Chapter 6 titled *Reading and Writing: New Applications of Language* was contributed by Dr. Tucker and edited by the senior author.

We want to express a special gratitude to our students, a group of young women and men who enriched our professional lives by their presence in our classrooms. Our students never allowed us to be complacent. They constantly challenged us to know more and understand better, just as we tried to challenge them to learn, integrate, and apply knowledge to the solution of real-life problems. They asked penetrating questions that required us to continue the process of learning. Their curiosity became our curiosity, and that is what makes teaching one of the most satisfying of human endeavors. We thank all Illinois State University students who shared time with us in our collective effort to understand more about communication development and disorders.

Finally, we want to thank the following people who reviewed the fourth edition of this book: Robert J. Ackerman, East Stroudsburg University of Pennsylvania; Bertha Smith Clark, Middle Tennessee State University; Ellen Stubbe Kester, The University of Texas at Austin; and Sharon M. Rogers, California State University, Fullerton.

Lloyd M. Hulit, Ph.D.
Merle R. Howard, Ph.D.

Born to Talk

1

A Connection of Brains

CHAPTER OBJECTIVES

This first chapter is designed to pique your interest in speech and language as processes within the broader process we call communication. We define and describe these processes, and we consider how speech and language interact to produce a form of communication unique to humans. We also consider how a speaker's thoughts are conveyed to a listener's brain through a series of communication transformations known collectively as the *speech chain*. Specifically, this chapter is designed to facilitate understanding of the following topics:

- Definitions of *communication, language,* and *speech*

- Speech and language as separate but related processes

- Design features of the human communication system

- The speech chain that connects the speaker's thoughts to the listener's understanding of those thoughts

1

The idea for *Born to Talk* was cultivated long before the first word of the original manuscript was written, and it was probably a good thing that there was a period of latency between the concept and the product. During that latency, I observed language development first hand in my two daughters, Yvonne and Carmen. I learned more about the power and wonder of language in observing them than I have in all the books and all the journal articles I have read over the course of my career because I witnessed their processes of discovery. I watched and listened as they made connections between the world in which they were growing up and the words and language forms that spilled out of them. They are now grown, and they have blessed my wife and me with five grandchildren, giving me five more opportunities to observe speech and language development close up and personal. The births of my grandchildren have spanned the time from the first edition of this book to the fourth. Each of them has reinforced my appreciation of language as one of humankind's greatest gifts and most powerful tools. As my colleague and I labor on the fourth edition, there is a new addition to my family—an eight-month-old eclectus parrot, named *Toby*. We are trying to teach Toby to talk. So far he says, "hello" and "step up." These are certainly not momentous utterances. They fall short of the magic of Abraham Lincoln's "Four score and seven years ago . . ." and John F. Kennedy's "Ask not what your country can do for you . . ." and Pee-wee Herman's "I meant to do that," but they are the beginning of speech, or at the very least, the beginning of speech-like behavior. What is fascinating about observing Toby is that the process of acquisition is so different than the process in human children, and it will always be different. His utterances, no matter how many he produces over his lifetime, will always be conditioned responses, and there is no way we will ever know if there is any connection between what is going on inside his parrot brain and what we believe in our human brains he is saying, which leads us to the power of ESP in speech and language.

Have you ever wished you could read someone's mind or ever wished or worried that someone could read your mind? Probably all of us at one time or another have at least wondered about mental telepathy, and perhaps some of you reading this page believe you have that gift. We would like to suggest that every person reading this page who is able to speak is capable of a form of mental telepathy, because human speech allows one human brain to communicate with another human brain in a wondrous and almost magical manner.

Most people give very little thought to the magic of speech because it is acquired so naturally and used by humans so effortlessly. It is the purpose of this book to explore the miracles of speech and language, to examine the marvelous anatomic structures and physiological processes we humans have adapted for speech, to unravel the layers of language from sounds to words to elaborate sentence structure that together make up speech, to investigate the dialectal differences in our own language, and to consider the problems that occur when speech and language do not develop properly or when something goes wrong after communication skills have been normal for a while. By the time you have turned the final page in your journey through this book, we believe you will be convinced that words such as *magic* and *wondrous* and *miraculous* in reference to speech and language are accurately descriptive, but before we go any further, we need to address some basic terminology.

Separate but Related Processes

In the preceding paragraphs we have used the words *speech* and *language* in a manner implying they are not the same thing, which is correct. They are separate but related processes in the larger process called communication. To understand any of these processes, you must understand all of them and how they are interconnected.

Communication is the sending and receiving of information, ideas, feelings, or messages. To appreciate the breadth of communication, consider just some of the methods by which human beings communicate. We transmit messages of all kinds by speech, the written word, Morse code, semaphore flags, Braille, facial expressions, gestures, art, music, dance, the distances we maintain when we interact, vocal variations, the clothes we wear, hairstyles, our natural and purchased odors, and the list goes on. We communicate hundreds, perhaps thousands, of messages every day. Some of our communications are intended, but many are not. We hope that most of what we send is received according to our intent, but unfortunately this is not always the case. The fact is, we humans cannot stop communicating even when we want to. You may decide to say nothing, but your saying nothing may be saying more than your saying something. Even when you are asleep you may be sending messages. You may talk in your sleep, of course, but even in the silence of unconsciousness, you may communicate restlessness by the way you thrash around in your bed, or you may communicate a basic insecurity by the way you curl into the fetal position, or you may transmit a message of utter tranquility by the relaxed and peaceful expression on your sleeping face. Do you get the point? Communication is so much a part of the human experience that we are constantly sending and receiving messages.

Language is an infinitely more difficult phenomenon to describe, so we will build a definition by first looking at some of the characteristics of language and then trying to piece them together. Most people think of language as "words strung together by grammar," but that captures only a part of language and only what appears on the surface of what we read or hear.

Language is an expression of an ability that is innate in all humans. We are born with the capacity to use language in the same way a spider is born with the ability to weave webs, and a bird is born with the ability to make a nest. To use language is instinctive in humans, but the capacity is realized differently in people according to the specific languages to which they are exposed. A child reared in a family of English-speaking adults, who hears only English during the language acquisition period, *will* speak English. You might be surprised that the logic of that observation escapes some people. My youngest sister, abandoned by her natural Korean parents, was adopted by the Hulit family when we lived in Korea. When we returned to a small town in rural Ohio two years later, some people were amazed that she spoke English without a Korean accent. Children do not know they are German, French, Russian, or Japanese when they are born. They speak the language they hear, but the innate capacity for that language is the same, no matter where they are born.

It is important to understand that language and the expression of language are two very different things. Language exists in the mind, and it exists whether it is expressed or not. It is useful to understand language as a system of abstract symbols organized according to basic rules that seem to be common to all the languages known to humankind. In other words, at the deepest, most basic level, all languages share common structural rules.

The fact that we do not all speak the same language suggests that some aspects of language are learned. Languages are different in many ways. They use different words. They have different rules for organizing words into grammatical sentences. English, for example, stresses word order in its grammar system, but other languages, such as Latin, place greater emphasis on word endings than on order to indicate grammatical relationships. That is, all languages have rules for making sentences grammatically correct, but the means by which correctness is achieved vary. We can conclude, therefore, that although the capacity for language is innate and although certain very basic rules are shared by all languages, the specific conventions of any given language are learned. The child who will speak English, for example, must learn the sounds of English as well as its vocabulary and grammar.

Now let us put some of these pieces together into a definition. **Language** is a system of abstract symbols and rule-governed structures, the specific conventions of which are learned. The symbols of language may be sounds that are combined into spoken words, or letters that are combined into written words, or even the elements of sign language that are combined into larger units. It is important to note that whatever the symbols, they are arbitrarily established by the conventional usage of a given people. Furthermore, the symbols or their combinations will change over time because language is a constantly evolving phenomenon. Much more needs to be added to this definition (and will be in the chapters that follow), but this will serve as a starting point.

We can now define speech, a relatively simple task if we understand communication and language. Very simply, **speech** is the oral expression of language. Sometimes people use the terms *language* and *speech* as though they are interchangeable, but they are clearly not. If they were interchangeable, one could not exist without the other because they would be one and the same thing. In fact, speech can and does exist in the absence of language, and language exists in the absence of speech. Consider the parrot or mynah, birds that can mimic human speech, often with remarkable clarity. These birds produce speech, but they do not have language. That is, they can produce strings of sounds with the acoustic characteristics of human speech, and human listeners recognize the sequences of sounds as words, but the speech of these birds is devoid of meaning and, therefore, is not the oral expression of language. They have speech but no language. Some human beings, most notably severely mentally retarded individuals, may have the ability to imitate speech perfectly even if they do not fully understand the language underlying the speech. They have speech that reflects language abilities they do not have. Even normal children, between the ages of eighteen to twenty-four months, often produce a form of speech known as **echolalia,** which is an imitation of words, phrases, or even whole sentences in the absence of an understanding of what they are saying.

Language can also exist independently of speech. Children who are born deaf, for example, may never learn to speak, but their deafness does not preclude language. If these children have no other problems and receive proper stimulation and appropriate educational opportunities, they can develop language abilities just as sophisticated and complete as the hearing child who speaks. The deaf child who does not have speech must learn a different way to express language, most likely through signs and gestures. In addition, of course, the deaf child can receive and express language through the written word.

We can best understand speech as a highly complex physiological process requiring the coordination of respiration, phonation, resonation, and articulation. Some of the movements involved in producing even the simplest of utterances are simultaneous and others are successive, but the synchronization of these movements is critical.

Consider just some of what happens in the production of the single word *statistics*. The tip of the tongue is lifted from a resting position to an area on the roof of the mouth just behind the upper teeth called the **alveolar ridge** to produce the "s" sound. The tongue is pressed against the alveolar ridge hard enough to produce constriction, but not so hard as to stop the airflow altogether. As the speaker slowly contracts the muscles of exhalation under precise control, air is forced between the tip of the tongue and the alveolar ridge. Leaving the tongue in the same area, the speaker now presses a little harder to stop the air flow and then quickly releases the contact for the production of the "t" sound. The tongue drops to a neutral position and the vocal folds in the larynx vibrate to produce the vowel "a." The speaker turns off the larynx and lifts the tongue to the alveolar ridge for the next "t," then vibrates the vocal folds for the vowel "i" while the tongue stays in a forward but slightly lowered position. The speaker turns the larynx off again and moves the tongue to the alveolar ridge yet again to produce the controlled constriction for the next "s," followed by increased pressure to stop the air flow and release it for the "t." The larynx is turned on one more time and the tongue lowered to a neutral position for the "i," and then turned off as the tongue arches to the back of the mouth where it contacts the velum, or fleshy part of the roof of the mouth, for the "k." Finally, the tongue tip darts to the alveolar ridge for the production of the final "s" sound.

All of this occurs in the production of *one* word! Imagine what occurs in the production of a long sentence produced at an average rate of speed. When you consider how many intricate adjustments are made so quickly in the speech mechanism, it is difficult to imagine that anyone learns to speak at all. But we do learn to speak, and we do it easily and naturally over a very brief period of time.

Speech and Language Rejoined

Now that we have established that speech and language are separate, although related, parts of the communication process, we will reconnect them for the remainder of our analysis. For practical purposes, in people with normal communicative abilities, they are not separate. Speech is commonly understood as oral language, and that understanding will serve our purposes well. It is certainly clear to anyone who has studied the development of communication in children that speech and language develop together, but we should always remember that they do not develop at the same pace. Most of what a child will ever know about language is acquired before entering school, but some speech sounds are not mastered until age seven or eight. Even within language itself, not all dimensions are acquired according to the same schedule. Rules pertaining to the structure of language are acquired early and most of the basic vocabulary of a language is learned early, but we may continue to add vocabulary as long as we live, and most of us are developing our knowledge about how to use language, a dimension called **pragmatics,** well into adulthood.

From this point on, however, we will consider speech and language as integrated parts of the same process in the same way that pictures and sounds are integrated parts of television. You can certainly have television without pictures: It's called radio. And you can have television without sound: That's called network difficulty. But television as we expect it includes not only pictures but also sound. Speech as we expect it in normal human beings combines phonated and articulated noises and the rule-governed structures of language.

The Unique Characteristics of Human Speech

To appreciate the powers of oral language, we can compare it to the communication systems of other animals. Other animals do communicate, of course, but there is much we do not understand about their systems. Some animals seem to communicate very general messages in simple ways. The beaver, for example, slaps its tail when it senses danger. Dogs bark when they are frightened or excited. Other animals are able to communicate more elaborate messages. Bees dance to tell their fellow bees where the flowers are. Other insects use their antennae to instruct or inform. There is a great deal of interest in the communication systems of dolphins and singing whales because they seem to be much more elaborate than the systems of most other animals (Herman & Forestell, 1985; Janik, 2000; Schusterman, 1986; Tyack, 2000). No matter how much we discover about the abilities of other animals to communicate, however, we remain convinced that no animal has a communication system as powerful as human speech.

One of the first linguists to take a detailed, analytical look at the characteristics of human speech in comparison to the communication systems of other animals was Charles F. Hockett (1960), who wrote a classic essay entitled "The Origin of Speech," in which he describes what he calls "thirteen design-features" of language. Although many animals share some of these features in their communication systems, Hockett believed that when his thirteen features are taken together, they effectively separate human speech from other forms of animal communication. Since Hockett wrote this essay, many of his assumptions and conclusions have been dismissed as the result of research data and new theoretical interpretations. Nevertheless, "The Origin of Speech" remains an important part of the literature on human language, because it challenged linguists to think about language and those who use language in revolutionary ways.

From Mouths to Ears

Hockett's first design-feature is the **vocal-auditory channel.** That is, human beings communicate by forcing air through the vocal folds of the larynx and breaking the vibrating air stream into sounds of speech, which are organized into words and sentences. These sounds are received by the listener's ears. This feature is so obvious that we may need to note that other channels can be used in communication and are used by other animals. Bees, for example, communicate by dancing, and that can be described as the visual channel. In fact, human beings who cannot hear use the visual channel when they produce and receive sign language. Still other animals communicate by touch or by odor. The primary advantage of the vocal-auditory channel for humans is that it leaves our hands free to do other things while we are communicating. We can build or repair, for example, while giving or receiving instructions. Imagine what it would be like for a construction crew building a house if everyone had to put down their tools every time one person needed to communicate with another through the gesture-visual channel. There is no question that vocal-auditory communication is convenient and allows us to be efficient in all tasks that involve communication in conjunction with other physical activities.

Sending and Receiving Signals

The second design-feature is **broadcast transmission and directional reception,** which is obviously related to the first feature. Two characteristics of speech are involved in this feature. When speech is produced, it radiates in all directions and can be received by any listener who is in range. In addition, a listener with two good ears can compare the loudness and timing of the signals reaching each ear and can determine the direction from which the sound is coming. If communication is visual, reception is much more limited. Deaf sign language, for example, can be received only by someone who is close enough to the sender to see the details of the gestures, some of which are quite subtle, and the receiver must directly face the sender.

Hear Today, Gone Immediately

Rapid fading means that speech signals are transitory. They do not linger. Humans have developed writing to put language information into a more permanent form, but writing is a relatively new ability for human beings, in comparison to speech. We have also developed electronic means for preserving speech, but each time a sample of speech is produced live or on tape, the signals are broadcast and rapidly fade. We cannot freeze-frame speech and study it in the same way we can read and study the written word or primitive paintings on the cave walls of prehistoric people.

If You Can Say It, I Can Say It

One feature of human speech that we may take for granted is **interchangeability.** This means that any human being can say anything that is said by any other human being. Children can and do imitate the speech of adults. Female humans can produce the same speech forms as are produced by males. Among other animals, this feature is rare. In courtship rituals, for example, the male of many species produces gender-limited communications, and the female produces gender-limited responses. Interchangeability removes communication barriers and is largely responsible for the unlimited exchange of information that characterizes human speech for both sexes and all ages.

Did I Say That? . . . Did I Mean That?

Total feedback means that human speakers have the capacity to monitor what we say and how we say it. We hear ourselves, of course, but we also receive information from the musculature of speech about what we feel as the articulators move and contact one another. This feedback component allows the speaker to make constant adjustments so that output is as finely tuned as possible in terms of conveying thoughts accurately. Feedback also provides controls for the mechanics of speech in the sense that speech errors are caught and corrected or even anticipated and avoided. The fact that the feedback system includes information from several sensory sources also protects the speaker from communicative disaster if part of the system fails. Adults who lose hearing, for example, can maintain reasonably good speech by attending more closely to how speech feels. If we lose some of our ability to monitor the motor aspects of speech, we can concentrate more intently on what our speech sounds like.

Speech Is for Talking—What Else?

The feature **specialization** suggests that speech is specifically designed for communication and serves no other purpose. In the appendix, you will discover that the physical processes of speech are actually the secondary functions served by the structures involved. That is, human beings have adapted structures that serve more basic biological purposes for speech. Nevertheless, it is true that speech itself is a specialized human function. People speak to communicate and for no other purpose, although we may speak when no one is listening, and sometimes when we speak, we do not successfully communicate.

Sending Messages Loud and *Clear*

Most other animals communicate fairly general messages, whereas humans can convey very specific messages with words having relatively stable relationships with the people, things, events, and concepts they represent. This feature of human speech is called **semanticity.** When the beaver slaps its tail against the water and fellow beavers scurry in fear, they do so because they have heard the message "Danger!" The danger could be a fire, an approaching bear, or a human hunter. Humans can both warn that danger is present and also name the danger.

Because We *Say* So!

One of the reasons languages differ so broadly across groups of people on Earth is that the words used to refer to the people, things, events, and concepts in human experiences do not directly reflect their referents. There is an **arbitrariness** about language. That is, there is nothing inherent in a spoken word to account for its meaning. We call the piece of furniture on which a person may sit a *chair*, not because it screams out to be called a chair, not because there is a connection between the nature of chairness and the word, but because someone at some time, for reasons of no interest to most people living today, arbitrarily decided to call it a *chair*. The obvious advantage of arbitrariness is that there is absolutely no limit to how language can describe anything and everything. Languages have different vocabularies because the arbitrary naming of the bits and pieces of the world has been done by different people at different places at different times.

The Limits of Speech

Discreteness is a feature that can be applied to human speech in at least two ways. Although the speech mechanism can produce an incredibly wide range of noises, each language is limited to a finite or discrete number of sounds. Furthermore, each sound used in one or more human languages has very specific characteristics so that each sound is discrete. Adult speakers adapt so completely to the specific sounds of a given language that they often have great difficulty breaking out of these patterns to produce sounds found in other languages but foreign to their own. Speakers whose native languages do not contain *l* or *r*, for example, struggle to produce these sounds when they are learning to speak English, and many of us who speak American English almost choke trying to produce some French vowels. The flexibility we have as infants to produce virtually all sounds known to all languages is quickly lost when we begin to narrow our range to the discrete sounds of our own language.

Back to the Future

One of the most intriguing features of human speech is **displacement.** That is, humans can talk about things that are distant in time or space. We can talk about what is going on in places across vast oceans or even across the infinite expanses of space. We can talk about events that occurred hundreds or thousands of years ago, and we can talk about things that have not yet happened. Although this feature may not be absolutely unique to human speech, we have no evidence that other animals have communication systems with this feature as fully developed as it is in human speech.

The Creativity of the Mind and Mouth

According to Hockett, **productivity** is one of the most important design-features of human speech. Humans have the amazing ability to be creative in their communication efforts. We can say things that have never been said before, or we can put old messages in brand new language forms. We use words in speech in much the same way the sculptor uses clay. The sculptor can take one mass of clay and make everything from an ashtray to a bowl or a bust. We can use a finite collection of sounds and words to shape an infinite variety of messages, some simple, some profound, some old, some new. No matter what the message is, however, if we obey the rules of our language, the message will be understood by anyone who shares the language we speak. Just imagine that on this very day you may say something that no one has ever said before and perhaps no one will ever say again in exactly the same way. The productivity or creativity of language gives human speakers a communicative power that is not shared by any other animal.

Many Wholes from a Few Parts

Part of the creativity that is characteristic of human speech is made possible by another design-feature, **duality of patterning.** Although a given language is restricted in the number of sounds it uses, these sounds can be combined in an infinite number of ways to produce an infinite variety of words, and the words of a language can be combined into an infinite variety of sentences. Every year of your life you will be witness to the creation of new words that are the product of this duality of patterning. Many of these new words reflect neverending advances in science and technology. Before there were telephones, there was no word *telephone,* but the sounds making up the word have existed for as long as human language as we know it has existed. It remained for someone to arrange this particular collection of sounds into this specific word to refer to that object. Just think for a moment about all the words that have been invented as a result of the explosion of computer-related technology. The patterning of sounds into words and words into sentences will end only when humankind ceases to communicate, and that is likely to happen only when humankind ceases to exist.

Born to Talk

The final design-feature Hockett describes is **traditional transmission.** Hockett was on the leading edge of a new view of human speech and language, which will be described in more detail in the next chapter. The suggestion in this feature is that speech is instinctive in humans. We have a genetic or biological capacity for language so powerful that few environmental factors can stop the acquisition of speech, although they may affect the rate at which it is acquired and they may affect the quality of the language we use. Although the capacity for language is genetic, the details of a language, including vocabulary and structural rules, are learned.

Not All Features Are Created Equal

Any reasonably informed observer would conclude that not all of Hockett's thirteen features are equally important in describing human language, and they do not all carry the same power to separate human languge from animal communication. As we have already acknowledged, much of what Hockett postulated on this subject in 1960 has been discounted by research and rejected on the basis of new theoretical ruminations about human communication. Even if we consider these thirteen features in the context of Hockett's original essay, however, we should understand that some of these features are more prominent than others. Four of the thirteen, in fact, might be described as most important or differentiating: (1) semanticity, (2) displacement, (3) productivity, and (4) traditional transmission. That is, while most animals communicate general messages, human communications are quite specific. Human communications exceed the boundaries of time and space. We can talk about events in the past and in the future, and we can talk about places far removed from ourselves physically, places we have never even visited. Human beings can say things that have never been said or heard before, and they will be understood by anyone using the same language conventions. It is certainly true that communication abilities are innate in all species that communicate, but it is especially important to note the innateness of language in human beings, because too many people assume that language is as much learned as say, canasta, and that is just not true. Even though language experts today continue to argue about the relative influences of nature and nurture on speech and language development, they would all agree that Hockett was absolutely on target in suggesting that language is genetically coded into human beings. In the next chapter, we will examine attempts to teach apes to use human language. The results of these attempts suggest that some other animals can be taught to communicate in ways that approximate human language, but these communications are limited and rudimentary by any standards. Based on the research conducted to date, it is still reasonable to conclude that only humans are born with a capacity for language as we know and understand it. Only humans, it seems, have such a strong biological drive to acquire language that they develop the ability to express language, especially through speech, even when the environmental odds are against them.

Speech: The Tale of Two Brains

We are now ready to return to the query that opened this chapter or, more specifically, to a more complete response to that question. All human beings who are able to speak are capable of using a kind of mental telepathy because speech allows two human brains to connect.

This connection is described in another portrait of human speech contained in a book entitled *The Speech Chain* (Denes & Pinson, 1993, pp. 1–9). A summary of this description will show how the brains of a speaker and a listener connect in a communicative sense.

The speech chain (Figure 1.1) has six steps or links. In the first step, you the speaker sort through your thoughts, decide which of these thoughts to express, and make some decisions about how to express them. Although this process occurs very quickly, within seconds or fractions of a second, it is actually a very complex process.

FIGURE 1.1 The Speech Chain

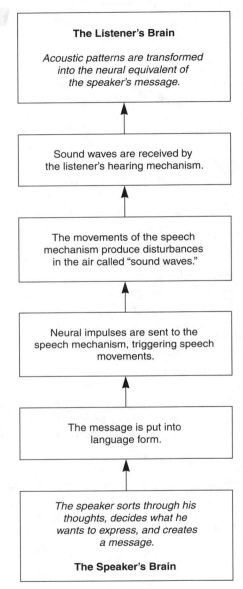

If, for example, a friend wearing the most atrocious dress you have ever seen asks you, "What do you think of my new dress?" you have some serious decisions to make. Your brain is filled with conflicting thoughts as you consider your response. You know that this article of clothing is an affront to anything resembling good taste.

You must also consider that your friend must have liked it because she did, in fact, actually give someone real, government-green money for it. You want to be honest, but you do not want to hurt her feelings. What do you do? What do you say? Well, you sort through all your thoughts. You make a decision about the relative merits of honesty and compassion, and you finally decide what to say. Incidentally, this step is much easier for very young children, who typically spend very little time arranging and editing their thoughts. The three-year-old is likely to say the first thing that comes to mind, which may be tactless and unintentionally hurtful. One of the aspects of communication acquired most slowly is the ability to make good decisions in the first step of the speech chain.

Regardless of how the decisions are made in the first step or whether they are appropriate decisions, the second step remains the same. You as speaker put your message into language form by leafing through your mental dictionary to pick out the right words and by selecting the appropriate rules of grammar to create the correct word forms and place them into the right order. This step also occurs so quickly that you cannot monitor yourself doing it, unless you cannot think of the right word. Only when the process is interrupted by this kind of failure do we begin to appreciate just how easily and naturally we translate thoughts into language. Notice that the first two steps are confined to the brain. We may think of speech as flapping lips and a wagging tongue, but the beginning of even the simplest utterance begins in the gray matter of the brain.

In the third step, the brain sends instructions, in the form of neural impulses, to the muscles of speech. Keep in mind that these are not just the muscles of the structures in the mouth. The brain must send instructions to the muscles of respiration, to the muscles of the larynx and pharynx, as well as to the muscles of the face that support speech with nonverbal expressions, and even to the muscles of the arms, hands, fingers, perhaps even the legs and torso, which provide additional nonverbal support to the speaker's words. The complexity of this operation is unbelievable and becomes even more amazing when you consider the speed at which all the parts are made operative.

In the fourth step, the movements of the structures of speech interrupt and constrict the flow of vibrating air from the larynx, setting up minute pressure changes in the air surrounding the speaker's mouth. These patterns of air pressure changes are called **sound waves.** Sound waves cause air particles to bump into each other, creating compression between some particles and spaces or rarefactions between others. The bumping, compression, and rarefaction of air particles continue until the sound waves reach the listener's ears.

As the air particles bump into the listener's eardrums in the fifth step, the listener's hearing mechanism is activated. As you will discover in more detail in the Appendix, the ear has the capacity to transform the mechanical energy of vibrating air particles into hydraulic energy in the fluids of the inner ear, and eventually into neural energy that travels along the acoustic nerve to the brain.

Finally, in the listener's brain, the neural impulses are analyzed and interpreted so that the listener recognizes the speaker's message. Consider what has happened in the speech chain. Thoughts have been transformed into language forms, which have been transformed into neural signals, which trigger the structures of speech, which by means of their movements disturb air particles into sound waves, which bombard the listener's ears, which transform the sound waves into neural patterns, which are received and decoded by the listener's brain. Incredibly, the message is not lost or changed. The listener may not always successfully understand what you intended to communicate, but if he is within hearing range and if you speak clearly, he will receive precisely the same pattern you sent.

Speech does indeed give us the power of mental telepathy. It allows brains to connect. Speech is so much a part of the human experience that we truly take it for granted, but it is a wondrous human gift. The next time you engage in a conversation with one or more people, consider the speech chains that connect speakers and listeners. Marvel at the speed involved in the sending and receiving of messages. Notice how quickly speakers become listeners and listeners become speakers in a ballistic communication give-and-take that almost defies understanding. Now consider that human beings know much of what they will ever know about language and have the basic skills involved in speech by the time they are just four or five years old! How does this happen?

In the remainder of this book, you will take a closer look at many of the elements in the speech chain. You will consider what the child must know to be a competent language user, and explore the acquisition process along all important dimensions of speech and language. You will learn that there is much still unknown about human language. The experts argue about almost every major topic, but much more is known about speech and language today than was known just thirty years ago. It is the purpose of this book to help you understand what is known, to recognize what is not known, and, most important, to appreciate the almost mystical nature of this uniquely human talent.

Review Questions

1. Define *communication, language,* and *speech.*
2. How are speech and language "separate but related" aspects of communication?
3. Which of Hockett's design-features most effectively separate human communication from animal communication, and why?
4. Trace the six steps in the speech chain that transforms the speaker's thoughts into the listener's understanding.

References and Suggested Readings

Bohannon, J. (1982). Close encounters of the primate kind. *American Journal of Primatology, 3,* 353–358.

Denes, P., & Pinson, E. (1993). *The speech chain* (2nd ed.). New York: Freeman.

Fillmore, C., Kempler, D., & Wang, S. (Eds.). (1979). *Individual differences in language ability and language behavior.* New York: Academic Press.

Gardner, R., & Gardner, B. (1980). Two comparative psychologists look at language acquisition. In K. Nelson (Ed.), *Children's language* (Vol. 2). New York: Gardner.

Geschwind, N. (1982). Specializations of the brain. In W. Wang (Ed.), *Human communication: Language and its psycho-biological bases* (pp. 110–119). San Francisco: Freeman.

Herman, L. (1981). Cognitive characteristics of dolphins. In L. Herman (Ed.), *Cetacean behavior* (pp. 363–429). New York: Wiley.

Herman, L., & Forestell, P. (1985). Reporting presence or absence of named objects by a language-trained dolphin. *Neuroscience and Biobehavioral Reviews, 9*, 667–681.

Herman, L., Hovancik, J., Gory, J., & Bradshaw, G. (1989). Generalization of visual matching by a bottlenosed dolphin (*Tursiops truncatus*): Evidence for invariance of cognitive performance with visual and auditory materials. *Journal of Experimental Psychology Animal Behavior Processes, 15*, 124–136.

Hockett, C. (1960). The origin of speech. *Scientific American, 203*, 89–97.

Janik, V. (2000). Whistle matching in bottlenose dolphins. *Science, 289*, 1355–1357.

Lane, H. (1979). *The wild boy of Aveyron.* Cambridge, MA: Harvard University Press.

Nelson, K. (1981). Individual differences in language development: Implications for development and language. *Developmental Psychology, 17*, 170–187.

Quigley, S., & King, C. (1982). The language of deaf children and youth. In S. Rosenberg, (Ed.), *Handbook of applied psycholinguistics: Major thrusts of research and theory* (pp. 429–475). Hillsdale, NJ: Erlbaum.

Schusterman, R. (1986). Cognition and intelligence of dolphins. In R. Schusterman, J. Thomas, & F. Wood (Eds.), *Dolphin cognition and behavior: A comparative approach* (pp. 137–139). Hillsdale, NJ: Erlbaum.

Slobin, D. (Ed.). (1985). *A cross-linguistic study of language acquisition.* Hillsdale, NJ: Erlbaum.

Tyack, P. (2000). Dolphins whistle a signature tune. *Science, 289*, 1310–1311.

Von Frisch, K. (1967). *The dance language and orientation of bees* (L. E. Chadwick, Trans.). Cambridge, MA: Belknap.

2

Language Acquisition:
A Theoretical Journey

One can only guess when the first nature-versus-nurture argument occurred, but whenever human behaviors are discussed, this argument is sure to arise. It is not surprising, then, that language experts have debated the relative influences of genetics and the environment on speech and language development. Is the child genetically predisposed to talk, or taught to talk? This chapter presents the implications of this question and some of the answers experts have suggested. The answers, as you will discover, cover the entire nature–nurture continuum.

This chapter is designed to facilitate comprehension of the evolutionary changes that have occurred over the past four decades in the theories of language acquisition. It considers the contributions made by each major theoretical view along the evolutionary continuum to furthering an understanding about how the various components of language emerge. Specifically, this chapter addresses the following topics:

- The general character of the *nature-versus-nurture* argument and its potential impact on an understanding of speech and language development

- The *behaviorist,* or nurture, interpretation
- The *nativist,* or nature, interpretation
- The *generative semantic* and *cognitivist* interpretations

- The *information processing* interpretation
- The *pragmatics* view and the *social interactionist* interpretation

---

People probably have argued about how human talents are acquired from the earliest days of our species. Is an artist born or made? Does the musician inherit talent, or is it shaped by hours of rehearsal? Is the great athlete destined to become a physiological virtuoso because of genes, or is athletic skill the product of teaching and practice? Even the casual observer must understand that in most nature-versus-nurture arguments, the truth does not come down on only one side. The master artist must surely be born with the ability to paint or sculpt, but it is only through study, training, and practice that an artist's skills are developed and refined. The child born with the genetic makeup to become a gifted athlete will realize that potential only when provided the opportunity to learn and perfect the skills of the game she chooses. In other words, most human talents are both born and made.

Even human traits widely considered to be purely genetic can be influenced by the environment. A child might be smaller than his genetically determined size because he is malnourished. A child born with great intellectual capacity might function at a normal or below normal level because she has not been provided adequate opportunities for learning. Sadly, if the poor diet continues long enough, the small child will remain undersized, and if the educational opportunities are withheld long enough, the intellectually gifted child will lose her gift. Sometimes, of course, environment can affect nature's outcomes in less dramatic and less permanent ways. A child born brown-eyed can have blue eyes by wearing tinted contact lenses. A short child can wear elevator shoes. The adult with naturally brown hair can have blonde hair by using peroxide. The list of environmental manipulations of natural conditions becomes longer with each generation of humans.

Theories designed to explain how language develops address the nature-versus-nurture debate at various points along the continuum, and you will note that each theoretical view addresses certain aspects of language more directly than others. Some theories, for example, focus primarily on the function of language. Others are more concerned with the structure of language. Others consider the connections between cognition and language, and still others attend to environmental factors as facilitators in the acquisition process.

Choosing Sides

Until about 1960, most people who studied the development of speech and language in children assumed that oral communication skills are learned. During the first half of the twentieth century, much emphasis was placed on parents teaching their children to talk, even though there was concern that parents were not very good teachers. Van Riper, as late as 1964, observed that "children learn to talk. Their parents do the teaching, and it is usually very poor" (p. 92). Many experts during this era believed that children learn to talk not because of their parents but in spite of them.

The nature-versus-nurture argument in speech and language became heated during the 1960s and early 1970s when theorists called *nativists* or *biological nativists* suggested that children are genetically predisposed to talk. That is, oral language is instinctive in humans and, like instincts in other animals, speech is a behavior the child produces with minimal environmental involvement. It is a genetically coded behavior and is as natural for the child as walking.

What is sometimes lost in discussions about this debate is that neither side completely discounts the other. Those who believe language is learned recognize that the child must have the right anatomic equipment and must be ready to acquire language in terms of cognitive, perceptual, and neuromuscular maturation. Their emphasis, however, is on environmental influences. They argue, for example, that a child reared in a stable home with parents who provide good language models has a distinct advantage over one reared in an economically, culturally, and socially impoverished home by parents who provide few and inadequate language models. The nativists accept the fact that environment plays some role in the acquisition of speech and language. That is, the child must be exposed to language models, but the nativists view these models as mere triggers for a natural, biological acquisition process. They argue that the innate drive for the development of language in humans is so powerful that even a poor environment will not prevent the child from talking.

As the debate has continued, the extreme views have moderated, and there is a general understanding that what the child brings to language development genetically is important, but so is the environment into which he is born. Differences among theorists still exist relative to the importance they place on the nature or the nurture, and given the history of this ongoing debate in all aspects of human development, it is unlikely the experts will ever agree.

With the general nature-versus-nurture debate as a backdrop, we will take a closer look at a number of theoretical interpretations reflecting the evolutionary changes in thinking about language acquisition over the past half century. These theoretical interpretations include behaviorism, nativism and the government-binding theory, generative semantics and cognitivism, information processing theory, and the pragmatics revolution that gave birth to the social interactionist view.

The Behaviorist Interpretation

Several basic assumptions underlie the **behaviorist** or **empiricist** interpretation of language development.

It is assumed, for example, that attention should be focused on observable and measurable behaviors. Behaviorists do not emphasize mental constructs or internal mechanisms that generate language structures. The problem from this perspective is that since mental activities cannot be seen, they cannot be defined or measured. Behaviorists do not deny the existence of these mental processes. They acknowledge that observable behaviors are connected to internal or physiological mechanisms, but, they argue, we cannot study what we cannot observe. Behaviorists, therefore, look for the overt behaviors that occur together in language performance. On the basis of their observations and measurements, they draw conclusions about the relationships among co-occurring stimuli and make predictions about future behaviors based on these relationships (Bohannon & Warren-Leubecker, 1989, pp. 171–172).

Using Watson (1924) and Skinner (1957) as examples, Bohannon and Warren-Leubecker (1989, p. 173) make the point that behaviorists believe language is learned because they do not believe language is unique among human behaviors. Watson (1924) categorizes language in its earliest stages as a behavior no more complicated than a habit used to influence or control the behaviors of others. Behaviorists argue that language is something humans *do,* not something they *have,* and it should be understood, therefore, in the same context of learning as other behaviors humans do such as brushing their teeth or tying their shoes. They contend that language is learned according to the same principles used in training animals and that like trained animal behaviors, language behaviors are learned by imitation, reinforcement, and successive approximations toward adult language behaviors.

One of the more controversial aspects of the behaviorist view is that children are passive during the process of learning language (Bryen, 1982). That is, children begin life with their "language tanks" on empty. They become language users as their tanks are filled by the experiences provided by the language models in their environments. This is not to say that children are totally inactive, of course. They are active in the sense that they imitate language forms, but they do not initiate these behaviors on their own, and the shape of their emerging language is determined not by self-discovery or creative experimentation but by the selective reinforcements received from their speech and language models.

This leads us to the key assumption underlying behaviorist views of language development. Although behaviorists have differing opinions about exactly how the process of learning occurs, they all agree that environment is the critical and most important factor in the acquisition formula. While nativists stress the *similarities* that occur in the language development of children, the behaviorists stress the *differences* that are explained by the widely varying environments of children during the language acquisition period. The behaviorists focus on the external forces that shape the child's verbal behaviors into language. They see the child simply as a reactor to these forces (Bryen, 1982).

Speech and Language as Operant Behaviors

The theorist most closely associated with the behaviorist interpretation of speech and language development is B. F. Skinner. It is not surprising that Skinner (1957) viewed speech as learned behavior, because he viewed virtually all behaviors as learned according to operant conditioning principles. To understand Skinner's explanation of speech and language development, therefore, one must understand the basic principles of operant conditioning.

An **operant** is any behavior whose frequency can be affected by the responses that follow it. If a target behavior's frequency of occurrence increases as a consequence of the response that follows it, **reinforcement** has occurred. If the frequency decreases, the target behavior has been **punished.** Very often people try to understand operant punishment in terms of aversiveness or unpleasantness, but these judgments may interfere with an understanding of the principle involved. If a target behavior's frequency of occurrence decreases as a consequence of the response that follows it, punishment has occurred whether or not the organism being conditioned perceives the response as unpleasant or aversive. In other words, reinforcement and punishment are defined on the basis of their effects.

In operant conditioning, the events that follow target behaviors are critical to learning, but the events preceding the target behaviors are also important, because they can come to control whether or not these target behaviors will be produced. Assume, for example, that a parent has conditioned a child to say "thank you" whenever he receives a gift by praising him (reinforcement) each time he remembers to say the words. If the "thank you" behavior increases as a result of the praise, we can conclude that reinforcement and learning have occurred. During the learning period, the parent may, consciously or not, give the child a certain look as he is receiving the gift, a look that reminds the child that he should say "thank you." We call this look a **discriminative stimulus.** Now notice the sequence. The child receives the gift. The parent gives the "look." The child says "thank you," and the parent praises him for his gratitude. Over time, the "look" or discriminative stimulus comes to control the frequency with which the child says "thank you."

There are other preceding events. The **delta stimulus** is a signal indicating that reinforcement will not follow a particular response, and an **aversive stimulus** warns that there will be an unpleasant consequence for a particular behavior. It is very important to remember, however, that these preceding events have only as much power to control behaviors as provided by the strength and consistency of the events that follow targeted behaviors. A parent might try to use an aversive stimulus by threatening to spank a child if she produces a certain behavior, but if that behavior is never followed by a spanking, the preceding event will have no power to control. This is why parents are counseled not to make empty threats. Behavior in children and all organisms can be managed by operant principles only if preceding events are connected to following events, at least part of the time. In other words, behavior management is effective only if efforts to manage are consistent and if the manager follows through on the promises or threats inherent in the preceding events.

Sometimes the behavior we want must be **shaped** in small steps that gradually approximate the target behavior. When the child is learning to say "water," she might begin by saying "wawa." The adult accepts this production as a step toward the target behavior and reinforces it, perhaps by giving the child a drink when she says "wawa." As the child gets older and expectations for her speech rise, she might be reinforced for saying "wada" but is no longer reinforced for saying "wawa." The next approximation might be "wata" and finally "water." In each step of the shaping process, what is reinforced is closer to the target. Productions that are not advanced or are perceived as regressions are ignored.

Many behaviors, including speech behaviors, occur in sequences. These sequences are learned through a procedure known as **chaining.** An example from Holland and Skinner (1961) makes the process more understandable than a definition: "At the same time sight of food is a discriminative stimulus for seizing food, it is a reinforcer for bending down to the food magazine and looking in. This sequence forms a chain: bending down, seeing food, seizing food" (pp. 161–162). This same procedure can be used to explain a sequence of behaviors involving language. A child sees his mother getting ready to go out and thinks she looks pretty. He says, "You sure look pretty, Mommy." The mother, flattered, responds, "Well, thank you! That was a nice thing to say." The child says, "You're welcome." Seeing his mother looking pretty is the discriminative stimulus for the child's initial comment, which is followed by the mother's response and the child's response to her response, each reinforcing the preceding utterance.

It is not too difficult to understand how Skinner and others have applied these basic principles to speech and language development. In general, the child acquires language as a result of selective reinforcements provided by his caregivers. The caregivers provide models. The child imitates the models. Imitations most closely resembling the models are reinforced by the caregivers when they give the child what he wants, when they respond with another comment, or when they give the child adoring attention. Over time, the child will cease to use productions that have not been reinforced and will continue to use those that have been reinforced. Stringing words together into sentences occurs as the result of chaining. Imitation, important throughout the learning process, undergoes a change as the child moves from single words to sentences. Staats (1971) suggests that this new version of imitation is introduced by the child's parents as their expectations for her speech increase. The child produces a single-word utterance. One of the parents, believing she can produce a longer utterance, expands this single word into a sentence and withholds reinforcement until the child imitates the expanded form.

Remember that behaviorists stress the idea that language is a doing or performing phenomenon more than a knowing phenomenon. Skinner (1957), for example, argues that verbal behaviors serve one of five specific functions defined according to what they do: echoic, tact, mand, intraverbal, and autoclitic. Perhaps the simplest of these behaviors is **echoic,** the imitation of a model in the presence of a nonverbal stimulus to which the word refers. For example, as a parent hands the child a dessert, she says, "Cookie." The child takes the treat and imitates the model, "Cookie." Eventually the child will associate the word with the object and will use the word to refer to or request a cookie, but in the beginning his production is simple, meaningless imitation.

After the child has established an association between an object and its corresponding word, an echoic becomes a tact. A **tact** is a verbal behavior used to name or label something, typically in response to things or events the speaker is discussing.

The next term sounds and looks something like the word *demand*, and that is not a coincidence. A **mand** is a verbal behavior used to request, command, or make a demand, and it identifies its own reinforcer. An utterance like "me want drink" indicates a request. If the request is granted, the drink becomes the reinforcement for the utterance.

An **intraverbal** is a production that often seems to have no direct connection to the utterance that precipitated it. A mother might say, "Daddy went to work," and the child might reply, "Go outside and play now?" Although there might seem to be no direct link between these two utterances, the child might be conditioned to go outside to play only after her father goes to work. In this context, the child's response makes sense. Intraverbals are used in the free association characteristic of conversation. In conversation, what one person says may not dictate the response received. In some cases, a person responds even when there is no request for a response. The free-associated and nonrequested responses in conversation and social gesture talk are intraverbals.

Autoclitic responses can be understood in two important ways. First, these responses influence and are influenced by the speaker's behaviors. Second, autoclitic responses account for the linking of words into sentences. Using operant terminology, each word serves as a discriminative stimulus for the following word. Another way to understand the linking of words into autoclitic responses is to consider how the child is combining isolated ideas. The child, for example, might be watching her brother, Billy, playing baseball, and she wants to comment on this observation. She knows the names for "Billy" and "ball," and she knows that striking the ball with a bat is called "hitting." She links the three ideas together to create the utterance "Billy hitting the ball." This is an autoclitic response.

As language structures become more complex, it is more difficult to explain them on the basis of learning alone. In reference to autoclitics, for example, Fey (1986) says there is the implication that only strings of words that have been specifically reinforced can be produced. We know, however, that all speakers, including young children, produce strings of words that have never been produced or heard before. In other words, operant principles cannot adequately account for the creativity that is a dominant characteristic of language. Additionally, operant principles alone fail to account for the acquisition of meaning in novel utterances.

Classical Conditioning in Meaning Acquisition

Staats (1971) believes we must include classical conditioning principles to explain language acquisition, especially the meaning component. In classical conditioning, an originally neutral stimulus is paired with an unconditioned stimulus that elicits an unconditioned response. In the famous Pavlovian experiment, the dog hears a bell just before seeing food, which elicits the unconditioned response, salivation. After a number of trials, the bell alone, now a conditioned stimulus, will elicit salivation, now a conditioned response. That is, the dog has learned or been conditioned to salivate upon hearing the bell. Staats argues that a word is, in the beginning, a neutral stimu-

The chaining of behaviors.

lus that acquires meaning only as responses are classically conditioned to it. The word *sit* develops meaning as it comes to represent the physical act associated with it through the process of conditioning. At first, when the child hears his parent say, "Sit!" there is no reaction, but if the word is paired with the physical act of being placed on a chair, the word alone, after enough trials, will elicit the act of sitting and will be understood to represent the act.

The Behaviorist Perspective in Review

The behaviorists stress the importance of environment. The child is viewed as an empty vessel to be filled by the experiences provided by the important people in his life. The child is typically viewed as having no knowledge about the rules of language. His parents and other speakers are credited for "teaching" language by providing models that the child imitates. By selective reinforcement, the parents shape the child's utterances into adult forms.

Obviously, the behaviorist perspective of language acquisition has not gone unchallenged. James (1990) provides an excellent and succinct summary of some of the problems and criticisms. The role of imitation has been questioned, for example. As noted earlier, children produce sentences they have never heard before. This may mean they produce sentences that are more creative and elaborate than their models, but it also means they produce utterances that are simply not produced by adults because such utterances are infantile. The child will typically say things such as "Daddy goed work" and "That mine milk," productions that are clearly not imitations of sentences produced by parents. Perhaps more importantly, the frequency of imitation decreases dramatically after the second birthday, but there is still a lot of language to be acquired beyond age two. Some children, even from the beginning, imitate very little. If imitation is as important as the behaviorists argue, we would expect to see imitations more consistent with the models provided, and we certainly would expect to see imitation play a major role in acquisition throughout the learning period. James also notes that since parents are more likely to correct children for the content of their utterances than for the grammatical accuracy of their sentences, syntactic development cannot be explained solely on the basis of selective parental reinforcement.

Whatever the problems with the behaviorist perspective, there seems little doubt that learning explains some aspects of language acquisition. We know that language changes over the course of a person's lifetime, well beyond the age range identified by the nativists as the critical acquisition period. These changes are best explained by general learning principles. An innate capacity for language, for example, cannot account for how humans learn the crazy nuances of language, such as when to use *who* and when to use *whom*, and environmental influences seem to be very important in changing a person from an adequate user of language into an exceptional user of language.

The Nativist Interpretation

If the behaviorist view represents the extreme nurture end of the nature–nurture continuum, the nativist perspective is the extreme nature end of the same continuum. As the name of this view suggests, nativists stress the idea that language is innate or biologically based. They argue that human beings are born with a species-specific capacity for language, a capacity that is realized with minimal assistance from the environment. While behaviorists seem solely concerned with performance, nativists stress competence or knowledge that leads to performance.

The theorist most closely associated with the nativist view is Noam Chomsky, a linguist. Chomsky (1968) expresses one of the basic assumptions of nativism in this declaration: "Anyone concerned with the study of human nature and capabilities must somehow come to grips with the fact that all humans acquire language" (p. 59). The idea that language is universal among humans and unique to humans is the foundation of the nativistic interpretation of language acquisition. These theorists point out that unless there are severe physical or mental limitations, human beings will acquire language, and that the innate drive to acquire language is so powerful that many humans talk in spite of what may seem to be insurmountable limitations. They also argue that only human beings are capable of acquiring and using language as we know and understand it.

One of the questions embedded in the larger issue of the relative influences of genetics and environment in language acquisition centers on whether animals can be taught to communicate using something comparable to human language. Among the strongest voices in the nativist movement of the 1960s was Eric Lenneberg (1964), who was so convinced that language is unique to humans that he asserted, "[T]here is no evidence that any nonhuman form has the capacity to acquire even the most primitive stages of language development" (p. 67). Although this seemed a reasonable conclusion at the time, some research conducted in the late 1960s and throughout the 1970s raised doubts about what other animals can and cannot do as users of language.

The earliest attempts to teach chimpanzees to speak failed, but when Gardner and Gardner (1969, 1971, 1975) began their research with Washoe, a ten-month-old female chimpanzee, they tried a different language avenue. They taught Washoe how to use American Sign Language, the manual communication system used by deaf people. Washoe eventually learned more than one hundred signs and, according to the Gardners, spontaneously produced combinations of signs to express basic requests such as "Listen dog" and "Give me food." The fact that Washoe brought her hands to a resting position only after a series of signs was produced was interpreted to mean that she intended to combine these signs. There is no question that what Washoe accomplished was beyond what Lenneberg would have imagined possible when he talked about language as a uniquely human ability, but even those most excited about attempts to teach apes to use language have recognized some important limitations. There is no evidence, for example, that Washoe learned any rules of grammar as reflected by consistent or meaningful word order. Some have suggested that this failure to acquire grammatical rules may be a function of American Sign Language, which is not bound by the strict word order rules used in spoken and written language. On the other hand, it may simply be that chimpanzees do not have the ability to learn syntax, a conclusion that seems to be supported by the findings of another researcher, Terrace (1980), who specifically analyzed his chimpanzee's signed utterances to determine whether there were any word order consistencies. He found none.

Efforts also have been made to teach language to pygmy chimpanzees (Savage-Rumbaugh, MacDonald, Sevcik, Hopkins, & Rubert, 1986). Pygmy chimpanzees are reportedly more intelligent and social than those used in earlier experiments, and the preliminary evidence suggests they have a greater capacity for language-based communication skills. According to their trainers, these chimpanzees have acquired symbols simply by observing their human trainers, and they have used these symbols spontaneously in apparent attempts to communicate with humans. There is also evidence that they can combine these symbols to create more complex utterances, and they seem to understand some spoken words. One of the more remarkable primates studied by Georgia State University researchers is Kanzi, a bonobo or pygmy chimpanzee, born in October of 1980. *Kanzi* is the Swahili word for *treasure,* an appropriate name for an animal that has been a treasure trove of discovery for those who care for him and study him. Kanzi is the first primate, other than human children, to acquire language, not by direct teaching, but by being reared in a language-rich environment. As is true of human children, all his interactions with his caregivers, from the time he was born, have been framed in language. It is significant to note that Kanzi understands not just words, but even word order. When given the instructions "Put jelly in the milk" and "Put milk in the jelly," Kanzi carries out the instructions appropriately, an accomplishment dependent on understanding word order (Rumbaugh & Beran, 2003; Savage-Rumbaugh, Shanker, & Taylor, 1998). As impressive as Kanzi's abilities are, it must be acknowledged that chimpanzees, including the pygmy variety, so far have not shown the ability to acquire adultlike syntax, but we must not overlook the fact that these primates seem capable of acquiring and using the kind of language expected of very young human children (Greenfield & Savage-Rumbaugh, 1984; Savage-Rumbaugh, 1990; Savage-Rumbaugh et al., 1986).

All the research conducted with apes must be understood in the context of the criticisms raised about the general methods used. Skeptics have noted that whatever "language" is learned is the result of extraordinary efforts to teach on the part of human trainers—the kind of constant and powerful teaching that is not necessary for humans to acquire language. Critics also suggest that the successes noted are more the result of imitation and prompting than any natural capacity for language (Terrance, Pettito, Saunder, & Bever, 1979).

Based on all the data now available, we have no reason to believe that nonhumans are capable of acquiring and using language, at least not a language directly and completely comparable to human language. Even if we accept that apes can acquire symbols and combine them, and that they can understand some spoken words, we have no evidence that they can acquire the rules for combining words into grammatical structures, engage in conversation, or use language creatively. If we believe that language goes beyond vocabulary to include structure, the layering of meanings, the transformations of word forms to indicate things such as plurality, possession, and tense changes, the use of language as a pragmatic tool, and the creativity that allows even young children to formulate utterances never produced or heard before, we must conclude that Lenneberg (1964) was more right than wrong—at least so far.

Another basic assumption of the nativist perspective is that since language is acquired so quickly and so early in the child's life, learning alone cannot adequately account for acquisition. Nativists argue that caregivers do not provide language models that are designed to "teach" progressive understanding of language forms. In fact, the nativist would question whether caregivers teach language at all. Children are exposed to language forms of enormous complexity, variety, and inconsistency, and they are never given specific feedback about whether their utterances are correct or incorrect (Pinker, 1984, 1987; Wexler & Culicover, 1980). If language is learned, the nativist argues, we would expect the teacher to provide models that allow children to develop progressively more sophisticated hypotheses about the rules and forms they are learning, and we would certainly expect the teacher to clearly indicate when a child's productions are right or wrong.

One of the most compelling arguments for the nativist perspective is that language is essentially the same experience for all human beings no matter what language they speak, where they live, or how they interact with their language models. As listeners and speakers of languages, we may be most impressed by their differences, but when languages are studied carefully, we discover many commonalities. All languages, for example, have rules for organizing words into grammatical sentence forms. They do not all use the same rules, of course. Some languages, like English, stress word order in developing grammatical sentences. Latin, on the other hand, allows more freedom in word order but stresses word endings to indicate the relationships among words. A given Latin noun, for example, has a different ending when it is the subject of a sentence than when it is a direct object.

Nativists stress the common ground, however. That is, all languages have rules to indicate the structural relationships among words in sentences. All languages distinguish between subjects and predicates and allow the embedding of one sentence structure into another to create an elaborated sentence representing both original structures. All languages have rules to indicate changes in tense and plurality, and draw sets of speech sounds from a common pool of sounds, and the list goes on. These commonalities or *linguistic universals* are evidence, say the nativists, that language is an ability humans possess, not by virtue of specific learning or teaching, but by virtue of their humanness. Spiders weave webs. Birds build nests. Humans speak. Enough said. Well, more needs to be said, of course, but you should be able to appreciate the form of this argument. If language were truly and solely learned, we would expect great differences among the languages spoken by people from different parts of the world. No matter which side of the debate you ultimately take, you must admit that language is a universal human experience and that there are startling similarities in the way people from widely varying cultures acquire and use language.

All of these assumptions led to the creation of a concept that underlies the nativist's understanding of language development: the **language acquisition device**, or **LAD** (Chomsky, 1965; Lenneberg, 1967). The LAD is an innate language reservoir filled with information about the rules of language structure. Nativists contend that it should be understood as a real part of the brain, that part specifically designed to process language. The LAD takes the syntactic information provided by the child's models and generates the grammar of that child's native language. Since no child is predetermined to speak any specific language, the LAD is driven by knowledge common to all languages. As you might imagine, the existence and certainly the nature of the LAD have been widely debated (Bohannon & Warren-Leubecker, 1989).

As you may have sensed in this discussion, nativists believe that the structure of language is somehow independent of its use. In fact, they view structure as being independent of meaning and almost every other aspect of the total language package. The rules for structuring sentences determine, for any given language, that some forms are grammatical and allowable and others are not. There is a finite, or specifically limited, number of rules for a given language. These rules allow the speaker to create an infinite number of grammatically acceptable sentences. The rules should not be understood in a prescriptive sense but in a descriptive sense. In other words, these rules do not tell the speaker what she should do but what she does do. They are rules that describe the regularities of a language. Once the speaker knows what these rules are, she can create an unlimited number of grammatical sentences, including the possibility of sentences that have never been produced by any other human. Language acquisition, therefore, is a matter of discovering and applying the rules or regularities of one's native language.

Transformational Generative Grammar

Chomsky (1957) devised **Transformational Generative Grammar** to account for the production of an unlimited number of grammatically acceptable sentences. This grammar suggests that language is processed at two levels, and two kinds of rules describe what is occurring at each level. **Phrase structure rules** describe the underlying relationships of words and phrases, the level of structure referred to as **deep.** These rules are universal and operate in all languages. **Transformations** are rules that describe the rearrangement of deep structures as they are moved to the next level of structure, referred to as **surface.** These rules are not universal. Each language has its own set of transformations, although the basic principles that operate in transformations are much the same in all languages. A complete description of Transformational Generative Grammar is beyond the scope of this book, but the reader should understand how the grammar works to appreciate Chomsky's point of view about language.

If we take a simple sentence such as "The little boy hit the white ball," we can identify three basic phrase structure rules that operate to create this kind of sentence:

1. *Sentence = Noun Phrase + Verb Phrase.* Our sample sentence consists of the noun phrase (*The little boy*) and the verb phrase (*hit the white ball*).
2. *Verb Phrase = Verb + Noun Phrase.* The verb phrase in our sentence consists of the verb (*hit*) and the noun phrase (*the white ball*).
3. *Noun Phrase = Modifier(s) + Noun.* There are two noun phrases in our sentence. In the first noun phrase, there are two modifiers (*The* and *little*) and the noun (*boy*). The second noun phrase also has two modifiers (*the* and *white*) and the noun (*ball*).

Keep in mind that Chomsky was devising a grammar to account for the production of an infinite number of grammatical sentences with a finite number of rules. By using just these three rules, it is possible to create an unlimited number of sentences. The example here is an English sentence, but these same rules can be used to describe the deep structure of similar sentences in any language.

Think of deep structures as the origins of a sentence in the brain before it is spoken or written. Phrase structure rules describe the relationships of the most basic elements of sentences while they are thoughts, before they become spoken or written sentences. To move these deep structures to the surface, we need transformations (rules that determine how words are shaped and organized to make sentences grammatical). Each language has its own set of transformations.

In English, for example, we can understand the creation of a grammatically correct question by understanding what happens as we move from the deep structure of a particular sentence to the surface. Let's assume that you want to know whether

Marco is going to the library. At the deep structure level, the origin of the question is something like this:

> "Marco is going to the library."—Question?

The rule in English for transforming this deep structure into a grammatically correct interrogative form is fairly simple. You rearrange the words, reversing *Marco* and *is* to create the surface structure "Is Marco going to the library?" The rule for rearranging the words to create a question is a transformation. If you are thinking:

> "Marco is going to the library."—No!

you can use a negative transformation to express that idea on the surface. In this case, you insert the word *not* between *is* and *going* to create the grammatically acceptable sentence "Marco is not going to the library." The transformation describes what you do on the surface to express what you have thought at the deep level.

It is also important to understand that every sentence has a deep structure and a surface structure. Notice, for example, that "The boy hit the ball" and "The ball was hit by the boy" mean the same thing. That is, they have the same deep structure. They differ only on the surface. The transformation used to change the first sentence into the second is called the **passive transformation.** Notice the reordering of words necessary to transform the active sentence into the passive sentence. Once you understand the rule, you can transform any active sentence into its correct passive version. Try it on sentences such as "The beautiful woman rode the aging horse" or "The vicious cat chased the frightened dog under the porch." If several people try the same transformation, assuming basic competence in English, the resulting sentences will be the same:

> The aging horse was ridden by the beautiful woman.
> The frightened dog was chased under the porch by the vicious cat.

How did you do? You have just demonstrated something many nativists believe supports their view. That is, you know what you know about language even if you do not know what you know. Think about that for a few seconds. The point is, you might not have known what the term passive transformation means, and if asked how to make a sentence passive, you might not have been able to explain it; but by changing active sentences that you have never seen before into passive versions, you have demonstrated your knowledge of not only the deep structures of these sentences but the rules for surface structure as well. The nativists would argue that if language were purely learned, you would have a more conscious understanding of what you are doing when you create sentences at the deep level and as you move them to the surface. Instead, they contend, your LAD provides you with innate knowledge of deep structures and the ability to easily acquire the rules for surface structures for your native language, an acquisition that comes by exposure to models, not direct teaching.

Chomsky (1981) has significantly expanded and extended his theoretical views regarding the acquisition of grammar with what is called the **government-binding theory.** One of the problems with previous theories of transformational grammar is that they were so powerful they could account not only for language patterns that are possible and realistic but also for language patterns that are outlandish. One of the primary emphases of the government-binding theory is "learnability." Chomsky suggests that there are limits on the possible hypotheses about language structure the learner can formulate. According to Leonard and Loeb (1988), the "government-binding theory is currently the dominant (though by no means the only) theory in linguistics" (p. 515).

While still allowing the language learner considerable latitude in terms of how language knowledge is processed and organized, the government-binding theory asserts that the learner's language knowledge must be consistent with the knowledge inherent in the grammars of presently existing and possible languages, and it must be possible to develop this knowledge from limited evidence. The internalized complex of rules and principles by which language knowledge meets these parameters is called **Universal Grammar.** Universal Grammar operates at four levels of representation: (1) deep structures, (2) surface structures, (3) phonetic form rules, and (4) logical form rules. In addition to these levels of representation, Universal Grammar also includes several subtheories.

Deep structures include the speaker's personal dictionary as well as rules for formulating sentences (rules comparable to those in Chomsky's earlier versions of phrase structure grammar). The personal dictionary specifies the meanings of words and also how words are to be treated syntactically. The sentence formulation rules are complex and versatile enough to explain how alternative sentences, such as question forms, are created from a basic form.

The **surface structures** of the Universal Grammar are similar to Chomsky's earlier versions. They differ in the sense that they come closer to spoken forms than the earlier versions, but they are still quite abstract and still derived from deep structures. **Phonetic form** and **logical form** rules operate at the same level of representation, but add differentiated information. Phonetic form rules are abstractions of the sound system and include the rules that govern the phonological shaping of words. Logical form rules are concerned with interpretation. If, for example, relationships between pronouns and antecedents in sentences are not clear based on structure alone, these rules, by the application of abstract logical interpretation, help clarify which pronouns are associated with which antecedents.

The subtheories of the government-binding theory are designed to explain the constraints and principles that allow language to be quickly acquired. According to the **bounding theory,** the movement of a grammatical constituent or component is limited. That is, no constituent can be moved out of a noun phrase and a sentence or clause by application of a single rule. *Noun phrase* and *sentence* are considered *bounding nodes* because they determine the extent to which constituents can move.

Government theory is concerned with the "privileged relations" among certain syntactic constituents. For example, in prepositional phrases, prepositions "govern," or exert influence over, the noun phrases that follow them. In a sense, the prepositions dominate and control their noun phrases.

Case theory is concerned with the rules by which meaning category or semantic case is assigned to noun phrases. Consider the assignment of nominative or objective case to noun phrases. For example, the active verb, *hit*, determines that the following noun phrase, *the ball*, will be objective case, whereas the preceding noun phrase, *The little girl*, will be nominative case. Even though case theory is a distinct subtheory, one can easily see government theory principles in operation.

Binding theory addresses the issue of "coreference," the idea that a given noun phrase may or may not refer to the same entity as one or more other noun phrases. For example, a reflexive clearly refers to the preceding noun phrase. In the sentence *"John made himself sick,"* the reflexive pronoun *himself* unambiguously refers to *John*. A pronominal such as *I, he,* or *she* may make an independent reference (as in the sentence *"Marco thinks she is pretty,"* in which the reference for *she* is not specified), or it may refer to a noun phrase (as in the sentence *"Mary thinks she is pretty,"* in which *she* refers to *Mary.*)

Thematic theory addresses the designation of roles such as *agent-of-action* and *goal-of-action.* The purposes of thematic theory and case theory are somewhat parallel. While case theory assigns grammatical case roles, thematic theory assigns semantic roles. In the sentence "Paul planted the tree," the grammatical case assigned to *Paul* is nominative, and the thematic role assigned to *Paul* is agent-of-action.

The last of the subtheories, **control theory,** is concerned with determining the possible references for pronouns or words used like pronouns when the references are not clear. The subject of an embedded infinitive phrase, for example, may be controlled by a noun phrase or it may make an independent reference. The sentence "Coach Smith considered what to do with the bases loaded" suggests that *Coach Smith* is the subject of the infinitive phrase. The subject of the embedded infinitive phrase is controlled by the noun phrase of the sentence. In the sentence "It is difficult to know what to do with the bases loaded," the reference is not controlled by the noun phrase and is not so clear. It is an independent reference to some unidentified *one,* as in a paraphrased version of the sentence "It is difficult for one to know what to do with the bases loaded."

The speaker who has acquired language presumably uses all of these components to decipher language and to create language forms. In the process, the Universal Grammar that forms the foundation for the acquisition of language is shaped to fit the specific and idiosyncratic characteristics of the speaker's native language. In closing this section on Chomsky's view of language acquisition, it must be emphasized that while Chomsky is certainly interested in the entire breadth of language, his primary focus has always been on language form or structure. He believes that the Universal Grammar is innate and that children master their native language by using the various components of the Universal Grammar to make sense of the language to which they are exposed.

The Nativist Perspective in Review

Nativists are clearly at the nature end of the nature-versus-nurture continuum. They believe human beings are born with a capacity for language—that given exposure to language, the human child will talk, even if environmental conditions are not favorable. Nativists contend that the universality of language among all human beings, the striking commonalities in how language is acquired, and the schedule by which it is acquired, regardless of cultural or other environmental variations, are evidence of the innateness of language. They believe children are born with a Language Acquisition Device, a neurophysiological entity filled with language knowledge. The LAD provides children with the knowledge they need to understand any language at the deep structure level and provides them with the ability to acquire easily and quickly the surface structure rules specific to the language they will speak.

James (1990, pp. 169–171) notes that it is difficult either to confirm or refute the nativist perspective, although several of its basic assumptions have been challenged. The assumption that language is unique to humans has been challenged, however inconclusively, by attempts to teach apes to use language. The assumption that language acquisition is essentially complete by the time the child is four or five appears to be overstated. There is evidence that significant language acquisition occurs well beyond five years and that some complex language forms are not mastered until adolescence. The argument that language must be innate because parents and others provide models that are too complex and ambiguous for progressive learning also appears to be incorrect. Although it is true that adults talk to other adults in language that is often confused, incomplete, and grammatically ambiguous, evidence indicates that adults use a different kind of language with children. That is, adults tend to use short, simple, and grammatically correct sentences when they talk to young children, the kind of models that could very well allow for approximations toward adult forms. Do not forget, however, based on the evidence gathered so far, that we have not ruled out the nativists' basic contention, which is that human beings are born with an innate capacity for language. What remains in the debate is to determine the relative importance of this innate capacity in comparison to the influence of environmental factors.

The Generative Semantics Interpretation

Not surprisingly, not all linguists accept Chomsky's views on language and language development. Some have made specific objections to his emphasis on syntax and his cursory attention to the meaning system of language. Chomsky does, of course, acknowledge the meaning level of language reflected in what he calls *deep structure*, but his primary focus is always on syntax and on how speakers generate syntax. Those who take the semantics view argue that for a language to be truly generative, it must generate meaning as well as structure, and that meaning in language is expressed not only in words but through the syntactic relationships among words. If we are to understand the acquisition of language, we must account for the expression of meaning.

One of the earliest and most often-cited generative semantics theories was developed by Fillmore (1968). Fillmore's **case grammar** is designed to explain the importance and influence of semantics on the form of language. Fillmore suggested that there is a deeper level of deep structure than that proposed by Chomsky. Beneath deep structure is a level composed of universal concepts that determine how nouns and verbs are related to one another. These are semantic concepts, not syntactic relations, and they are independent of surface structure. Even though these semantic concepts are universal, they are not necessarily innate. According to generative semantics theorists, these concepts are either genetic or environmental phenomena (Chafe, 1970).

Fillmore suggests that sentences have two components: modality and proposition. **Modality** is concerned with sentence characteristics such as verb tense or the expression of negation or interrogation. The second component, proposition, is more critical to the semantic theory. **Proposition** is concerned with the relationship between nouns and verbs in sentences. The relationship between the noun and verb in a given sentence determines the meaning underlying that sentence. Each proposition represents a type of sentence that includes a verb in combination with a *case* or a set of nouns. In the context of this view of language, certain categories of verbs require certain cases. Case refers to a specific semantic role or function that can be filled by a particular type of noun phrase.

Fillmore identifies seven universal cases. An **agentive** case noun phrase is the initiator of an action and, as you would expect, is usually animate. A **dative** case is a person, animal, or other animate being that is affected by the action or by the state of being ascribed by the verb. An **experiencer** is a person, animal, or other animate being that experiences an action or a mental or emotional state. A **factitive** is an object or a being that is the product of an action or state ascribed by a verb. An **instrumental** is an inanimate object that is not the instigator of an action but the means by which the action occurs. A **locative** is the place or location where the action or state ascribed by the verb occurs. An **objective,** considered the most neutral of the cases, is a noun phrase whose role in the action or state ascribed by the verb is determined by the specific meaning of the verb. A summary of these cases with sample sentences is displayed in Table 2.1.

Note that there are not exclusive sets of nouns for each case. A given noun may be used in any case if it meets the definition and requirements of that case. The word *boy* is agentive in the sentence "The boy broke the window." It is dative in the sentence "The woman gave a generous tip to the boy." It is experiencer in the sentence "The boy dreamed about owning his car," and it is objective in the sentence "The homecoming queen kissed the embarrassed little boy." In each case, the verb determines the case of the noun phrase, which means that structure can be explained on the basis of the semantic functions of nouns as determined by verbs. In short, structure is a product of semantic relations.

Chomsky and Fillmore share an important viewpoint relative to language production. Each believes that language production is a generative process and that any theory of language acquisition must account for how language is generated. The essential difference between Chomsky and Fillmore should be clear, however. Chomsky devised a theory to account for the generation of structure. Fillmore devised a theory to account for the generation of semantic relationships, which underlie and provide a foundation for structure.

Chomsky's ideas about generative transformational grammar led many linguists during the late 1960s to analyze children's emerging language from a syntactic point

Table 2.1 Fillmore's (1968) Seven Universal Cases

Case	Definition	Example
Agentive	The initiator of an action	*Tom* hid the present.
Dative	A being affected by the action or state of being ascribed by the verb	Sally gave *him* a generous tip.
Experiencer	A being who experiences an action or a mental or emotional state	*Jerry* enjoyed the concert.
Factitive	An object or being that is the product of an action or state ascribed by the verb	They built the *house.*
Instrumental	An inanimate object that is the means by which an action occurs	She made the fire with *charcoal.*
Locative	The place where the action or state ascribed by the verb occurs	He went camping in the *forest.*
Objective	A noun phrase whose role in the action or state ascribed by the verb is determined by the specific meaning of the verb	Dad kicked *the ball* to me.

of view. Lois Bloom joined this movement. She discovered that syntactic analysis provided valuable information about the early utterances of children, but she also concluded that it did not provide adequate information about the meaning system underlying early language production. Based on her experiences in analyzing the meanings of early utterances using contextual information, Bloom (1970) asserted that transformational generative grammar is more useful in explaining children's language if the analysis includes semantic information that can be used to help analysts draw conclusions about underlying structure. This shift from syntactic analysis to semantic analysis was the beginning of what has been called the *semantic revolution,* a point of view about children's language that suggests that we should study the structure of early language within the context of the speaker's intended message. This context must necessarily take into account linguistic and nonlinguistic information because the communications of children are not words, only events. This kind of analysis is described as a *richer* form of analysis than the transformational generative analysis precisely because it goes beyond the speaker's words to take into account environmental and other nonverbal factors that contribute to the total message.

Other linguists, including Schlesinger (1971) and Brown (1973), reached essentially the same conclusions as Bloom about the importance of semantics in the analysis of early language. Schlesinger went a step further when he concluded that the grammar of early language is semantic, not syntactic, and that early productions are best understood in terms of the semantic relationships expressed in these productions rather than in terms of abstract syntactic categories such as *subject, verb,* and *object.*

The Cognitive Interpretation

At about the same time as the semantic revolution was under way, there was renewed interest in Piaget's cognitive theory and its relationship to language acquisition. Theorists considered specific connections between Piaget's stages of cognitive development and stages of speech and language development, with special emphasis on Piaget's sensorimotor period. This stage of cognitive development extends from birth through two years, the period of time which, not coincidentally, is critical for early speech and language development. In other words, it is easy to understand why linguists would be intrigued by possible, and highly plausible, connections between cognitive development and language acquisition.

It should be noted that all theorists accept that a relationship exists between cognitive development and language development. What separates cognitive theorists from others is their belief that language does not hold an absolutely unique position in overall development. They believe that language itself is not innate, even though the cognitive precursors for language *are* innate. They also believe that language is not learned as behaviorists suggest it is learned. Language emerges, in the cognitive view, not because children are specifically genetically predisposed to produce language and not because language is shaped by learning principles. Language emerges as a product of cognitive organization and development. Language is one of several abilities the child develops for the purpose of conceptual representation and manipulation. All of these abilities emerge as a consequence of cognitive maturation. They emerge when there is imbalance between the child's existing cognitive structures and new information he is receiving from his environment. These theorists agree that the child's cognitive abilities differ from the adult's in terms of how much information is processed and how effectively it is processed. But no matter where a person is in cognitive development, he adds new information into existing cognitive categories, or, if the new information does not fit, he extends, combines, or creates new categories. The process of language acquisition, according to this view, is not separate from but related to cognitive development; it is one part of, and fully integrated into, cognitive development.

Cognitive theorists have noted a number of correlations between language and other cognitive behaviors, correlations that may help us understand how language is acquired. There certainly seems to be a relationship, for example, between the child's understanding that words represent people, places, things, and ideas and the cognitive behavior known as *symbolic play*. There seems to be a connection between understanding that language can be used to get things done and the cognitive behaviors involved in solving problems with tools. Imitation is an important behavior in overall cognitive development, and imitation is clearly an important behavior in speech and language acquisition.

The Information Processing Interpretation

To appreciate the **information processing theory,** one must first understand how it relates to other theoretical perspectives and how these other perspectives relate to one another. By way of a brief review of where we have been so far, the reader should understand that the behaviorist view stresses language function. Linguistic views, best represented by Chomsky's transformational generative grammar and government-binding theory, emphasize language structure. The cognitivist view stresses logical structure. Into this context, we bring the information processing theory. This theory shares with the behaviorist perspective a greater emphasis on *how* language is learned than on the abstract rule system that presumably underlies language, but it goes a step further by making a concerted effort to relate structure and function.

The information processing view is represented well in the *competition model* developed by Bates and MacWhinney (1987). The basic assertion of this theoretical view is that function, not abstract grammar, generates language structure. This view suggests that a human being processes information in much the same way a computer does. That is, a human being has an information processing system that gathers information from the environment and puts that information into symbolic codes, codes that include but are not limited to words and numbers. This internal information processing system interprets these symbolic codes, holds them in memory, and allows for the retrieval of stored information. Language acquisition occurs when a child experiences and gathers language evidence in the productions of her speech and language models and uses that evidence to make fundamental changes within her personal information processing system. The system is constantly adjusted to make its functions consistent with the language evidence the child is gathering.

According to this view, children are not born with an internally wired system for language. Rather, they are born with a potential for all kinds of connections between symbols and the things and ideas symbols can represent. Based on their experiences, some connections are firmly established because they are repeated over and over again. Other possible connections eventually fade away because children do not experience the evidence to activate them. Children internalize language and the connections between language symbols and the things and ideas they represent because there is a constant inpouring of language evidence.

The information processing theory suggests that the processing patterns responsible for the acquisition of language are *parallel* rather than *serial*. Parallel patterns occur at many levels at the same time. By contrast, serial patterns, which are suggested by Chomsky's linguistic view, occur in a kind of vertical sequence. That is, deep structures are generated and are then transformed in a highly predictable sequence into surface structures. Information processing theory suggests that the order in which language forms are acquired is determined by what these forms accomplish. Those language forms that show up most often in a child's language models and that tend to serve the same purpose are acquired first. If, for example, a child's earliest language evidence is filled with examples of structures that make requests, language structures that fill the requesting function will emerge early.

Those who take the information processing view try to explain what occurs in children's minds when they acquire language. They suggest, as already mentioned, that the child processes language information at a number of levels at the same time, a form of processing known as *parallel distributed processing*, or *PDP*. The competition model of Bates and MacWhinney (1987) is an example of a PDP system. A basic premise of this model is that children are not born with an innate understanding of language but with a powerful PDP device that has the capacity to process many different forms of information, including language information. In the earliest stages of language development, the PDP device does not differentiate among words, phonological patterns, and language forms in terms of their ability to represent communicative functions or meanings. This changes, however, as children's experiences with language increase and become more differentiated. Words, phonological patterns, and language forms that are experienced repeatedly activate and strengthen connections in the PDP device. Other connections weaken. As the name of the model suggests, the patterns or connections that are most consistent with the language evidence the child is gathering win the *competition.* They are retained within the child's communication system. Patterns that do not match the evidence lose the competition and are discarded.

So, is the information processing view (and therefore the competition model) a nature or a nurture view of language acquisition? You have probably already surmised, correctly so, that this view includes elements of both extremes. Bates, Bretherton, and Snyder (1988) suggest children are innately predisposed to acquire language just as they are innately predisposed to acquire other behaviors. In this sense, they believe that there is a biological, or innate, basis for language acquisition, though they do not believe that it necessarily accounts for language universals. In terms of nurture, they assert that each child uses biologically based abilities to learn language creatively. They point out, for example, that there are significant individual variations in language acquisition among children within the same culture as well as across cultures. Within the context of the competition model, these differences are the result of varying experiences resulting in differentiated connections within the PDP system.

The Pragmatics Revolution

The semantic revolution that was a reaction to Chomsky's narrow emphasis on structure eventually led to a focus on **pragmatics,** the study of the functions served by communication. Researchers became concerned with how the context of language influences meaning and how language serves different functions for speakers under varying circumstances. The pragmatics revolution of the 1980s and 1990s had its origins many years earlier in work completed by Austin (1962) and Searle (1969). Austin's primary assertion was that when speakers produce utterances, they are doing more than saying words organized by conventional language rules. They are also using these words to get things done. Searle, a student of Austin's, suggested that every speech act consists of three separate acts: (1) the locutionary act, (2) the illocutionary act, and (3) the perlocutionary act.

The **locutionary act** is the most obvious part of the utterance because it is the part that strikes our ears. It is the expression of the words. If you say to a friend, "You've lost some weight," the locutionary act is limited to the utterance itself. It is the sentence the speaker speaks and the hearer hears. The locutionary act, because it is a sentence, consists of a subject, or *referring expression,* and a predicate, or *predicating expression.* Beyond the words, however, consider the possible reasons for your making this observation, and you will get some sense that there may be more to your utterance than meets the listener's ears.

The **illocutionary act,** or **illocutionary force** (Searle, 1976), is concerned with the motive or purpose underlying an utterance. When someone says, "I know what you said, but I want to know what you meant," she is asking the speaker to identify his illocutionary act. Using the earlier example above, if you say to a friend, "You've lost some weight," you could be telling him that he looks good, but you could also be saying that he looks sickly. Your motive might be even more contrived. You might believe that your friend should be losing a lot of weight and hope saying that you have noticed some weight loss will motivate him to lose more. Consider the purpose that might be served by what Searle (1975) calls an *indirect speech act.* If a woman says, "It's a little drafty in here," it is not likely she is simply making an observation about the wind currents and the temperature level in the room. It is more likely that her comment is an indirect way of saying, "Close the window!"

The **perlocutionary act** takes the listener into account. It is concerned with the effect the locutionary act might have on the listener, an effect that may or may not be consistent with the speaker's communicative intention. If you intend to compliment your friend by saying, "You've lost some weight," but your friend knows that he has, in fact, gained a few pounds, he might be offended by the comment, believing you are being sarcastic. Communication works best, of course, when the listener's reactions match the speaker's intentions in terms of communicative content (locutionary act) and purpose (illocutionary act). When this happens, the speaker and listener agree that they are "on the same page," communicatively speaking. When they are not on the same page, communication can be very frustrating. The speaker may be frustrated because he knows what he is trying to say, but no matter how he tries to say it, the listener does not seem to get it. The listener may be frustrated by a sense of communicative paranoia that may or not be justified. The disconnection between speaker and listener, relative to communicative purpose, is not pleasant for either party, and it causes the process of communication to break down.

The Social Interactionist Interpretation

The evolution in theoretical interpretations relative to language acquisition eventually led theorists to explore a middle ground. This is what usually happens in nature-versus-nurture arguments, so the emergence of a compromise view was probably inevitable, although it has emerged later than some might have expected. This middle ground view is known as **social interactionism.**

According to the social interactionist interpretation of speech and language development, both biological and environmental factors are important in the acquisition process, although not necessarily equally. Some interactionist theorists are closer

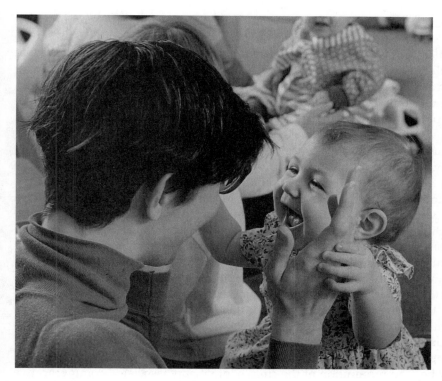

Language development is facilitated by social interaction.

to the nature end of the continuum in that they understand language development as a product of general cognitive development (Bates & MacWhinney, 1982). Others place more emphasis on the contributions of the environment, but all agree that the interaction of biological abilities with environmental influences accounts for language acquisition, and they note the importance of children's interaction with their parents or other caregivers. This basic assumption about the importance of both biology and environment has led to other basic interactionist assumptions about language development.

For example, these theories assume that language acquisition is a product of children's early social interactions with the important people in their life. They point out that children communicate and interact socially with other people before they are able to produce language forms. They believe that language develops as a natural consequence of these interactions. That is, children's attempts to communicate and socialize prompt their parents and other caregivers to provide the language appropriate for these exchanges. As children develop language, their communicative and social skills increase, allowing more mature and sophisticated interactions. These more mature interactions prompt more complex language forms from the parents, and the cycle continues until children's language system and corresponding social skills reach adult levels.

James (1990) provides an excellent example of this progression. She suggests that a nine-month-old child requests a cookie by reaching for it and vocalizing with an utterance such as "Uh, uh, uh," while making eye contact with her mother. The mother, recognizing the communicative intent, might provide a language form as she gives the child a cookie: "Do you want a cookie? Say, 'Cookie . . . cookie.' " By the time the child is two years old, she might make the same request by saying, "Mommy, want cookie," an utterance met with a cookie and an expanded language form modeled by mother: "Say, 'Mommy, I want a cookie.' " By the time the child is four, she will have learned, on the basis of her social and communication experiences, to ask for the cookie by hinting. She might say, "You know, Mommy, I haven't had a cookie for a long time." Notice what happens in this progression. The child is able to make a request from the beginning, before she has any language, and she certainly is able to interact with other people before she can speak. As she acquires language, however, her communicative and interactive abilities improve, and she is able to make her request known in more socially appropriate, more adultlike ways.

James's (1990) example illustrates another emphasis in the interactionist perspective. Unlike the nativists, who stress structure independent of communicative function or intent, interactionists focus on language use. The intent to communicate leads the child to interact with people who can respond to his intent. The intent shapes his initial attempts to communicate, no matter how crude or unsophisticated these attempts may be. The recognition of the child's intent and associated communicative attempt prompts the caregiver not only to meet the intent but to provide an appropriate language model to support the intent. It may be that the model is given only to provide the child an opportunity to confirm or deny the intent, but the model is provided nonetheless. Over time, even though a given intent remains constant, the child acquires more sophisticated language forms by which he can make the intent more immediately and clearly known to his caregivers.

Interactionists, like the behaviorists, emphasize the importance of parents or caregivers in the language acquisition process. Behaviorists, however, view children as passive recipients of language shaped by selective reinforcement. Interactionists believe children are active participants in language acquisition by virtue of their bidirectional involvement with their parents. That is, children initiate communicative and social efforts, perhaps as often as they receive them.

In comparison to the nativists, the interactionists would concede that children come to the language acquisition process with innate cognitive and linguistic abilities, but they do not believe these innate abilities are of greatest importance in language development. Children's interactions, socially and communicatively, with the important people in their environments are the most important factors in the acquisition of language.

Interactionists do not ignore structure or grammar in their understanding of language development. In fact, like the nativists, they try to discover common forms of structure in a variety of languages and cultures (DePaulo & Bonvillian, 1978). They believe, however, that these forms are fairly simple imitations of models to which children are exposed in social interactions (Moerk, 1975, 1983). It can be concluded, therefore, that although interactionists look for and try to explain structure, they are not as focused on structure as nativists. Since their emphasis, as already noted, is on the function of language within social-interactive contexts, they are concerned with how structure contributes to the use of language in getting things done.

Whereas nativists see structure or grammar as almost an end unto itself, interactionists view structure as a means to the end of accomplishing intent. This has led them to study language structure within the child–parent or child–caregiver interaction. In the beginning, these studies focused on the language forms of the caregiver (James, 1990), but more recent studies have examined the child's role and responses in these exchanges.

James (1990) notes that studies of caregivers' speech have revealed that the language forms adults use with young children are very different from the forms they use with other adults or even older children. According to James's review of the relevant research, when caregivers talk to young children, they do the following:

1. Use short, simple sentences.
2. Talk about objects that the child is attending to or actions being engaged in.
3. Repeat their own utterances.
4. Repeat the child's utterances.
5. Use a slightly higher pitch and an exaggerated intonation pattern.
6. Introduce significant pauses between utterances.
7. Use a lot of questions and commands. (p. 179)

This style of speech has been given several names, but perhaps the most popular and descriptive is **motherese.** It should be noted, of course, that this general style is used by all adults when they talk to young children, although there may be some gender differences. Ratner (1988) has found, for example, that although mothers and fathers use the same vocabulary in talking with young children, fathers are more likely than mothers to include the less commonly used words in that vocabulary.

Although no empirical data confirm the efficacy of any of the elements of motherese in facilitating language development, interactionists believe that motherese is ideally designed to help children in language acquisition. It can be argued that repetition, for example, provides multiple models and, depending on the nature of the communicative exchange, several opportunities for the child to practice a particular language form. The use of short, simple sentences seems to provide the child with models he can reasonably expect to imitate. The use of pauses may help him recognize where utterances begin and end. The use of emphatic prosodic patterns might direct the child to those words or structures that are most important. Talking about what is present and readily observable helps keep the communicative process concrete, which in turn probably helps hold the child's attention. The use of questions and commands seems to have the effect of keeping the child active in the communicative process.

On the basis of some research (Barnes, Gutfreund, Satterly, & Wells, 1983; Cross, 1978), one facet of motherese that seems to be related to language acquisition is the use of a technique known as **expansion.** Expansion occurs when the adult repeats what a child has said but adds additional words and/or structure (see Table 2.2). For example, the child might point to a passing vehicle and say, "Truck!" The parent might respond with "That's a fire truck." Parents and other caregivers frequently use expansions when they talk to young children, and they seem to do it naturally, without instruction. Because expansions are more frequently used by the caregivers of linguistically advanced children, and because the use of this technique seems to be associated with an increase in the mean length of children's utterances, it is reasonable to conclude that expansion probably facilitates language development. It is important, however, not to take the conclusion too far. There is, as yet, no evidence suggesting that this technique is essential for normal language development.

Remember that the interactionist view emphasizes the importance of the interaction between the child and her caregiver(s). What is known about the nature of this interaction, especially as it might be related to communication and language development? First, that many adults treat the child as a communicator from the time she is born and begins to cry. That is, when the infant cries, her caregivers try to figure out why. They want to know what she is communicating. Her caregivers also try to understand what the infant's cooing and babbling sounds mean and even what her facial grimaces and body movements mean. Even though the infant's vocalizations, grimaces, and body movements may be random and accidental, her caregivers assume that they have meaning and respond as though they are intentional communications. This is a bidirectional communicative exchange in which the child is treated as an active participant.

Table 2.2 Motherese in Action

Imagine a toddler walking through a zoo with her mother. She is seeing animals she has never seen before, and she is very curious about these new and different creatures. Imagine the rate, pitch, and intonational patterns of the child's speech as well as the mother's speech. In the following exchange, notice some of the typical characteristics of motherese: a topic selected by the child's attention; short, simple sentences; repetition of key elements of the child's utterances; the use of questions to prompt additional responses; and expansion of the child's utterances into more complete, adultlike productions.

CHILD (pointing to a monkey):	Mommy, what's that?
MOTHER:	That's a monkey. Can you say "monkey"?
CHILD:	Monkey!
MOTHER:	Yes, "monkey." What's the monkey doing?
CHILD:	Him eating.
MOTHER:	What's he eating?
CHILD:	Him eating banana.
MOTHER:	Do you eat bananas?
CHILD:	I like bananas!
MOTHER:	The monkey likes bananas, too. . . . What's he doing now?
CHILD:	Him swinging by his tail.
MOTHER:	Can you swing by your tail?
CHILD:	No. I don't gots a tail.
MOTHER:	No, you don't have a tail like the monkey.

As the child grows older, the interactions become a little more elaborate. Many parents, for example, read aloud to their children long before the children are producing language. Why do parents read to speechless children? They may assume that their children are receiving something of linguistic value in the exercise even if they cannot express anything in language form. They may assume that the interaction itself is valuable because it is establishing a bond that will facilitate more meaningful learning when their children are old enough to talk. Parents and other caregivers also play speech-related social games, such as peekaboo, with children. This kind of routine is highly structured, allows the child to participate by predicting what is going to happen (Bruner, 1978), and is a simple but comfortable communication activity. It is, after all, a game. It is nonthreatening and fun, but it provides children with an opportunity to experience all aspects of oral and nonverbal communication, and it gives them a chance to experiment with some of the components of language they are acquiring.

When a young child interacts with a caregiver, his nonverbal communications contribute to the fun and pleasure of the activity, but his nonverbal signals may also be helpful to the caregiver. When the adult uses a language form that the child cannot understand because it contains unfamiliar words or because it is too long or syntactically complex, the child will very likely send some kind of signal, perhaps verbal, but more often nonverbal, to indicate that he is confused and needs help. He might simply look puzzled, or he might shrug his shoulders. When the adult receives this kind of signal, he offers another utterance, which he adjusts toward what he believes is necessary to facilitate the child's understanding. In this way, the verbal and nonverbal interaction allows the adult to simplify and reformulate language forms in ways that certainly facilitate improved communication and may facilitate language development.

Once again, be careful not to read too much into what is happening in these interactions. If, as has been suggested, adults adjust their language to facilitate child–adult communication, it is probably not because adults are making conscious efforts to "teach" their children how to talk. Keep in mind that when adults talk to other adults and an obvious failure to communicate occurs, the listener lets the speaker know that the message has not been received, and the speaker tries again by creating a new version of the original message that is more carefully crafted, in terms of vocabulary and/or structure. When adults talk to children, they make exactly the same kinds of adjustments, and, interestingly, when children talk to adults, they sometimes have to adjust in ways that help the adults understand. Are these adjustments essential in helping children acquire language? As tempting as it may be to let common sense answer yes, there is no data to draw that conclusion.

Consider a specific example of the social interactionist view. One of the most recent formulations of this interpretation of early language acquisition is the **Child Talk** model proposed by Chapman, Streim, Crais, Salmon, Strand, and Negri (1992). Chapman and her colleagues have developed a model that purports to address the diversity of everyday conversational experiences observed in young children during the language acquisition period. This model fully incorporates the most recent evidence researchers have gathered demonstrating the essential contributions of context and world knowledge to language understanding and production. **Context** includes the physical characteristics associated with a communication experience: the nature of events the child is experiencing at the time of the communication, the child's social relationships with other people involved in the communication experience, and all utterances previously produced during the communication. **World knowledge** includes the speaker's past and present knowledge about those aspects of context that might be used to facilitate understanding of or to formulate an utterance. The Child Talk model suggests that language develops as the child becomes increasingly expert in using context and world knowledge.

According to Chapman and her colleagues, "classical accounts" of language acquisition make a number of assertions that need to be challenged. Specifically, these accounts claim that early language formulation is creative, that early productions consist of linguistic units, that language development essentially involves learning rules for how to combine linguistic units, and that language development involves the generation and application of hypotheses about linguistic rules. Each of these assertions, according to Chapman and her colleagues, is problematic.

To argue, for example, that an utterance such as "He runned fast" is evidence that a child is creative in his language production is not wrong but too simplistic. Nelson (1986) and Peters (1984), among others, have shown that while children are sometimes creative in their language productions, they often repeat what they have heard others say in a given circumstance, or they say what they themselves have said in the same or similar situation. The Child Talk model suggests that children sometimes do create utterances, but they also sometimes reproduce utterances. A child needs to have a history of being exposed to conversations associated with a variety of interactions to create a kind of language reservoir. The history she develops will result in a compilation of the utterances the child has heard and understood in all these conversational situations. It constitutes what is called a **lexical script,** a kind of linguistic background the child uses in the process of formulating her own utterances.

The classical accounts of language development suggesting that children learn linguistic units arrived at this conclusion based on two observations: (1) when children learn to talk, they acquire one word at a time and their single-word productions are devoid of prosody; and (2) the measure of average length of utterances, using morphemes as the basic linguistic unit, is a reliable indicator of grammatical complexity and early language competence. The problem with this view, according to Child Talk proponents, is that it oversimplifies what actually occurs in early productions. During the early stages of language acquisition, children produce phrases as whole units, with no apparent understanding of the constituent parts. Children typically include utterances such as *Night-night, Allgone, Wannago,* and *Sobig* among their first meaningful productions. These are single-unit productions, not adultlike combinations of morphemes. Even adults, Chapman and her colleagues note, do not always formulate sentences by drawing linguistic units from a morpheme-restricted well. The adult, when producing idioms, proverbs, or other common expressions, probably gives no attention to the individual morphemes in these utterances. The adult says, "The more you know the more you know you don't know," or "You can lead a horse to water, but you can't make it drink," without paying attention to the morphemes in these words. In fact, the adult probably gives little attention to the individual words or their meanings in these productions. The focus, whether linguistic or semantic, is on the whole unit, not on its parts. Child Talk people argue that units of language production can range from syllables to sentences. The only criterion that must be met for a unit to be considered a unit is that it must be connected, in a general sense, to meaning.

The third assumption derived from classical structural models is that when children acquire language, they acquire rules by which they formulate sentences. The Child Talk people note, however, that since the 1970s, theorists have revised the nature of these rules. Early models, including pivot grammar, focused on syntactic category rules. These models gave way to case grammar models that describe rules based on the semantic roles or functions of noun phrases, and then to models that identify rules based on semantics and pragmatics. Language theory has progressed, therefore, from views of language development that narrowly focused on rules based on linguistic structure to views that take into account how words are used in reference to one another, what they mean, and for what communicative purposes they are used. Slobin (1986) and Nelson (1986), for example, suggest that rules for selecting and structuring words and their morphemes into productive utterances are based on the roles of referents in events as children conceptualize these referents and events. In other words, you cannot separate children's language productions from children's real-life experiences and their understandings of these experiences. The idea that children organize language based on what they experience and on how they conceptualize the people, things, and events in their experiences suggests that language is organized not by linguistic universals but by conceptual universals. Conceptual universals refer to the shared views children have about what is happening around them, a phenomenon Nelson (1986) calls *event knowledge*.

Finally, there is the classical account assertion that during language acquisition, children acquire rules by developing and testing hypotheses. The suggestion is that children apply principles of scientific inquiry to the acquisition of language, an idea the Child Talk people believe challenges the limits of plausibility. Beyond the plausibility issue, however, is a more practical concern. The classical view suggests that children develop and test language hypotheses without getting specific affirmations or denials from their environment. In other words, children operate independently in developing hypotheses and in either retaining or rejecting them. This assumption had its origins in the work of Brown and Hanlon (1970), who found very few specific and explicit reactions from parents in reference to the syntactic accuracy of their children's utterances. They found that parents reacted to the accuracy of their children's observations rather than the syntactic correctness of their utterances, and even these reactions were limited. The Child Talk people wonder how children determine which hypotheses are valid and should be retained and which hypotheses are incorrect and disposable. Chapman and her colleagues acknowledge that other studies, utilizing a more liberal view of negative feedback in reference to children's language errors, have generated evidence of more negative feedback from parents in their exchanges with their children than suggested by Brown and Hanlon. Even these studies, however, do

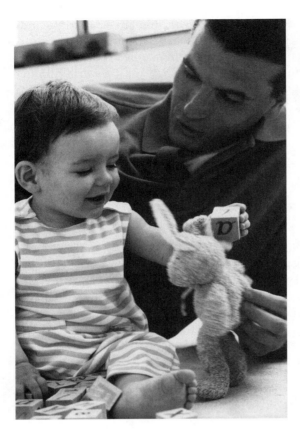

Language acquisition occurs within the child's total environment.

not make clear how this kind of negative reaction leads children to accept, modify, or reject their hypotheses about language production. Child Talk proponents further argue that even if children's productions can be described as analogous productions or as overextensions, we have still not explained why the child does not dispose of these forms when adults try to correct them.

To this point, we have identified the assumptions of the classical view that have been refuted by Child Talk theorists. But what assumption underlies the Child Talk view of language acquisition? They assume that early language acquisition occurs as the child is introduced to his world, becomes acquainted with the social and physical characteristics of his environment, learns about the people and objects to be found in his environment, experiences the sounds, sights, and movements associated with all these things, and learns that he can make things happen by means of his own vocalizations and nonverbal actions. The basic assumption, then, that underlies the Child Talk model is that language acquisition occurs in context, broadly defined. The child's developing knowledge of everything in the life that swirls around him helps him establish goals for getting things done and develop strategies for suc-

Table 2.3 Tracing the Evolution of Language Acquisition Theories

Theory	Primary Architect/ Date(s)	Essential Idea	Primary Focus
Behaviorist	Skinner/1957	Language is learned by selective reinforcement.	General
Transformational generative grammar	Chomsky/1957	Language is processed by universal and innate rules governing deep and surface structure.	Syntax
Government-binding theory	Chomsky/1981	Extended version of TGG, but with emphasis on *learnability*.	Syntax
Case grammar	Fillmore/1968	There is a level beneath deep structure composed of universal semantic concepts that determines the relationships between nouns and verbs.	Semantics
Information processing theory	Bates & MacWhinney/ 1987	Function, not abstract grammar, generates language structure.	Structure by function
Child Talk model	Chapman et al./1992	Context and world knowledge drive language acquisition.	Interaction of all language components

cessfully meeting these goals. According to the Child Talk view, the child formulates utterances because he has goals in mind that can best be met by using these utterances. Drawing on the linguistic and nonlinguistic experiences of his own past, however brief that past is, the child uses his language knowledge in combination with his knowledge about other relevant aspects of his world to formulate utterances that will serve as means to today's ends. Consistent with other interactive models of language production, the Child Talk model suggests that a variety of language components, including semantics, syntax, and phonology, interact as the child formulates and interprets language. (See Table 2.3 for a brief summary of language acquisition theories.)

And the Evolution Continues

Where does the evolution in theories of language acquisition stand as we enter the twenty-first century? It would be inaccurate to say that the experts have reached consensus about how children acquire language, but it would also be erroneous to conclude that we have not made progress in our considerations. Some are still convinced that language is a uniquely human and innate ability that only needs an environmental trigger to emerge, almost magically, according to a biologically predetermined schedule. Some still believe that language is almost entirely the product of environmental influences and that human children do not "develop" language as much as they "receive" language from their caregivers by virtue of their selective reinforcement and shaping of their initially random language-like behaviors. There seems to be growing support, however, for the middle ground in this nature-versus-nurture argument. As suggested in the opening of this chapter, this kind of compromise was almost inevitable. The interactionist perspective, therefore, is likely to have an increasingly greater voice in how theorists describe language acquisition and in formulating the questions researchers will attempt to answer about human language and its development.

Chapters 3–5, tracing the development of language from the preparation stage through late childhood, are written primarily from the interactionist point of view, with references to other explanations where appropriate. For people who are just beginning to explore language and its development in children, it is particularly important to take the broadest possible view. Humans are complex beings who do not live in vacuums and certainly do not grow up in vacuums. To a large extent children are shaped by their environment, especially by parents and other significant caregivers. At the same time, do not lose sight of the enormous power of genetic talent. Who does not marvel at world-class musicians and athletes? These people have worked hard to develop their considerable skills, but without the right genetic stuff a woman cannot high-jump seven feet, no matter how much she practices, and without the appropriate genetic gift, a pianist will never do justice to great music, no matter how many hours he spends at the keyboard. Language, like many other human abilities, is acquired by way of genetic gift shaped by environmental forces. Which is the greater factor, heredity or environment? Let's not go there!

Review Questions

1. What is the general nature-versus-nurture argument, and how does it apply to language development?
2. Summarize the behaviorist interpretation of speech and language development.
3. What do behaviorists mean when they describe language as a doing or performing phenomenon as opposed to a knowing phenomenon?
4. How can classical conditioning principles be used to explain the acquisition of *meaning* in language?
5. What have we learned about language development from experimental attempts to teach chimpanzees to use language?
6. What is the *Language Acquisition Device (LAD)*, and what is its role in language development, according to the nativist interpretation?
7. In Transformational Generative Grammar, what is the difference between *surface* structure and *deep* structure?
8. How does the issue of *learnability* separate government-binding theory from Chomsky's earlier versions of transformational generative grammar?

9. Identify the four levels of representation at which Universal Grammar operates, and briefly explain what each level contributes to language production.

10. Briefly explain the following sub-theories of the government-binding theory: bounding theory, government theory, case theory, binding theory, thematic theory, and control theory.

11. In the context of Fillmore's case grammar, what is meant by *modality* and *proposition?*

12. Briefly define and provide an example for each of Fillmore's seven universal cases.

13. What is the essence of the *cognitive* interpretation of language development?

14. What is meant by *parallel distributed processing* (PDP), and how does a model based on PDP, such as the competition model, explain language acquisition?

15. Compare and contrast the LAD and the PDP.

16. What are the three parts of the *speech act*, according to Searle, and what does each part contribute to the whole speech act?

17. Discuss the objections of Child Talk proponents to the assumptions underlying the so-called "classical accounts" of language acquisition.

18. What assumptions underlie the Child Talk view? Explain why proponents of this view believe these assumptions are more valid than the assumptions underlying the classical interpretations of early language development.

19. How does the social interactionist interpretation fill the gap between the nativist interpretation at one end of the nature-versus-nurture continuum and the behaviorist interpretation at the other end of the continuum?

20. Based on your understanding of the twists and turns in the evolution of theories regarding language development over the past fifty years, what kinds of theoretical interpretations do you think language experts will be considering fifty years from now?

References and Suggested Readings

Austin, J. (1962). *How to do things with words.* London: Oxford University Press.

Barnes, S., Gutfreund, M., Satterly, D., & Wells, G. (1983). Characteristics of adult speech which predict children's language development. *Journal of Child Language, 10,* 65–84.

Bates, E., Bretherton, I., Beeghly-Smith, M., & McNew, S. (1983). Social basis of language development: A re-assessment. In H. Reese & L. Lipsitt (Eds.), *Advances in child development and behavior* (Vol. 16, pp. 8–75). New York: Academic Press.

Bates, E., Bretherton, I., & Snyder, L. (1988). *From first words to grammar: Individual differences and dissociable mechanisms.* New York: Cambridge University Press.

Bates, E., & MacWhinney, B. (1982). Functionalist approaches to grammar. In E. Wanner & L. Gleitman (Eds.), *Language acquisition: The state of the art* (pp. 173–218). Cambridge, MA: Cambridge University Press.

Bates, E., & MacWhinney, B. (1987). Competition, variation, and language learning. In B. MacWhinney (Ed.), *Mechanisms of language acquisition*. Hillsdale, NJ: Erlbaum.

Berko-Gleason, J. (Ed.) (1989). *The development of language* (2nd ed.). Columbus, OH: Merrill/Prentice Hall.

Bloom, L. (1970). *Language development: Form and function in emerging grammars*. Cambridge, MA: MIT Press.

Bloom, L., Hood, P., & Lightbown, P. (1974). Imitation in language development: If, when and why? *Cognitive Psychology, 6*, 380–420.

Bohannon, J., & Hirsch-Pasek, K. (1984). Do children say as they're told? A new perspective on motherese. In L. Feagans, C. Garvey, & R. Golinkoff (Eds.), *The origins and growth of communication* (pp. 176–195). Norwood, NJ: Ablex.

Bohannon, J., MacWhinney, B., & Snow, C. (1990). Negative evidence revisited: Beyond learnability or who has to prove what to whom? *Developmental Psychology, 26*, 221–226.

Bohannon, J., Padgett, R., Nelson, K., & Mark, M. (1996). Useful evidence on negative evidence. *Developmental Psychology, 32*, 551–555.

Bohannon, J., & Warren-Leubecker, A. (1988). Recent developments in child-directed speech: You've come a long way, baby-talk. *Language Science, 10*, 89–110.

Bohannon, J., & Warren-Leubecker, A. (1989). Theoretical approaches to language acquisition. In J. Berko-Gleason (Ed.), *The development of language* (pp. 167–213). Columbus, OH: Merrill/Prentice Hall.

Brown, R., & Hanlon, C. (1970). Derivational complexity and order of acquisition in child speech. In J. Hayes (Ed.), *Cognition and the development of language*. New York: Wiley.

Brown, R. (1973). *A first language: The early stages*. Cambridge, MA: Harvard University Press.

Bruner, J. (1978). Learning the mother tongue. *Human Nature, 1*, 42–49.

Bryen, D. (1982). *Inquiries into child language*. Boston: Allyn & Bacon.

Cameron-Faulkner, T., Leiven, L., & Tomasello, M. (2003). A construction based analysis of child-directed speech. *Cognitive Science, 27*, 843–873.

Chafe, W. (1970). *Meaning and the structure of language*. Chicago: University of Chicago Press.

Chapman, R., Streim, N., Crais, E., Salmon, D., Strand, E., & Negri, N. (1992). Child talk: Assumptions of a developmental process model for early language learning. In R. Chapman (Ed.), *Processes in language acquisition and disorders*. St. Louis, MO: Mosby-Year Book.

Chomsky, C. (1969). *The acquisition of syntax in children from 5 to 10*. Cambridge, MA: MIT Press.

Chomsky, N. (1957). *Syntactic structures*. The Hague: Mouton.

Chomsky, N. (1965). *Aspects of a theory of syntax*. Cambridge, MA: MIT Press.

Chomsky, N. (1968). *Language and mind*. New York: Harcourt, Brace & World.

Chomsky, N. (1979). Human language and other semiotic systems. *Semiotica, 25*, 31–44.

Chomsky, N. (1981). *Lectures on government and binding*. Dordrecht, Holland: Foris.

Chomsky, N. (1997). *Language and mind: Current thoughts on ancient problems* (Part 1). Available online at http://fccl.ksu.ru/papers/chomsky1.htm

Chomsky, N., & Place, U. T. (2000). The Chomsky–Place correspondence 1993–1994 (T. Schoneberger, Ed.). *The analysis of verbal behavior, 17*, 7–38.

Clark, E. (1977). Strategies and the mapping problem in first language acquisition. In J. MacNamara (Ed.), *Language learning and thought* (pp. 147–168). New York: Academic Press.

Corballis, M. (2002). *From hand to mouth: The origin of language.* Princeton, NJ: Princeton University Press.

Cross, T. (1977). Mother's speech adjustments: The contribution of selected child listener variables. In C. Snow & C. Ferguson (Eds.), *Talking to children: Language input and acquisition.* Cambridge, MA: Cambridge University Press.

Cross, T. (1978). Mother's speech and its association with rate of linguistic development in young children. In N. Waterson & C. Snow (Eds.), *The development of communication.* New York: Wiley.

DePaulo, B., & Bonvillian, J. (1978). The effect on language development of the special characteristics of speech addressed to children. *Journal of Psycholinguistic Research, 7,* 189–211.

Derwing, B. (1973). *Transformational grammar as a theory of language acquisition.* Cambridge, MA: Cambridge University Press.

Elman, J., Bates, E., Johnson, M., Karmiloff-Smitt, A., Parisi, D., & Plunkett, K. (1996). *Rethinking innateness: A connectionist perspective on development.* Cambridge, MA: MIT/Bradford.

Enard, W., Przeworski, M., Fisher, S., Lai, C., Wiebe, V., Kitano, T., Monaco, A., & Paabo, S. (2002). Molecular evolution of FOXP2, a gene involved in speech and language. *Nature, 418,* 869–872.

Fey, M. (1986). *Language intervention with young children.* San Diego, CA: College-Hill.

Fillmore, C. (1968). The case for case. In E. Bach & R. Harmas (Eds.), *Universals in linguistic theory.* New York: Holt, Rinehart & Winston.

Gardner, R., & Gardner, B. (1969). Teaching sign language to a chimpanzee. *Science, 165,* 664–672.

Gardner, R., & Gardner, B. (1971). Two-way communication with a chimpanzee. In A. Schrier & F. Stollnitz (Eds.), *Behavior of nonhuman primates* (Vol. 4, pp. 117–184). New York: Academic Press.

Gardner, R., & Gardner, B. (1975). Early signs of language in child and chimpanzee. *Science, 187,* 752–753.

Gleitman, L., Newport, E., & Gleitman, H. (1984). The current status of the motherese hypothesis. *Journal of Child Language, 11,* 43–79.

Gleitman, L., & Wanner, E. (1982). Language acquisition: The state of the state of the art. In E. Wanner & L. Gleitman (Eds.), *Language acquisition: The state of the art* (pp. 3–48). Cambridge, MA: Cambridge University Press.

Greenfield, P., & Savage-Rumbaugh, S. (1984). Perceived variability and symbol use: A common language-cognition interface in children and chimpanzees (*Pan troglodytes*). *Journal of Comparative Psychology, 2,* 201–218.

Hirsh-Pasek, K., & Golinkoff, R. (1993). Skeletal supports for grammatical learning: What the infant brings to the language learning task. In C. Rovee-Collier & L. Lipsitt (Eds.), *Advances in infancy research* (Vol. 8, pp. 299–338). Norwood, NJ: Ablex.

Hirsh-Pasek, K., & Golinkoff, R. (1996). *The origins of grammar.* Cambridge, MA: MIT Press.

Hoff-Ginsberg, E. (1986). Function and structure in maternal speech: Their relation to the child's development of syntax. *Developmental Psychology, 22,* 155–163.

Hoff-Ginsberg, E., & Shatz, M. (1982). Linguistic input and the child's acquisition of language. *Psychological Bulletin, 92,* 3–26.

Holland, J., & Skinner, B. F. (1961). *The analysis of behavior.* New York: McGraw-Hill.

James, S. (1990). *Normal language acquisition.* Austin, TX: PRO-ED.

Lenneberg, E. (1964). A biological perspective of language. In E. Lenneberg (Ed.), *New directions in the study of language.* Cambridge, MA: MIT Press.

Lenneberg, E. (1967). *Biological foundations of language.* New York: Wiley.

Leonard, L., & Loeb, D. (1988). Government-binding theory and some of its implications: A tutorial. *Journal of Speech and Hearing Research, 31,* 515–524.

Link, J., & Bohannon, J. (2003, April). *Negative evidence in Spanish.* Paper presented at the biennial meeting of the Society for Research in Child Development, Tampa, FL.

Lovaas, O. (1977). *The autistic child: Language development through behavior modification.* New York: Irvington.

MacWhinney, B. (1987). *Mechanisms of language acquisition.* Hillsdale, NJ: Erlbaum.

Maratsos, M., & Chalkley, M. (1980). The internal language of children's syntax: The ontogenesis and representation of syntactic categories. In K. Nelson (Ed.), *Children's language* (Vol. 2). New York: Gardner.

Maratsos, M., Kuczaj, S., Fox, D., & Chalkley, M. (1979). Some empirical studies in the acquisition of transformation relations: Passives, negatives, and the past tense. In W. Collins (Ed.), *Children's language and communication.* Hillsdale, NJ: Erlbaum.

McClelland, J., Rummelhart, D., & PDP Research Group. (1986). *Parallel distributed processing: Explorations in the microstructure of cognition* (Vol. 2). Cambridge, MA: Bradford.

Menyuk, P. (1977). *Language and maturation.* Cambridge, MA: MIT Press.

Moerk, E. (1975). Verbal interactions between children and their mothers during the preschool years. *Developmental Psychology, 11,* 788–794.

Moerk, E. (1983). *The mother of Eve—As a first language teacher.* Norwood, NJ: Ablex Publishing Corporation.

Moerk, E. (1989). The LAD was a lady and the tasks were ill-defined. *Developmental Review, 9,* 21–57.

Nelson, K. (1986). *Event knowledge.* New York: Academic Press.

Newport, E. (1976). Motherese: The speech of mothers to young children. In N. Castellan, D. Pisoni, & G. Potts (Eds.), *Cognitive theory* (Vol. 2). Hillsdale, NJ: Erlbaum.

Owens, R. (1992). *Language development: An introduction* (3rd ed.). Upper Saddle River, NJ: Merrill/Prentice Hall.

Owens, R. (2001). *Language development: An introduction* (5th ed.). Boston: Allyn & Bacon.

Owens, R. (2005). *Language development: An introduction* (6th ed.). Boston: Allyn & Bacon.

Palermo, D. (1978). *Psychology of language.* Glenview, IL: Scott, Foresman.

Penner, S. (1987). Parental responses to grammatical and ungrammatical child utterances. *Child Development, 58,* 376–384.

Peters, A. (1984). *The units of language acquisition.* New York: Cambridge University Press.

Pinker, S. (1979). Formal models of language learning. *Cognition, 7,* 217–283.

Pinker, S. (1984). *Language, learnability and language development.* Cambridge, MA: Harvard University Press.

Pinker, S. (1987). The bootstrapping problem in language acquisition. In B. MacWhinney (Ed.), *Mechanisms of language acquisition* (pp. 399–439). Hillsdale, NJ: Erlbaum.

Pinker, S., & Prince, A. (1988). On language and connectionism: Analysis of a parallel distributed processing model of language acquisition. *Cognition, 28,* 73–193.

Ratner, N. (1988). Patterns of parental vocabulary selection in speech to very young children. *Journal of Child Language, 15,* 481–492.

Ritchie, W., & Bhatia, T. (1999). Child language development: Introduction, foundations, and overview. In W. Ritchie & T. Bhatia (Eds.), *Handbook of child language acquisition* (pp. 1–33). New York: Academic Press.

Rumbaugh, D., & Beran, M. (2003). Language acquisition by animals. In L. Nadel (Ed.), *Encyclopedia of Cognitive Science.* London: Macmillan.

Savage-Rumbaugh, E. (1987). A new look at ape language: Comprehension of vocal speech and syntax. In D. Leger (Ed.), *The Nebraska symposium on motivation.* Lincoln: University of Nebraska.

Savage-Rumbaugh, E. (1990). Verbal communication in the chimpanzee. In N. Krasnegor, D. Rumbaugh, R. Schiefelbusch, & M. Studdert-Kennedy (Eds.), *Biobehavioral foundations of language development.* Hillsdale, NJ: Erlbaum.

Savage-Rumbaugh, E., MacDonald, K., Sevcik, R., Hopkins, W., & Rubert, E. (1986). Spontaneous symbol acquisition and communicative use by pygmy chimpanzees (*Pan paniscus*). *Journal of Experimental Psychology: General, 115,* 211–235.

Savage-Rumbaugh, E., Sevcik, R., Brakke, K., & Rumbaugh, D. (1990). Symbols: Their communicative use, combination, and comprehension by bonobos (*Pan paniscus*). In L. Lipsitt & C. Rovee-Collier (Eds.), *Advances in infancy research.* Norwood, NJ: Ablex.

Savage-Rumbaugh, S., Shanker, S., & Taylor, T. (1998). *Ape language and the human mind.* New York: Oxford University Press.

Saxton, M. (2000). Negative evidence and negative feedback: Immediate effects on the grammaticality of child speech. *First Language, 20,* 221–252.

Saxton, M., Kulcsar, B., Marshall, G., & Rupra, M. (1998). Longer-term effects of corrective input: An experimental approach. *Journal of Child Language, 25,* 701–721.

Schlesinger, I. (1971). Production of utterances and language acquisition. In D. Slobin (Ed.) *The ontogenesis of grammar.* New York: Academic Press.

Searle, J. (1969). *Speech acts.* Cambridge, England: Cambridge University Press.

Searle, J. (1975). *Indirect speech acts.* In P. Cole & J. L. Morgan (Eds.), *Syntax and semantics 3: Speech acts.* New York: Academic Press.

Searle, J. (1976). The classification of illocutionary acts. *Language in Society, 5,* 1–24.

Shatz, M. (1982). On mechanisms of language acquisition: Can features of the communicative environment account for development? In E. Wanner & L. Gleitman (Eds.), *Language acquisition: The state of the art.* Cambridge, MA: Cambridge University Press.

Skinner, B. F. (1957). *Verbal behavior.* Upper Saddle River, NJ: Prentice Hall.

Slobin, D. (1986). Cross-linguistic evidence for the language-making capacity. In D. Slobin (Ed.), *The cross-linguistic study of language acquisition: Theoretical issues.* Hillsdale, NJ: Erlbaum.

Snow, C. (1981a). Social interaction and language acquisition. In P. Dale & D. Ingram (Eds.), *Child language: An international perspective.* Baltimore: University Park Press.

Snow, C. (1981b). The uses of imitation. *Journal of Child Language, 8,* 205–208.

Snow, C. (1999). Social perspectives on the emergence of language. In B. MacWhinney (Ed.), *The emergence of language* (pp. 257–276). Mahwah, NJ: Erlbaum.

Staats, A. (1971). Linguistic-mentalistic theory versus an explanatory S-R learning theory of language development. In D. Slobin (Ed.), *The ontogenesis of grammar.* New York: Academic Press.

Staats, C., & Staats, A. (1957). Meaning established by classical conditioning. *Journal of Experimental Psychology, 54,* 74–80.

Stine, E., & Bohannon, J. (1983). Imitation, interactions and acquisition. *Journal of Child Language, 10,* 589–604.

Tager-Flusberg, H., & Calkins, S. (1990). Does imitation facilitate the acquisition of grammar? Evidence from a study of autistic, Down syndrome, and normal children. *Journal of Child Language, 17,* 591–606.

Terrace, H. (1980). *Nim: A chimpanzee who learned sign language.* New York: Knopf.

Terrance, H., Pettito, L., Saunder, R., & Bever, J. (1979). Can an ape create a sentence? *Science, 206,* 891–902.

Van Riper, C. (1964). *Speech correction, principles and methods* (4th ed.).

Upper Saddle River, NJ: Prentice Hall.

Watson, J. (1924). *Behaviorism.* Chicago: University of Chicago Press.

Wexler, K., & Culicover, P. (1980). *Formal principles of language acquisition.* Cambridge, MA: MIT Press.

Wexler, K. (1999). Maturation and growth of grammar. In W. Ritchie & T. Bhatia (Eds.), *Handbook of child language acquisition* (pp. 55–110). New York: Academic Press.

Whitehurst, G., & Vasta, R. (1975). Is language acquired through imitation? *Journal of Psycholinguistic Research, 4,* 37–59.

Wilbur, R. (2003). What studies of sign language tell us about language. In M. Marschark & P. Spencer (Eds.), *The handbook of deaf studies, language, and education* (pp. 332–346). Oxford: Oxford University Press.

Zimmerman, B., & Whitehurst, G. (1979). Structure and function: A comparison of two views of the development of language and cognition. In G. Whitehurst & B. Zimmerman (Eds.), *The functions of language and cognition.* New York: Academic Press.

Zukow-Goldring, P. (2001). Perceiving referring actions: Latino and Euro-American infants and caregivers comprehending speech. In K. Nelson, A. Aksu-Koc, & C. Johnson (Eds.), *Children's language* (Vol. 11, pp. 140–163). Mahwah, NJ: Erlbaum.

3

Cognitive Development: Building a Foundation for Language

What is the role of intellectual development in language development? This is one of the most interesting and challenging questions to be addressed in a study of human communication development. Since language is a means by which people express what they are thinking, the relationship between cognition and language is important, but does the development of one precede the development of the other? Do cognition and language develop in a parallel manner, and if they are connected, how are they con-

nected? This chapter addresses these and related questions and, in the process, shows that theorists hold widely varying views about whether language and thinking depend on one another and how.

Then two major theoretical views of cognitive development are presented, one proposed by Jean Piaget and the other by Lev Vygotsky. We consider how these two interpretations account for early intellectual development, with special attention to the implications relative to child language development. Finally, we consider the perceptual bases that underlie early cognitive and language development. Specifically, this chapter is designed to facilitate understanding of the following topics:

- Jean Piaget's theory of cognitive development, with emphasis on the first of the four stages of intellectual development he describes

- *Distancing*, a basic perceptual principle critical to early intellectual development

- Concepts and behaviors central to intellectual functioning and development, including *object permanence, causality, means-ends, play,* and *communication*

- Challenges to Piaget's theory as the result of recent research

- Lev Vygotsky's theory of cognitive development, which emphasizes the role of language in intellectual and social development

- The perceptual preparation for communication development, focusing on visual perception, auditory perception, and the child's early interest in the human voice and speech

Chapter Two examined a number of theories of language development that can be arranged along a continuum representing the possible influences of nurture and nature on the language acquisition process. The basic question that has driven the writers of these theories can be framed as follows: "Is language genetically or environmentally determined?" The answer, as you discovered, is not to be found in any simple extreme, but the question provides an appropriate segue into this chapter.

Are you ready for another question about language for which there is no answer or, more accurately, no easy answer? Well, ready or not, here it is. Does thought shape language, or does language shape thought? It is important to know whether the development of thought, or *cognition,* precedes the emergence of language, follows the emergence of language, or develops concurrently with language.

Since language is used to express thoughts, common sense would certainly suggest that thought shapes language, at least in the early stages of human development. Common sense would also suggest, however, that at some point in development, language begins to shape thought. In this case, common sense is probably correct on both counts. The important point is that, for many thought processes, it is not possible to separate thinking and language. As you read the words on this page, you are processing language to interpret the intended thoughts of the writers, and as you consider what the messages on this page mean, you are manipulating your thoughts in some kind of language form. You might not use complete sentences in your inner language, and your cognitive sentences may not always be grammatically correct, but they are in language form.

At the same time, human beings can and do think in ways that do not involve language. When Beethoven wrote his music, he *thought* music. When artists paint, they think in colors and forms and visual messages. When a football coach designs plays, he thinks in Xs and Os. Mathematicians think in numbers and formulas. Thinking takes many forms other than language. We all think emotions, and sometimes these emotions cannot even be expressed in language. We all think images and sounds and smells, and even though these sensory experiences can sometimes be described in words, words often fail to do them justice. If a picture is worth a thousand words, a thought, even a simple thought, has the potential to bankrupt the vocabulary.

What then, is the relationship between thought and language? We can conclude that thought does shape language because thought determines what we will say and how we will say it. We can conclude that language shapes thought because we often use language in our thought processes and manipulate our thoughts in language forms. And we can conclude that some thoughts are expressed in forms other than language, such as musical tones and chords, mental images, or even mathematic abstractions.

To facilitate an understanding of the critical relationship between cognition and language, we will examine two highly regarded theories of cognitive development. We will consider the research evidence that supports each view and the scholarly ponderings these theories have generated, and we will determine what each theory suggests about the role of language in cognitive development.

Before we examine each of these theories in some detail, a few general observations are in order. First, it must be emphasized that Piaget did not specifically propose a theory of language development. He treated language as just one of a number of symbolic functions children develop as they interact with their environment. Piaget viewed cognitive development as an essential prerequisite for the development of all symbolic functions.

Also note that while Piaget's theoretical views are widely respected among those who study human intellectual development and language development, several aspects of his theory have been challenged. One aspect of particular interest to us is the theory's failure to account adequately for how children assign words to their referent (Owens, 1996, p. 148). Both Piaget and Vygotsky asserted that children are active players in the process of acquiring knowledge about their world, but beyond this general agreement, there is a crucial difference. Piaget believed that the child is an independent operative in cognitive development. His theory is considered a **constructivist approach** because he believed the child, in the process of actively searching and discovering, *constructs* essentially everything she knows about her world.

Vygotsky believed that during cognitive development, the child maintains a cooperative relationship with the environment and culture. In his view, this cooperative relationship is a vitally important component in the process of achieving cognitive competence.

Piaget's Theory of Cognitive Development

Jean Piaget is well known in the United States, where he is usually thought of as a child psychologist. Although his work has certainly been applied to child psychology and education, Piaget was actually a genetic epistemologist. **Genetic epistemology** is the study of how knowledge is acquired, so Piaget devoted his life to understanding cognitive or intellectual development. This science has rather obvious applications to both education and psychology. Piaget moved easily in these disciplines, and his ideas have been influential in both.

Piaget's original passion was biology, a passion born and cultivated at a young age. By the time he was ten years old, he had already published an article describing a partly albino sparrow. This intellectually gifted child earned his bachelor's degree at eighteen and his doctorate at twenty-one, by which time he had already published twenty-five professional papers. Piaget's early studies of mollusks caused him to believe that development was not just the product of biological maturation guided by genetics but was also affected by environmental factors. Over the years of his professional career, this conclusion led him to understand that cognitive development is the result of biological maturation in interaction with the environment (Wadsworth, 1971, pp. 2–3).

This conclusion about the interaction of heredity and environment can be clearly observed in Piaget's stages of cognitive development. We will begin our examination of Piaget's theory by identifying and describing several basic concepts underlying the theory. Using this understanding as a foundation, we will consider the overall framework of the theory. We will briefly describe the four stages before examining the first stage, the **sensorimotor period,** in detail. This discussion will reflect Piaget's theory as he originally proposed it, but we will follow this discussion with a review of recent research evidence that calls some aspects of Piaget's theory into question.

The Elements and Processes of Cognitive Organization

It is important to remember what Piaget learned from his work as a biologist. He came to understand that many actions of living creatures are *adaptations* to their environments and that these actions help creatures *organize* their environments (Wadsworth, 1971, p. 9). He applied this understanding in explaining children's cognitive development by assuming that cognitive acts *organize* children's environments and are the result of children's *adaptation* to their environments. According to Piaget (1952), four basic concepts underlie cognitive organization: schema, assimilation, accommodation, and equilibrium. As you will discover, it is difficult to understand one of these concepts without considering the others because they are related. We will begin by defining and explaining *schema,* but your understanding of schema will not be complete until you understand how the other three concepts relate to schema and to one another.

A **schema** can be understood as a concept, mental category, or cognitive structure. The plural of schema is **schemata,** so as a child develops intellectually, she develops many schemata by which she organizes and adapts to her environment. Think of a schema as a computer file of the brain. A personal computer's memory bank might be filled with a number of specific files for things such as business expenses, addresses, letters, appointments, checking account, and so forth. When you process new information on the computer, you save that information in the appropriate file. In much the same way, adults use many schemata to process, identify, and store information. Even if you see a dog unlike any dog you have ever seen before, you have no difficulty processing that stimulus as a dog. Your dog schema is so well developed that you can put the smallest Chihuahua and the largest Great Dane in the same category. You know what dogness is. You may encounter a rat bigger than a Chihuahua or a horse smaller than a Great Dane, but you do not misfile these stimuli into your dog schema because you have a rat schema and a horse schema, and you know the differences among these three animals. If, however, you see an animal unlike any animal you have ever seen before, you will scan all your schemata and find no place to fit this new stimulus. You will either modify an existing schema to make the new stimulus fit or create a new schema so that you can put this new creature into its proper file. This brings us to the next two concepts: assimilation and accommodation.

Return to the computer file analogy for a moment. If a person has a letters file in his computer's memory, any letter he composes will be saved into that file. Other things he may write, such as recipes, memos to professional colleagues, lyrics for songs he is composing, or material for what he hopes is the next great American novel, go in other files, but every letter he writes is saved into the letters file. In much the same way, each time you encounter a new stimulus, you scan your schemata to decide where this stimulus fits. **Assimilation** is the cognitive process whereby a person includes a new stimulus into an existing schema. Until a few years ago, I had never seen a sharpei, the cuddly and wrinkled Chinese dog that has become popular. I recognized this stimulus as a dog, however, and assimilated it into my existing dog schema, right there with Chihuahua, Great Dane, German shepherd, schnauzer, and all the other dog stimuli. As we experience life, our existing schemata are constantly being expanded by the inclusion of new stimuli that fit these categories.

What happens when some new stimulus just does not fit into an existing schema? Return once more to the computer file analogy. The man in the example may be a prolific letter writer, so after months or years of producing and saving letters, his letter file becomes very large. Because he writes many different kinds of letters, it also becomes unmanageable and virtually meaningless. He may have family letters, letters to friends, business letters, and love letters in the same file, and it becomes clear they do not all belong in the same computer file. What does he do? He creates new files, of course. He might develop a file for personal letters, another for business letters, and another for love letters. In other words, he accommodates the diversity of letters by creating separate categories for them in his computer's memory. When people develop new schemata to allow for the organization of stimuli that do not fit into existing schemata, we say that **accommodation** has occurred.

A person's dog schema may be well developed as an adult, but for the young child this schema presents some organizational problems. You have probably known a child who has pointed to a horse, cow, perhaps even an elephant or giraffe, and said, "Doggie!" What is going on here? The child is observing a stimulus she has never experienced before. She searches her schemata for a category into which to place this new stimulus. She sees a creature with four legs. Her "doggie" schema includes animals with four legs. Eureka! This must be a doggie, she thinks, so she assimilates the horse, cow, elephant, or giraffe into her existing doggie schema.

Unlike a computer file, which has a size limit based on a computer's memory capacity, a schema has no size limits. No matter how many new dogs a person may see in his lifetime, he will always have room for new varieties of dogs in his dog schema. If, however, he assimilates stimuli into a schema that he gradually recognizes as not fitting the shape of the schema, he must accommodate either by reshaping an existing schema or by developing new schemata. As a child, he might understand dogness as "any animal with four legs," but as he has more experiences with his environment, he begins to reshape his dog schema to include "any animal with four legs, fur, a wet nose, a wagging tail, within certain size limitations, that barks." As this understanding of dogness develops, he begins to separate dogs from other animals that might share some traits with dogs but that differ in other important ways. As a result of experiences with his environment, he adapts and reorganizes by developing new schemata to accommodate stimuli that do not belong in his reshaped dog schema. Eventually, he will have schemata for horses, cows, elephants, giraffes, and all other animals with which he becomes acquainted in a cognitive sense.

The dog example illustrates an important difference between children's and adults' schemata. When the child is young, her schemata tend to be very large and, in comparison with adult schemata, imprecisely defined. As the child develops intellectually, her schemata become more adultlike in that they become more narrowly and more accurately defined.

It should be noted here that some schemata, even for the most intelligent adults, are never completely accurate. An adult, for example, who has little interest in football, might have a schema for football player as incompletely formed as the young child's doggie schema that includes all four-legged animals. This adult might not understand the specialized responsibilities of the various players on offense and defense. He might not understand the difference between a nose guard and an outside linebacker, between a cornerback and a safety, or between a slot back and a wide receiver. He might not understand that the punter is considered a defensive player and the place kicker is considered an offensive player even though they both kick when their team possesses the football. To the person who knows little or nothing about football, these players all fit into one large, undifferentiated schema called "football player." The point is, we are all ignorant in our own ways, and our ignorance is reflected in how our schemata are shaped and cataloged.

We are now ready to consider the final basic concept, equilibrium. Think of **equilibrium** as a balance between assimilation and accommodation. Cognitive development can be understood as a process resulting from assimilation and accommodation, but if these cognitive strategies are not in balance, problems arise. If, for example, a person *assimilates* all new stimuli she experiences, she will have relatively few schemata—but these schemata will be so broadly defined that she will be unable to recognize important differences among the things she is trying to categorize. But if she *accommodates* all new stimuli, she will have many narrowly defined schemata and will be unable to recognize the commonalities among the things she is trying to categorize. Too much of either strategy results in an inadequate understanding of the parts and wholes of life and life's experiences. Each person is constantly in the process of finding a balance between assimilation and accommodation to create a kind of cognitive peace.

Each time the child encounters a new stimulus, he either assimilates or accommodates, but he places the stimulus somewhere. He might assimilate a new stimulus for a short time before he accommodates by creating a new schema more appropriate for that stimulus, but he does not leave his cognitive organization in disarray. Unlike the retailer who might be a few pennies short or a few pennies over at the end of the day, the child balances his cognitive account every day. It does not matter that his schemata are right or wrong in comparison with adult schemata. In fact, you should not understand assimilation and accommodation in cognitive development as right or wrong. The child places stimuli according to *his* understanding of the world at any given moment in his intellectual development. As he grows older, his schemata become more and more adultlike, but they are always right, within the context of his understanding. In other words, he always finds his **equilibrium,** his cognitive peace, even though his balance might represent **disequilibrium** in an adult's cognitive organization.

When does a person stop assimilating and accommodating? These processes cease only when a person no longer has new experiences or new understandings of old experiences. As long as the brain continues to function, existing schemata accept new stimuli, existing schemata are reshaped, and new schemata are created. One of the marvelous aspects of intellectual development is that it continues throughout life. You may reach your maximum height when you are nineteen or twenty, and you may reach your athletic peak in your late twenties or early thirties, but you can continue to grow intellectually by assimilating and accommodating into your eighth or ninth decade and beyond.

The Stage Concept of Cognitive Development

Throughout our discussion of language acquisition, we will encounter stages and substages of development. It is important to remember that these stages are *not* like stair steps, in which moving from a lower step to the next higher step means leaving the lower step behind. In language development, what is acquired in one stage is carried over and integrated into the next stage. The same is true in cognitive development. Piaget's stages of intellectual development are not discrete. Each stage builds on the preceding stage so that development is a continuing process of qualitative changes in a person's schemata. As children grow intellectually, they do not discard schemata. They accommodate by reshaping a schema and by creating new schemata, but schemata are not disposable any more than stages of development are passed through and forgotten. Intellectual growth is a cumulative, integrative, expanding process. As the child comes to understand that not all four-legged animals are dogs, she does not throw away her dog schema. She accommodates this schema to make it more doglike, and she acquires new schemata to allow for other four-legged animals. She might for a time put horses, cows, donkeys, and zebras in her horse schema, but she eventually sorts out all the four-legged animals into adultlike schemata.

Piaget compares the progression through the stages of cognitive development to the building of a pyramid, which may be a helpful way to understand the progression of one stage to the next and the interdependence of the stages. Just as the structure of a pyramid is layered, each stage of cognitive development lays the foundation for the following stage, but what is acquired in each stage is not forgotten. The child's schemata are corrected and refined, and he continually adds schemata. Cognitive development should be understood as an improving and adding process, like remodeling and adding on to an existing house as opposed to destroying it and building a new one.

The Big Picture

Piaget (1963) described four stages of intellectual development from birth through late adolescence, briefly summarized here:

1. *Sensorimotor intelligence* (birth to two years). Most of the child's behaviors during the sensorimotor intelligence stage are reflexive and motor. That is, he interacts with his environment in physical and mostly unlearned ways, especially early in the stage. He does not manipulate ideas in a conceptual sense, although cognitive development occurs in this stage, and it occurs rapidly. The child at two is a very different creature intellectually from the child in infancy.

2. *Preoperational thought* (two to seven years). The most rapid period of language development occurs during the stage of preoperational thought. The child begins to think conceptually, is able to categorize things in his environment, and can solve physical problems.

3. *Concrete operations* (seven to eleven years). The child develops the ability to think logically in dealing with concrete or physical problems. He is able to place stimuli into categories based on order and levels.

4. *Formal operations* (eleven to fifteen years). Cognitive abilities become fully developed. The child is able to think abstractly, to solve problems mentally, and to develop and test mental hypotheses. He reasons and thinks logically.

Remember, *these stages are not independent.* They are cumulative and integrated into one another. The ages attached to these stages are not absolute. They simply represent the ages when most normal children are experiencing the cognitive developments indicated. One child might show signs of preoperational thought at fourteen months, but another child ten or eleven years old might still be demonstrating characteristics of preoperational thought, and both children could be normal. There is a great deal of variability among children in terms of when and how quickly they pass through each stage, but, as Piaget insists, each child must pass through the stages in the order listed, and a child will not skip a stage.

With this overview of cognitive development in mind, we will now direct our collective attention to the first stage, sensorimotor intelligence. During this stage, according to Piaget, the child develops those intellectual abilities that lay the foundation for symbolic behaviors such as dreaming, drawing, and language. Within the larger context of symbolic behaviors, therefore, this stage of cognitive development prepares the child for the challenges and expressive opportunities inherent in speech and language development.

The Principle of Distancing in Sensorimotor Development

The primary focus of this chapter is on the intellectual and perceptual prerequisites experts assume are necessary for the development of early language. Note, however, that as important as these factors are to language development, the acquisition of language is an extraordinarily complex process that depends on factors other than cognition and perception. This complexity being established, we will consider how perception works with cognition in helping establish a foundation for language. To understand this relationship, we must go back one step further to sensory input.

A person receives stimuli through his senses: touch, taste, smell, hearing, and vision. **Perception** refers to the processes by which the person selects, organizes, integrates, and interprets sensory stimuli. It should be obvious, therefore, that the child must be able to receive and perceptually process sensory stimuli to put this information into manipulable thought forms. Later in this chapter, we consider some of the child's earliest perceptual abilities, which appear to be related to his first attempts to communicate.

Before we can continue our explanation of the sensorimotor stage of cognitive development, however, we must identify and describe **distancing,** a basic perceptual principle affecting those cognitive changes that apparently precede and lay the foundation for language acquisition.

The infant relates to her environment in a very physical way. She grasps things with her hands and puts things into her mouth. In fact, parents often believe that everything goes into the infant's mouth. The infant is trying to understand her world primarily through touch, taste, and smell.

Now consider how you relate to the world, especially to new stimuli. The first time you saw a laptop or iPod, you did not put these new things into your mouth. You looked at the laptop. You looked at and listened to the iPod. You used senses that placed you at a greater distance from these new stimuli than if you had explored them by touch, taste, or smell. One can reasonably assume that you would eventually touch these items, but, unless you are very strange, you probably would not taste or smell an iPod during your first encounter. One thing that happens during perceptual development, therefore, is that the child relates to stimuli from a greater and greater distance. Moerk (1977) believes that the child's long-range visual and/or auditory images of new stimuli are the forerunners of representational meaning. That is, she first relates to an object by putting it into her mouth—immediate and maximal contact. As she develops, she creates a kind of mental picture of the object based on what she sees. The visual image represents the real thing, and the child recognizes the real thing based on that image.

Consider what happens as distancing progresses. A toy truck represents a real truck. A block of wood might be used by the child to represent a toy truck, which represents a real truck. The child will then recognize a truck in a picture. Eventually, the word *truck* represents the real thing. In each progression, the distance between the child and contact with the actual object becomes greater. Language represents the ultimate perceptual distance, and consider the advantages gained in the use of language. Linguistic symbols allow the child to mentally manipulate objects more quickly and easily than the objects themselves can be physically manipulated, and the mental manipulation of symbols representing things, people, places, and ideas is unfettered by time or space. Distancing moves the child's experiences with her environment from her hands and mouth to her brain. This is a short trip when measured in feet and inches, but when understood in the context of cognitive development, it is a journey spanning an intellectual universe.

Concepts and Behaviors Central to Early Cognitive Development

As we progress through the six substages of the sensorimotor phase of cognitive development, we will encounter three concepts (object permanence, causality, and means-ends) and three behaviors (imitation, play, and communication), which account for increasingly advanced intellectual functioning as they change. Consider these concepts and behaviors the principal players in the unfolding sensorimotor drama. Although the roles of these six characters in our cognitive drama change from scene to scene or substage to substage, these concepts and behaviors are the forces that together, in an interactive manner, shape the child's intellectual growth during this rapidly evolving first stage of cognitive development. And now, before the curtain goes up, let's meet the players.

A common bond shared by all six players in our drama is **representation,** the idea that a stimulus can stand for or represent something else. A stop sign itself does not prevent you from driving a car through an intersection, but the sign represents the law, which says a person must stop before proceeding. The whistle of an approaching train will not destroy your car, but the distinctive sound of the whistle causes you to approach the railroad crossing cautiously because you know the whistle represents the train, which can destroy your car and you if you put yourself in its path. As you drive down the road, you watch the rear lights of the car in front of you. If the brake lights go on, you slow down because these lights represent the driver's intention to slow down or stop. If the right turn signal flashes, you assume the driver is about to turn right because that signal represents the driver's intention to turn. All day, every day, we are bombarded by stimuli representing ideas, people, things, and directions. An important and basic part of cognitive development is the evolutionary understanding of the concept of representation. Without this understanding, language is not possible because words are symbols that direct our thoughts to the things for which they stand.

The first player in our drama is a concept clearly related to representation, **object permanence.** It would not be accurate to say that the infant is not aware of objects, because even the youngest child will grasp or suck the things in his environment with which he has direct contact. When an object is removed, however, the infant pays no attention to its removal and does not look for it. When an object is out of sight, it is literally out of mind. As cognitive development proceeds, the child understands that objects exist even when they are not being touched, tasted, smelled, seen, or heard. Only when the child understands that things are permanent can he represent them cognitively, perhaps first in mental pictures, but eventually in words.

The next member of our cast is **causality.** In the beginning, the child has no concept of cause and effect. As she develops intellectually, she realizes that certain events cause other events, and she understands that she can produce behaviors that have predictable effects. According to Bates, Benigni, Bretherton, Camaioni, and Volterra

The child's first contacts with his world are physical and sensory.

(1979), the development of causality is a significant factor in the child's social and communicative maturation. Communication is a process driven by intentions. We do things or say things to produce desired and predictable results. An early understanding of causality might be reflected in the child's pushing a spoonful of strained carrots out of her mouth with her tongue. As she develops language, she might simply say "No!" She uses a word to represent her intention to cause the carrots to not be delivered to her stomach.

Means–ends can be understood as a concept that extends causality. As this concept develops, the child learns to use the cause–effect concept to solve problems. The young infant's first behaviors are random and unintentional. Perhaps she sees a cookie she would like to consume. She reaches out to grab it, but it is beyond her reach. Her mother sees the child reaching, figures out what she wants, and gives her the cookie. Although the child got what she wanted, she stretched out her arms not to communicate intent but to reach the cookie. As she becomes more cognitively sophisticated, she is able to establish goals and to figure out *means* by which to accomplish these goals or *ends.* She will eventually reach for an object she knows is beyond her reach because she is intentionally signaling by this gesture that she wants the targeted object. In terms of language development, means–ends is important because language is used to get things done. It becomes a means by which many ends are accomplished. The child must learn not only that language is a means–ends phenomenon but that adjustments in language must be made depending on who the listener is and what kind of relationship the child has with the listener. If she wants a cookie from her younger brother, she might simply demand it. If she wants a cookie from her mother, she will likely ask for it—and say, "Please!" In both cases, the end is thoughtfully targeted, and the means is carefully created to maximize the possibility of success.

The fourth principal player is **imitation.** Anyone who observes young children will quickly and comfortably conclude that imitation is an important factor in cognitive development and in language development. Most of what children learn, and much of what adults learn, appears to be the result of attending to models and trying to duplicate them.

The research data concerning the acquisition of communication skills support the conclusion that imitation is an important developmental factor (Moore & Meltzoff, 1978; Rees, 1975; Snyder, 1978). It is assumed that imitation facilitates children's ability to internalize models of the behaviors of others, which they can then duplicate. Early imitations are crude, imprecise, and always immediate, but over the course of development, imitated behaviors become more accurate and sophisticated, and they occur in a delayed manner. **Delayed or deferred imitation** is important because it allows children to produce a desired behavior even when the model is not present. Without deferred imitation, language would not progress beyond the kind of parroted productions accomplished by talking birds. Even before children can imitate language forms, they imitate movements and gestures. Imitations of behaviors associated with objects seem to suggest some understanding of the objects themselves. For example, if the child, with or without a real comb in his hands, imitates a combing motion, we might reasonably assume he knows something about the function of the comb. Bates and Snyder (1987) suggest that imitation is a primitive kind of labeling. That is, the child labels a comb by imitating, immediately or on a deferred basis, the action of combing. In the sensorimotor drama, imitation is a major player, as you will see.

Our next player is **play** itself. Many adults think of playing as a frivolous activity, but play is viewed by professionals concerned with child development as fairly serious business. Play is certainly a fun and entertaining activity, but it also provides children with many opportunities for learning about the things and people in their world, as well as concepts ranging from colors, numbers, and simple prepositions such as *in* and *on,* to more complex things such as sharing and social interactions. As the children grow older, language and other forms of communication become increasingly prominent and important components in play activities. Experts in cognitive and language development are especially interested in **symbolic play,** an activity in which one object represents another object. How many times, for example, have you watched children play for hours in a big box, pretending it was a house or a fort. A child might use a block as a truck. My youngest daughter, when she was about two years old, used rubber bands as bracelets and often had ten or twelve on her wrist at one time. All of these are examples of symbolic play. This kind of play has a rather obvious connection to language. In symbolic play, the child might use a stick to represent a nail-driving tool. In language, he can use the word *hammer* to refer to the same object. Both are representational activities. It is probably not a coincidence, then, that

Bates, Bretherton, Snyder, Shore, and Volterra (1980) found that children who are able and willing to use objects to represent other objects progress more quickly in language development than children who are more rigid in their use of objects.

Sixth, **communication** is the leading character in our version of the sensorimotor drama, because speech and language are the focus of this book. The development of the concepts we have identified are reflected in the child's increasingly sophisticated communication system, and few would argue with the conclusion that imitation and play are important in helping children acquire greater conceptual understandings and more advanced communicative skills by which to express their understandings. It is also reasonable to assume that, at some point, children use their communication abilities, especially language, to facilitate advances in their cognitive development. As we proceed through the substages of sensorimotor development, we will track changes in communication as well as changes in the other concepts and behaviors we have identified. For the sake of convenience and to allow for direct comparison of the substages, we discuss the players in the same order in each substage; however, keep in mind that the order signifies nothing about the importance of these players. The interactions among the players are more important than the individual players themselves. The further into cognitive development we proceed, the more inextricably connected the players become.

The cast is set. The curtain is rising. Let the play begin.

The Sensorimotor Period (Birth to Two Years)

Scene 1—Substage 1 (Birth to One Month)

Piaget believed the understanding that objects are permanent is not innate. That is, the newborn infant reacts to objects as though they no longer exist when they are not in sight. The concept of object permanence develops in stages as the child gets to know the things in his environment (Piaget, 1954, p. 4; see also Table 3.1). At birth, the

Table 3.1 Concepts and Behaviors Central to Early Cognitive Development

Concepts	Behaviors
Object permanence—knowing that objects exist in time and space even if you can't see or act on them	***Imitation***—duplication of models you hear and see
Causality—the understanding that events can cause other events	***Play***—provides the child with opportunities for learning
Means–ends—a conceptual extension of causality; the understanding that there are ways (means) to attain a goal (end)	***Communication***—conceptual development contributes to the ever-increasing development of a child's language ability

child has no concept of objects. He gives no indication that he understands the difference between himself and the things around him. He reacts to objects only by looking, grasping, and sucking them, and even these reactions are reflexive, or unlearned, and they are undifferentiated. That is, he does not demonstrate preferences for some objects over others based on an understanding of meaningful differences. The world, to the newborn, consists of unexplored and relatively uninteresting things that pass, with little notice, in and out of his sensory fields.

At birth and through the first three substages of the sensorimotor period, the child is egocentric. As Piaget used the term, **egocentrism** means that the child sees and understands the world only as an extension of himself. He has no other point of view. He does not understand that he is one thing among many other things in the environment. This means that the newborn infant has no concept of causality. He is so far removed from this concept, in fact, that he does not understand that there is a difference between himself and other objects. It will be some months before we glimpse even the beginning of cause–effect understanding. From the newborn's perspective, there are not even parts to act on one another. Everything in the newborn's world is a member of a whole, and the whole is **him!**

If the newborn sees the world as one undifferentiated mass of himness, it should not be surprising that he shows no understanding of means–ends. One cannot identify an objective and plot a strategy to obtain it if the world is ensconced in one tightly bound, leakproof package. Imagine what it would be like to have no goals, no tasks to be done, no chores to complete, no responsibilities to fill. Since there are no identifiable ends, the newborn does not need to devise any means.

The substage 1 infant is not capable of imitation but does produce behaviors that seem to be imitative. McCormick (1990) refers to one example of this behavior as "vocal contagion." That is, when one newborn begins to cry, other newborns in the same room are likely to cry, too. Piaget believed that what happens in this case is not imitation but the stimulation of an already established response by an external stimulus. In other words, the newborn has already established the ability to cry. His crying is usually triggered by pain or hunger, but in the case of vocal contagion his crying is triggered by another newborn's cries.

The newborn infant does not play. He exists. He sees, hears, grasps, sucks, eats, sleeps, and relieves himself—often—but he does not play. Playing must wait until the time when he knows there are other people and other things in the world.

Not much communication exists during the first substage. There is certainly nothing we can call language. The newborn child produces reflexive cries, usually in response to stimuli of discomfiture, and fairly early in his life he makes sounds of pleasure, sounds we might interpret as sighs, but the communicative effects of these behaviors are limited. Parents quickly learn to identify the conditions under which cries and sighs are produced, and in that sense, there is communication, but there is no communicative intent on the part of the child in substage 1.

As dramas go, this has not been the most exciting opening scene one might imagine. What do we have here? We have a living organism with enormous cognitive and communicative potential, but he is just sitting on the stage crying, grasping, and sucking. He pays little or no attention to the audience and is constantly falling asleep. This drama builds in excitement, so hang in there. It gets better.

Scene 2—Substage 2 (One to Four Months)

During this substage, the child begins to show some awareness of objects, but the awareness is sensory rather than conceptual. She reacts to objects visually and auditorially, and, more significant, she is able to coordinate her visual and auditory contacts with objects. That is, when she hears a noise, she searches for the source with her eyes, and if the sound source moves within her field of vision, she follows its movement. Piaget (1954, pp. 10–11) reported that one of his daughters during this substage not only visually located objects but was also able to look away from an object and then locate it again. Whether a child reacts to this visual and auditory hide-and-seek activity with disappointment and expectation as Piaget suggested, it is reasonable to conclude that the child is developing an interest in objects and is using her senses to make and maintain contact with them.

Even though there is sensory interest in objects during this substage, the child still does not demonstrate an understanding that objects are separate from her. She makes few, if any, meaningful differentiations among objects and does not differentiate objects from herself, even when the objects move in and out of her sensory fields. In other words, she is still very much egocentric. As was true in the first substage, there are no parts; therefore, there is no possibility for a demonstration of causality.

Since the child has not yet developed the concept of causality, we should not be surprised that there is no evidence of means–ends in the second substage. Even though we see sensorimotor behaviors in this substage that we did not see earlier, such as visually locating and following a moving object or grasping and looking at an object, we should not conclude that these behaviors reflect intentionality. These are still essentially reflexive behaviors even though they can be modified by other people who cause objects to move or make noise. Piaget (1952) contended, "Even when the child grasps an object in order to look at it, one cannot infer that there is a conscious purpose" (p. 143). In this example, it might be tempting to think of looking as the end and the grasping as the means, but since grasping is a reflexive behavior, we cannot conclude that the sequence of behaviors from grasping to looking is intentional. It just happens, and the looking is part of the reflexive sequence.

We see the beginning of imitation in this substage, although it is a specialized kind of imitation. The child produces a behavior that someone, perhaps a parent, imitates. The child then repeats the behavior. What we have then is the child imitating a behavior that she produced, but only after someone else imitated her. Got it? These behaviors might be gestural but are usually vocal. In a common example, the child says, "Goo-goo." The parent mimics the child, saying, "Goo-goo." The child, terribly excited by this insightful communicative exchange, repeats her original production, "Goo-goo." Piaget called this behavior "pre-imitation," suggesting it is behavior that sets the stage for true imitation. McCormick (1990) calls the same behavior "mutual imitation," which describes the nature of the exchange.

It would be a real stretch to call anything the child does in the second substage *play*, but she is engaging in sensorimotor behaviors that are preliminary to play. She is not only grasping objects but holding them for brief periods of time and looking at them, and she is showing some interest in the sensory characteristics of objects. Even the primitive imitative responses we see in this substage are preparing the child for play activities seen in later substages. Early play activities involve very basic motor and sensory behaviors, and they often involve imitation, so the child is getting ready for play.

During the early weeks of this substage, most of the child's communications are still in the form of reflexive cries, but as the substage progresses, the child cries less frequently and develops distinctly different types of cries. According to D'Odorico (1984), at about four months the child produces three differentiated cries to signal discomfort, to call, and to request. Noncrying vocalizations signaling pleasure develop during this substage. The child begins to coo, especially when interacting with someone else. These productions are described as vowel-like to indicate that there are no consonant approximations and to suggest that the sounds produced are not true vowels. They are random, undifferentiated productions of sounds with vowel characteristics. Toward the end of this substage, at about four months, the child is also laughing (Stark, 1979), a delightful development for child and parents. The child may not be receptive to political humor or satire at this point, but she does laugh. It is, in fact, often difficult to figure out what makes a four-month-old child laugh, but if gentle pokes in the belly accompanied by funny faces and silly vocal noises make her laugh, parents will enjoy it! They have made communicative contact with their child about subjects other than hunger and soiled diapers.

Scene 3—Substage 3 (Four to Eight Months)

In the third substage, the child begins to develop the concept of object permanence, the idea that objects exist even when they are not in view or in physical contact with the child. The concept at this point is limited, however. The child watching an object move will anticipate its future position. If he is sitting in a high chair, he might drop food and watch it fall onto the floor, and he will react to the general direction of the fall, anticipating the food's final resting position on the newly scrubbed vinyl floor. As in the previous stage, he will grasp an object and look at it, but now he seems to examine it with greater interest. If a toy is partially hidden by a piece of paper, he might reach for it, but if the same toy is out of sight, he will not search for it. This is what Flavell (1977, p. 43) calls the "essential limitation" of substage 3. That is, the child will briefly look for an object that is hidden, but will not conduct a physical search for it. Even though the child in this substage has not yet developed the concept of object permanence, he is rapidly moving toward this understanding.

To appreciate what this child understands about causality, one must remember that he is still very much egocentric. The child will repeat actions he finds interesting or pleasurable, and in that sense, he knows he is causing the action that precipitates the pleasure. There are two important limitations, however. First, the child pays little attention to the effects of his behaviors, especially in a cognitive sense. For the

Where did this light come from, and where is it going?

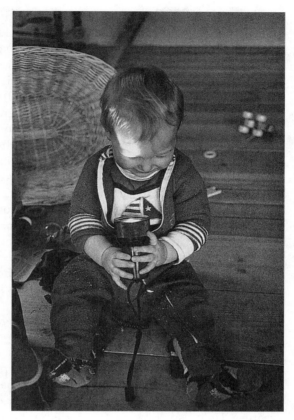

concept of causality to be truly developed, the child must understand cause *and* effect. Second, the child in this substage behaves as though he is the cause of all actions. He does not recognize that other people or objects cause actions. If, while holding the child, Dad rings a bell, he might throw his arms up or push Dad's face to cause the bell to ring again. He does not understand that it is his father's hand, moving in a specific manner, that causes the bell to ring. The child believes it is *his* action that causes bell ringing and all other events because he is still the master of his universe.

The sophistication of means–ends in this stage matches the child's understanding of causality, as we would reasonably expect. In the first two substages, we saw no evidence of intentionality. In the third substage, there is a limited but important progression in means–ends development. The child might pick up a new rattle, for example. In the course of examining the rattle, she shakes it and it makes a noise she finds interesting. She continues to shake the rattle. This can certainly be construed as intentional or goal-oriented behavior, but the goals in this substage are established only after the activity has begun (Wadsworth, 1971, p. 46). Behavior based on a complete understanding of means–ends is initiated in an intentional manner after a goal has been identified and a strategy for reaching that goal has been developed. At this point, the child is engaging in intentional behaviors but is not yet a planner.

Interesting changes in imitation occur in the third substage, but as with the other concepts we have described in this substage, it is important to stress the limitations as we identify the progressions. McCormick (1990) refers to substage 3 imitation as "systematic imitation." The most significant progressions are that the child imitates a wider range of behaviors, and she will imitate the behaviors of others. Most imitations are of sounds and physical actions, but the child will not imitate an action she herself has not performed spontaneously at an earlier time. She will imitate only complete sequences of behaviors, not isolated parts of a sequence. The child must be able to see herself perform the activity she is imitating, and if it involves sound, she must be able to hear herself. If we put these limitations together, they mean the child will imitate making and releasing a fist if she has previously done this on her own. If, in releasing her fist, the child spontaneously spreads her fingers, she will spread her fingers when she imitates the fist-making/fist-releasing sequence, but she will not imitate only the spreading of her fingers. She will imitate fist making/fist releasing if she can watch herself, but she will not imitate this sequence of behaviors while holding her hand behind her back.

In the third substage, we see the child engaging in activities that more closely resemble play. The child is interacting with other people. Even though his imitations are limited to his repertoire of behaviors, he does respond to models of physical and vocal activity. He is finding toys more interesting and repeats actions on toys that may or may not be appropriate. That is, he might shake a rattle, but he might also bang it on the floor or on Mom's forehead. He is still very much a sensory creature. He grasps toys, ears, nostrils, and dog's paws, and he still tries to put all objects, including the coffee table leg, into his mouth. The child is deriving pleasure from his play activities, and they provide him opportunities for developing concepts and elaborating behaviors important for later cognitive and communicative development.

Few dramatic changes in communication occur in this substage. The child continues to produce vowel-like utterances, but we do notice the emergence of consonant-like sounds. Keep in mind that the *-like* qualification affixed to *vowel* and *consonant* means that these productions are random and not meaningful, but they are sounds that have characteristics of true sounds. Toward the end of this substage, at about six to eight months, the child begins to produce productions referred to as **babbling.** These are combinations of vowel- and consonant-like sounds, resulting in utterances such as "gagaga" or "mamama." As you might imagine, parents often interpret these babbled productions as "words," but until a production is used in a consistent, intentional, and meaningful manner, it cannot be considered a word. It will be a few months before the child is producing true words, but she is laying the groundwork at this point by establishing control over the components of her speech mechanism (Sachs, 1989, p. 45). It would certainly be a mistake to assume that the child in substage 3 is not communicating. She is using her vocalizations and gestures to communicate many things, from "I'm not a very happy person right now because my diapers are wet—again" to "I would like very much to have that cookie in your hand, and if you don't mind, I am going to grab it while distracting you with my devastating smile."

Scene 4—Substage 4 (Eight to Twelve Months)

As the child moves into the last few months of his first year, he seems more curious about his world. Part of what adults might perceive as curiosity is the further development of the object permanence concept. In the first two substages, if an object was out of sight, it was out of mind. In the third substage, the child would reach for an object if it was partially hidden but would not physically search for it if it was completely out of sight. In the fourth substage, the child shows evidence that he remembers objects. If a playful adult hides his favorite pacifier under a pillow, he will lift the pillow to find it. In addition to understanding that objects are permanent, the child demonstrates an understanding that the shape and size of objects are constant. If a familiar object, such as his bottle, is given to him upside down, he knows that the business end has a nipple on it, and he will turn the bottle around. In other words, he knows the shape has not changed even when his perspective of the bottle is different. He will also recognize his bottle when viewed from a distance, even though the bottle appears smaller from thirty feet away than from six inches. The object concept is not yet fully developed, however. For example, the child will look for an object that has disappeared, but often only if he sees it disappear. Piaget (1954, p. 51) observed that his daughter, Jacqueline, in the fourth substage, would search for hidden objects where they usually disappeared, not necessarily where she saw them disappear. The object concept is fairly complete by the end of this substage, but some gaps still exist, and we will not see a thorough understanding of object permanence until the sixth substage.

In the fourth substage, we encounter a child who is far less egocentric than in earlier substages. This shift from an egocentric view of the world is most noticeable in the child's more sophisticated understanding of causality. In the third substage, the child had a limited understanding of causality but behaved as though she was the cause of all actions. She now externalizes causality. That is, she understands that other people and other objects can cause activities. Using the same example of bell ringing we employed in the preceding substage, we can create a very different scenario. Earlier the child believed she was responsible for causing the bell to ring even though she did not touch the bell. Now when the child watches Dad pick up the bell and ring it, she will push Dad's hand toward the bell to indicate that she wants him to ring it again. She understands that Dad caused the action.

In the third substage, the child showed evidence of a very elementary understanding of means–ends. She used goal-oriented behavior, but the goals were set only after behavior was in progress. In the fourth substage, the child plans behavior. She devises a means or strategy before initiating a behavior, and there is a clear connection between the strategy and the goal. Wadsworth (1971, p. 48) suggests that this behavior is one of "the first clear acts of intelligence" we observe in the developing child. Many of the child's behaviors are now intentional, and they reflect thoughtful planning. In an earlier example related to object permanence, the child searched for her pacifier under a pillow. This same example demonstrates her more sophisticated means–ends understanding. The problem is a missing pacifier. The end is to find the pacifier. The means is to move the pillow. Eureka! There is the pacifier!

Imitation undergoes some interesting and significant changes in the fourth substage. The child now imitates behaviors he has not produced himself, although he is likely to imitate only actions or vocalizations similar to those he has produced on his own (McCormick, 1990). It is not necessary in this substage that he be able to see or hear himself while he is imitating. For example, if while holding the child on my lap, I stick out my tongue, he might imitate this behavior even though he cannot see his own protruding tongue. Owens (2001, p. 141) suggests that this kind of imitation requires some short-term motor memory, which has obvious relevance to the speech skills he will acquire in the near future.

It should be apparent by this point in our drama that play provides children with opportunities to use their developing concepts in activities that are pleasurable. More important perhaps, it is through play that children discover new aspects of these concepts and demonstrate these new understandings to those who observe them. While playing with her toys, the child in the fourth substage will look for toys that are not in sight. She might demonstrate means–ends by pulling the string on a toy that makes animal sounds, but if this action is too difficult, she might encourage someone else to pull the string, demonstrating her understanding of external causality. She might use a few objects in a manner that suggests an understanding of function. For example, she might roll a ball or bang on a toy drum, although it will be some time before she is able to build a small nuclear device or create havoc by making contact with NASA's computer system.

In the early months of the fourth substage, the child is still babbling. By the end of the substage, she may actually produce her first meaningful words. Whether or not there are true words during this time, it is evident that the child is communicating, vocally and gesturally, in an intentional manner. Even without speech, children in the latter months of this substage link gestures and vocalizations to convey fairly specific messages. Bates, Camaioni, and Volterra (1975) studied a girl in this substage who, on one occasion at least, vocalized "ha" to her mother while looking in the direction of the kitchen. When her mother carried her into the kitchen, the girl pointed at the sink, prompting her mother to give her a drink of water. The child did not use words, but she certainly communicated.

Scene 5—Substage 5 (Twelve to Eighteen Months)

The child in this substage is tantalizingly close to having a complete understanding of object permanence. In the last scene, the child would search for an object if he saw it disappear, but even if he saw it disappear, he would look for it where it is usually hidden, not always where he actually saw it hidden. In the fourth substage, he cannot accommodate sequential displacements (Wadsworth, 1971, p. 55). If Mom usually hides his pacifier under a pillow, but she now hides it under his blanket, he will look for the pacifier under the pillow, even if he watches Mom hide it under the blanket. This seems strange from an adult point of view, but remember the developing child's perspective. He is a physical and sensory creature who only gradually acquires the ability to deal with objects in an abstract sense. For him, what you see is what you get, and through the fourth substage, what you see is what you get only if what you get is where you expect it to be! In the fifth substage, we see a giant step forward. He is now capable of following sequential displacements. If Mom hides his pacifier under the pillow, he will look under the pillow. If Mom then hides it under his blanket, he will look under the blanket, and if Mom puts it in her shirt pocket, he will search for his pacifier in her pocket, undoubtedly ripping the shirt in the process. Why, then, is the concept not complete? Although the child can handle sequential displacements if he can see them, he cannot handle a displacement he cannot see. If, for example, Mom hides his pacifier under the pillow, and while she has her hand under the pillow, she slips the pacifier between the sofa cushions, the child will look for the pacifier under, over, and around the pillow but will not search between the sofa cushions. The object permanence concept becomes complete in the sixth and final substage when the child is finally able to move an object from its place in the restricted physical world to the mind, where it is represented abstractly and is free of all time and space limitations.

The change in causality in substage 5 is subtle but important. In the last substage, the child was aware that people and things other than herself can be agents of cause, but she demonstrated this understanding only in relation to people, things, and actions with which she was familiar. In this substage, the child's understanding of causality becomes more sophisticated in that she sees other people and objects as agents for causality in new situations. If, for example, the child is given a new toy unlike anything she has seen before, she might examine it carefully and, deciding she does not know what to do with it, push it into an adult's hand. She is seeking the adult's assistance as an agent of causality. In essence, the child is saying, "Show me what this thing does!" In another example, we have a child who, when playing with his mother's lipstick got the sticky red goo all over his fingers. He now approaches a fire hydrant painted the same bright red as the lipstick. He touches the hydrant and examines his fingers, expecting to see them colored red. In this example, the child is able to transfer his understanding of causality from one situation to another, and in the process learns that red does not always icky fingers make. In both examples, we see evidence that the child's understanding of external causality has increased.

Means–ends in the fifth substage can be characterized as more creative or experimental in comparison to the fourth substage. The child is becoming a problem solver, and in the process of learning to solve problems, she experiments with objects and actions. The child, for example, has a toy workbench. She uses a play hammer to drive a large wooden peg through an opening in the bench. Banging the hammer is the means by which to reach the end, defined as making the peg move. She now picks up a banana. It weighs about the same as the hammer, and it has a convenient "handle," so the child hits the peg with the banana. The banana breaks, and the peg does not move. This means did not accomplish the desired end because, as the child learned

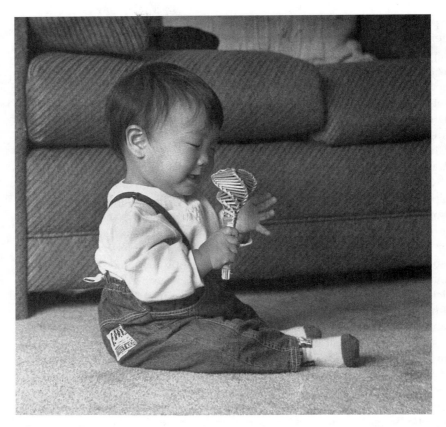

My, look at the intricate detail in this thing.

through trial and error, the banana is too soft. As her experimentation proceeds, she will learn that things other than the hammer can be used, like Dad's shoe, or Mom's skillet, to drive the peg through the bench because, like the hammer, they are hard. As you might imagine, this experimentation business can be interesting and dangerous. Parents are well advised to observe their children carefully as they identify their goals and map their strategies for attaining them. A peanut butter sandwich might be approximately the same size as a VHS cassette, but pushed into the loading device of the VCR, the peanut butter sandwich has a markedly different effect than the cassette. Yech!

The same willingness, perhaps eagerness, to experiment observed in means–ends experiences is observed in imitation. The child is an excellent and uninhibited imitator in this substage. The accuracy of his imitations is limited only by his motor abilities (Owens, 2001, p. 142), but he will try almost anything. According to McCormick (1990), this child imitates to better understand his world and the things in it. He will imitate animal noises, for example, and will attempt to imitate even complex speech productions. When my own children were in this substage, I modeled words such as *encyclopedia, electroencephalographic,* and *diadochokinesis,* which they gladly tried to imitate. Their productions of these words were not accurate, but they produced excellent imitations of words and actions that were within their motoric capabilities.

The child's play in this substage clearly reflects his cognitive advances. He thoroughly examines his toys and quickly figures out the operative pieces. If the toy is relatively simple to operate, he figures out how to make it work through trial and error. If there is a string, he pulls it. If there is a lever, he pushes it. If there is a dial, he turns it. If he cannot figure out what to do with the toy, as mentioned in the causality discussion, he hands it to someone else for consultation and demonstration. The child also combines toys in a functional manner. He might, for example, use his toy hammer to make a ball roll across the floor.

It is during this substage that we typically see children producing their first meaningful words. These words are monosyllabic (e.g., *go, no*) or duplicated disyllabic forms (e.g., *mama, wawa*). There is no question that communication during this substage is intentional. For example, the child might say "bye-bye" to indicate that she wants to leave or wants someone else to leave. Toward the end of this substage, it is not uncommon for the child to say "nite-nite," while shaking her head from side to side, to suggest that she has no intention of going to bed now, under any circumstances, not until *Monday Night Football* is over or until the popcorn is all gone, whichever occurs first. Communication continues to be heavily dependent on nonverbal messages in the voice, face, and gestures, but there is very little of importance, as defined by the child's own needs and desires, that she cannot communicate.

As scene 5 closes, we leave the last of the truly sensorimotor substages. The child is now ready for an important transition. Through the first five substages, he has evolved from a creature tied completely to his physical world by his senses and his oral and manual manipulation of objects to a creature who has gradually distanced himself from direct contact with objects. In the fifth substage, we have seen a child who understands that he is only one of many people in the world. He understands that other people and other things are agents of cause. He is a curious creature who tests and expands his understanding of causality and means–ends by exploration and experimentation. He freely and happily interacts with other people by imitating their vocalizations and their actions, including behaviors totally unfamiliar to him, and he communicates with other people. He sends and receives messages nonverbally and, for the first time, verbally. This has been an exciting scene in our drama, the transitional scene that sets the stage for the final scene, substage 6, during which we will see the completion of the concepts and the elaboration of the behaviors we have been following in the first five scenes.

Scene 6—Substage 6 (Eighteen to Twenty-Four Months)

The common denominator underlying all the significant changes in the sixth substage is representation. That is, the child's understanding of her world moves from the sensorimotor level to a level in which she is able to represent objects internally and to manipulate these internal representations of reality to solve problems. She is becoming, in a word, a cognitive thinker instead of a touchy-feely experiencer.

The child now has a fully developed concept of object permanence. Not only can she follow sequential displacements, but she can accommodate invisible displacements. If Mom moves the pacifier out of sight under the pillow and then slides the pacifier between the sofa cushions, the child will first look under the pillow, but not finding it, will continue to look in and around the area where it disappeared until she finds it. She now has a mental image of the pacifier that is entirely free of her senses and her physical contacts with it. She knows that the pacifier and all objects are permanent, do not disappear just because they are out of sight, and do not change in size or shape just because they are viewed from different angles or distances. When the object is out of sight, it is now firmly in mind. It is, in reference to the common denominator of this substage, *represented* in her mind.

The child's understanding of causality is also enhanced by this ability to represent objects and cause–effect relationships in her mind. A child in the early substages, for example, might simply react with frustration when trying to remove a play telephone from her toy box, the receiver of which is tangled on another toy at the bottom of the box. She cannot see what has tangled the receiver, and she does not have the ability to conceptualize the cause–effect relationship that is preventing the removal of the telephone. After tugging a few times, she might give up or cry, but she will not try to solve the problem by identifying and eliminating the cause. If we move this same child forward to substage 6, we see a much different performance when faced with the same problem. After tugging on the phone a time or two, she reaches into the toy box to discover what is tangling the receiver. She eliminates the tangle and removes the telephone. She was able to solve this problem because, even without seeing what was catching the receiver, she was able to mentally represent a physical obstacle of some kind. She understood the principle of cause and effect that was operating, and she applied this intellectual understanding to the solution of a physical problem.

Means–ends, in its fully developed form, is about intentionality. It is a process of identifying goals and planning strategies for attaining those goals. Obviously, the more fully the child understands causality, the more capable he is of creating sophisticated means–ends strategies. In the sixth substage, the child can represent the goal mentally, and can map out plans for reaching that goal in his mind's eye. In earlier substages, the child might get a cookie out of the unreachable cookie jar by pointing and grunting until someone gets the cookie for him. By the end of the sensorimotor stage, the child might push a chair to the counter, climb onto the counter, and stand on tiptoes to reach the cookie jar on the shelf his mother thought was safely beyond reach. He set a goal. He invented a means for reaching the goal, and he put the plan into action. This kind of creative planning is just part of what is waiting for parents during the stage of child development often called the terrible twos.

Imitation undergoes significant changes as we proceed through the six substages. In the early substages, the child imitates only those actions and vocalizations she produces spontaneously. In the fourth substage, she imitates behaviors that are similar to those she produces; in the fifth substage, she imitates new behaviors. In the sixth sub-

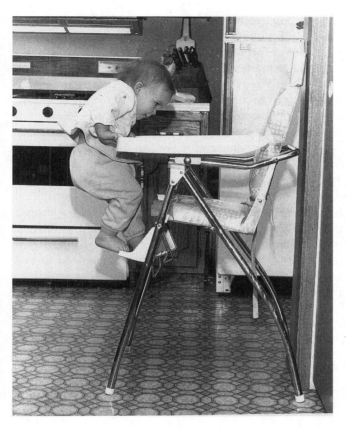

Executing an imperfect and perhaps dangerous plan
of action.

stage, the child produces what are called "deferred imitations" (McCormick, 1990). This means that the child can imitate a behavior modeled for her earlier, an action or vocalization that she has represented mentally and stored in her memory. Now when someone asks the child what sound the cow makes, she retrieves the model from her own mental catalog of animal noises and imitates that model by saying, "Moo!" When someone leaves the house, she does not need to have someone prompt a wave by demonstration and exhortation. She remembers the action and produces it spontaneously, a deferred imitation of a model she has stored in her memory.

In addition to seeing the child apply his more complete conceptual understandings in play, we observe some fundamental changes in the nature of the child's play in the sixth substage (Westby, 1980). Early in this substage, the child might pretend to drink out of a cup or glass or pretend to sleep, but all of his pretending behaviors are autosymbolic. That is, he limits pretending to his own actions. About midway through the final substage, he extends pretending to other objects during symbolic play, but the objects must be realistic. The child will pretend he is feeding a doll with a real or toy spoon, for example, but will not pretend that a Popsicle stick is a spoon. By the end of the sixth substage, the child will engage in play activities that represent real-life experiences. He might play house, but the toys used must still be realistic in terms of function and, to some extent, even in terms of size.

Even though the focus in this section is on Piaget's sensorimotor period of cognitive development, your understanding of *play* and *pretending* as precursors for the child's use of symbols in language will be enhanced if you project beyond sensorimotor intelligence to preoperational thought, a stage of development that typically covers the ages between two and seven years. During this age span, the child becomes increasingly proficient in what caregivers and child development experts call *make-believe play.* In make-believe play, the child develops, practices, and perfects pretend actions that represent what he observes people, including himself, execute in real life situations. Some of these behaviors are mundane, like eating, drinking, and grooming. Others are the products of exotic special features in movies and in television programs. In the earliest stages of make-believe play, the child's pretending is limited to real, or at least realistic-looking, objects. At eighteen months, for example, he will pretend to eat with forks and spoons—either actual forks and spoons or toy forks and spoons, but he will not pretend that a roofing plank from a set of Lincoln Logs is a fork. He is quite literal and rigid in what he uses and in the actions he performs. As he moves beyond his second birthday, he becomes more flexible. He might use a Lincoln Logs roofing plank as a fork or a knife, and he might put a bowl on his head, pretending it is a baseball cap (Tomasello, Striano, & Rochat, 1999). By the time the child is three years old, there need be no connection, even a visual similarity, between the object he is using in play and the object it represents (O'Reilly, 1995). He might, for example, use the bowl or the roofing plank as a car or truck.

As make-believe play evolves, the child moves from a self-only orientation to an increasingly other-directed form of play and pretending. The child pretends to feed herself, for example, before she pretends to feed someone else. As she approaches her third birthday, she might pretend that one Power Ranger action figure is feeding another Power Ranger action figure, so that her pretending is detached from reality, an important step in the kind of representational thought she will need when she manipulates language. She understands, at this level of make-believe play, that the agents of action and the objects of action are not rigidly connected to another, that given a set of actors and a set of actions, almost anything is possible (McCune, 1993).

As one would expect, we also observe that the actions in make-believe play become increasingly complex as the child matures. A child at eighteen months, for example, might pretend to eat, but does not combine that action with the actions involved in preparing the food and setting the table. As he moves through the preschool years, he will combine actions, and he will pretend in concert with playmates in an activity called *sociodramatic play.* The name is fairly self-explanatory. That is, the child acts out social situations in the context of play, as a way of developing not just his representational skills, but also developing his social skills. This kind of make-believe play is noticeable in the child at about thirty months and becomes an increasingly important component in his play repertoire over the next several years. By the time the child is five years old, his make-believe play with other children is truly interactive. A play activity is conducted within the context of an unfolding make-believe story, complete with roles to be played and a plot to play out (Göncü, 1993; Haight & Miller, 1993).

It is interesting and significant to note that the preschool child, certainly by the time she is four years old, not only engages in sociodramatic play, but she understands that it is representational, and her understanding becomes more sophisticated as she moves through the early primary grades (Lillard, 2001). Two of my grandsons were particularly enthusiastic about this kind of play. Lance, at the age of four years, in the back seat of our car would describe elaborate *Star Wars* scenarios, and he made sure that everyone riding in the car had a role to fill. His brother, Peyton, was a big fan of the Power Rangers. When he was three and four years old, he would lure me into the basement and identify me as a villain and himself as the *Red* Power Ranger. He would then establish a story line, but he told me exactly what I was supposed to do and say. If I strayed from the script, and especially if I got the upper hand in our battle, he would quickly rewrite the script in his head and adjust the action so that his character would prevail. Children at this age understand pretending. They talk about pretending. They write their own mental pretending scripts, and they try to write mental pretending scripts for their playmates. They are, in a very real sense, thinking about thinking, and that is an important step toward using language to effectively represent thought.

As we return to our discussion of the sixth substage of the sensorimotor period, remember that the development described in the preceding paragraphs regarding make-believe and sociodramatic play actually occurs during the preoperational period that follows the sensorimotor period, but it's important to understand that these advanced stages of pretending and representational activity are extensions of the cognitive development that occurs during the sensorimotor period. With that in mind, we will emphasize that all the changes we have identified in the sixth substage of the sensorimotor period have direct implications for what is happening to the child as a communicator as she completes this phase of her cognitive development and prepares to move forward. Until the child has some understanding that objects are permanent, she cannot represent them in words. Only when the child understands that all people and many objects can be agents of cause will she be ready to use communication as an agent for causality. If intentionality is the key to means–ends, it is clearly the key that opens the door of communication, both verbal and nonverbal. As the sensorimotor stage unfolds, the child learns that gestures can be used to make needs and desires known, and she eventually learns that words can be even more effective because they allow greater specificity.

Language has been described as a tool for many years, and in the context of means–ends, that is an apt description. As the sensorimotor stage comes to a close, the child is using words and combinations of words to get things done. Imitation, especially deferred imitation, is critical to the development of communication. The child learns gestures by imitation and, as mentioned earlier, will use a gesture to label an object "by carrying out an action typically associated with it" (Bates & Snyder, 1987).

Imitation also plays a role in the acquisition of speech. By the end of the fourth substage, the typical child is producing her first meaningful words that, although they may be only approximations of adult utterances, are evidence of internalized models. In the fifth substage, the child is imitating adult utterances unlike anything she has produced on her own, and by the end of the sixth substage, she is imitating and spontaneously producing multiple word utterances. The essential contribution of imitation is that it helps the child develop the ability to represent behaviors internally, and eventually to produce these behaviors even when the models are not present. This is the essence of language, a system of communication based, in part, on a huge inventory of internalized models. As the child's play progresses from a solitary, physically limited activity to a more interactive and representational activity, language plays a more important role. We have to go beyond the sensorimotor stage to observe speech as a primary play activity, but in the latter months of this first stage of cognitive development, we see communication becoming an increasingly important part of play.

As the curtain slowly falls on the sensorimotor drama, remember that this is but the beginning of the cognitive development story. Piaget's theory has three more stages, which might be viewed as sequels to the sensorimotor drama. Unlike sequels to bad movies, which typically only compound the badness of the original, however, the cognitive sequels are improved dramas, because each stage is based on and incorporates the preceding stage. We are pausing after the sensorimotor phase, not to indicate intellectual closure but to indicate that the stage has now been set for the part of the child development story that is the primary focus of this book—speech and language acquisition. (Table 3.2 reviews the highlights of the child's sensorimotor development.) We will provide closure to our discussion of Piaget's theory of cognitive development, however, by reviewing reservations about some of his views precipitated by research data gathered in recent years.

Recent Research: A Critical Review of Piaget's Sensorimotor Stage

Because the Piagetian view of cognitive development was so widely accepted and so heavily influenced the understanding of many aspects of early child development (with direct and indirect connections to cognitive development), researchers have tried to verify Piaget's observations about what happens during the sensorimotor stage and when. The results of this research suggest that children exhibit some cognitive abilities at much earlier ages than Piaget indicated. Note, however, that reservations about what Piaget proposed should not be construed as criticisms of the man. Today's researchers understand that Piaget did not have access to modern research methodologies that would have allowed him to conduct the kind of carefully designed and rigorously implemented studies the human behavioral research community demands today. Piaget suggested, for example, that the infant shows evidence that he is exploring his world and making preliminary efforts to control aspects of his

Table 3.2 Highlights of Sensorimotor Development

Substage (and Months)	Object Permanence	Causality	Means–Ends	Imitation	Play	Communication
1 (0 to 1)	Out of sight, out of mind	No concept of causality	No understanding of means–ends	None	None	No communicative intent
2 (1 to 4)	Uses senses to make and maintain contact with objects	No concept of causality	No understanding of means–ends	Pre-imitation. Repeats her own behavior that has been imitated by someone else	Produces behaviors preliminary to play, including grasping and looking at objects	Cries, coos, and laughs
3 (4 to 8)	Watches object move and anticipates its future position, reaches for partially hidden object	Does not understand cause–effect, behaves as though she is the cause of all actions	Produces goal-oriented behaviors but only after activity has begun	Imitates only behaviors she has spontaneously produced at an earlier time	Still very sensory but begins to interact with other people	Babbles
4 (8 to 12)	Looks for an object if he sees it being hidden	Externalizes causality, knows other people and objects can cause activities	Evidence of planning and the production of intentional behaviors	Imitates behaviors he has not spontaneously produced	Uses developing concepts in his play activities	Links gestures and vocalizations to convey fairly specific messages
5 (12 to 18)	Follows sequential displacements to find hidden object	Sees other people and objects as agents for causality in new situations	Uses experimentation to solve problems	Uninhibited imitation to facilitate her own understanding	Play reflects cognitive growth. He figures out how to make toys work	Produces first meaningful words. Communication is intentional but still heavily nonverbal.
6 (18 to 24)	Fully developed concept of object permanence, can now accommodate invisible displacements	Causality enhanced by ability to represent objects and cause–effect relationships in his mind	Can mentally represent a goal and his plan for achieving the goal	Deferred imitation, imitates a behavior he has represented mentally and stored in his memory	Progresses from autosymbolic to symbolic play	Imitates and spontaneously produces multiple word utterances

environment when he is about four to eight months old. Using basic operant conditioning principles, researchers have demonstrated that the child is displaying this level of cognitive awareness immediately after birth. This conclusion is drawn from evidence that the neonate will enthusiastically suck on a nipple in order to produce a wide range of sounds and sights he finds interesting. This experiment demonstrates that the newborn child is aware of these auditory and visual stimuli and that he is able to exercise rudimentary control to make them happen. Similar research strategies, based on operant conditioning principles, have been used to reveal what the sensorimotor-stage child knows about object permanence and mental representation and when he knows it.

Object Permanence

You may recall that during substage 3 of the sensorimotor period, when the child is four to eight months old, she is beginning to demonstrate an awareness of *object permanence*, the idea that even if an object is out of sight, it still exists. At this point, however, the child does not try to locate an object that is hidden. According to Piaget, trying to locate a hidden object is a behavior that provides evidence that the child knows object permanence. The suggestion from Piaget is clear. Until the child is older than eight months, she believes that an object that is out of sight has ceased to exist, an idea so widely accepted that we often use a maxim based on this assumption: "Out of sight, out of mind." Is Piaget's assertion about when the child's knowledge of object permanence emerges supported by research? It is not.

Baillargeon (1987) and Baillargeon and Devos (1991) provide evidence that children may have object permanence as early as three and a half months. The method used to make this determination involves what is called the *habituation–dishabituation response.* The subjects were first habituated to two events. The first event involved a picture of a short carrot moving from left to right behind a yellow screen. This event was alternated with a second event, which involved a tall carrot moving from left to right behind a yellow screen. After the subjects were *habituated* to these events, which essentially means that they paid attention to them, two test events were introduced. Two changes were made to the test event scenes: (1) each scene now had a wall with an inserted window in the middle of the visual field, and (2) the color of the screen was changed from yellow to blue to help draw the subjects' attention to the wall and window. The two test events involved a *possible event* and an *impossible event.* In the *possible event,* the short carrot moved from left to right behind the wall and below the lowest margin of the window and reappeared on the other side. In real life, this is exactly what would happen. That is, an object shorter than the bottom frame of the window could be seen before reaching the wall, would be out of sight as it crossed behind the wall and below the window sill, and would reappear only when it reached the right side of the wall. In the *impossible event,* the tall carrot moved from left to right behind the wall, and even though the tall carrot was higher than the window sill, it also disappeared until it reached the right side of the wall. In real life, any object taller than the lowest boundary of the window would be visible when it moved by the window, so what the subjects saw in this second event was not possible, not realistic. Although it seems incredible, subjects as young as three and a half months habituated to the possible event and dishabituated to the impossible event, suggesting that they understood object permanence.

It is reasonable to wonder why there is such an age discrepancy between what this research indicates about when the child understands object permanence and what Piaget asserted. Baillargeon, Graber, DeVos, and Black (1990) conclude that it is possible that the child understands object permanence even if she is not yet capable of implementing the means–ends strategies necessary for locating an object when it is moved out of sight. It is one thing, after all, to know that an object still exists even when it is no longer visible, and it is quite another to push aside, lift up, or reach behind whatever is hiding the object. The child might know object permanence, therefore, even if she is not yet demonstrating that knowledge in her searching or locating behaviors.

According to Piaget, when the child is in substage 4 of the sensorimotor period, which extends from about eight to twelve months, she begins to search for objects when they are hidden. When an object is hidden several times in different locations, however, she sometimes looks in the wrong place. At one time, there was general agreement that these searching errors reflected the child's inability to remember where an object is hidden if it is hidden in several places. Baillargeon, DeVos, and Graber (1989) offer an alternative explanation based on their finding that the child at eight months does remember the last location of an object that is hidden in several different places. That is, prior to her first birthday, the child might look in the wrong place because she has difficulty incorporating what she knows about an object's being moved from location to location into a viable searching strategy. We must remember that there are two different factors operating here: (1) knowing that an object is permanent and that it is being moved from place to place, and (2) developing a strategy for finding the object. Baillargeon et al. (1989) suggest that prior to twelve months, the child has a pretty good handle on *knowing* but is still struggling with *finding*.

Mental Representation: Deferred Imitation and Categorization

According to Piaget's cognitive theory, the child cannot represent experience until she is about eighteen months old. Meltzoff (1988a) has demonstrated, however, that deferred imitation occurs in children as young as nine months. In this study, nine-month-old subjects were introduced to three toys they had not seen before, three toys that could be manipulated in specific ways. They included a bendable L-shaped piece of wood, a box equipped with a button that could be depressed, and a plastic egg containing metal nuts that could be shaken like a rattle. These actions were modeled for the experimental subjects. Control subjects were introduced to the toys but did not receive the modeling exposure. When all the subjects were tested the next day, those who had observed how the toys functioned demonstrated the toys' actions much more frequently than those who did not have the benefit of modeling. The subjects who reproduced the actions modeled for them were demonstrating deferred imitation, a form of mental representation, and they exhibited this behavior almost one year earlier than Piaget suggested it should be produced.

Meltzoff's findings went even further, however. He found that the child at nine months can retain several actions in memory at the same time. By the time the child is fourteen months old, according to another Meltzoff (1988b) study, she can hold in memory as many as six modeled actions over the course of a week. In view of these findings, Piaget's predictions relative to deferred imitation are much too conservative.

According to Piaget's theory of cognitive development, we do not see evidence of mental representation, including deferred imitation and categorization, until the end of the sensorimotor period. Recent evidence indicates that mental representation is probably not the end product of sensorimotor development, as Piaget's theory suggests. Mandler (1992a, 1992b) believes it is more plausible to conclude that sensorimotor schemes and symbolic schemes develop simultaneously. This view would certainly be consistent with research findings relative to categorization. Hayne, Rovee-Collier, and Perris (1987), for example, have found that infants as young as three months can categorize the physical characteristics of mobile elements, and they are able to distinguish one mobile from another based on the categories they have developed. In one of the experiments that led to this conclusion, three-month-old subjects were introduced to a mobile constructed of blocks, each of which was marked with the letter *A*. The subjects discovered that they could make the mobile move by kicking the blocks. When this activity was interrupted and then resumed, the subjects would enthusiastically kick the blocks only if they were marked with the letter *A*. If the mobile was changed so that each block was marked with *2*, the subjects' kicking behavior was drastically reduced in frequency and vigor. The investigators concluded that during their first experiences with the mobile, when the subjects kicked the mobile to make it move, they grouped the elements of the mobile together into an A category, and they associated their kicking with this category. When the elements of the mobile were changed to 2, they differentiated between the A category and the 2 category by kicking the A elements and by not kicking the 2 elements. This is a rather primitive application of categorization, but there is no question that these children were exhibiting behaviors based on their abilities to mentally group and differentiate.

The same habituation–dishabituation strategy that was used in the short carrot–tall carrot study has been used in experiments designed to determine whether infants can categorize. Using this strategy, subjects might be shown a series of pictures of different kinds of birds. After reasonable exposure time to pictures of members of the bird category, the subjects are shown pictures of birds along with pictures of things that clearly do not belong to this category. These might include pictures of buildings or trains. The investigators then observe the subjects to determine whether they pay greater or lesser attention to pictures of things outside the bird category than to pictures of birds. Using this habituation–dishabituation strategy, researchers have found that children as young as nine to twelve months habituate, or look longer, at pictures of things within the category to which they have been exposed than to pictures of objects foreign to that category. They have found that children in this age range can place things into a wide range of categories, including birds, food, and stuffed animals (Oakes, Madole, & Cohen, 1991; Roberts, 1988; Sherman, 1985). By the time children are just eighteen months old, they can categorize objects into two classes (Gopnik & Melt-zoff, 1987). This means that an eighteen-month-old child, given a mixture of blocks and dolls, has the ability not just to know that there is a block category and a doll category but to physically group all the blocks together and all the dolls together. All of these mental representation abilities are manifested at ages far earlier than Piaget predicted, suggesting to those who question Piaget's theory that the emergence of these abilities cannot be explained solely within the context of sensorimotor development.

What Does All This Suggest about the Sensorimotor Stage?

The findings of current research on the cognitive abilities of young children make it impossible to escape the conclusion that many essential and basic cognitive abilities, at least in preliminary form, are exhibited by children considerably earlier than Piaget predicted. To some, this might seem grounds enough to dismiss Piaget's theory, but we should react cautiously to the apparent contradictions between what Piaget proposed theoretically and what researchers have found in actual behavior. Berk (1994) notes, for example, that "when these (cognitive) capacities first appear, they may not be secure enough to make a large difference in the baby's understanding of the world or to serve as the foundation for new knowledge"(p. 231). It is also important to affirm, as Berk and others have, that the general developmental time line established by Piaget's sensorimotor stage holds in terms of when many basic cognitive abilities are fully emerged even if Piaget did not accurately predict the earliest manifestations of these abilities.

The most significant differences between what Piaget proposed and what researchers have found center on the emergence of specific cognitive abilities, such as object permanence, and on how early cognitive development takes place. That is, some cognitive abilities do emerge earlier than Piaget asserted. These include the abilities we have highlighted in this discussion, object permanence and mental representation. A more important gap between the theory and current research focuses on *how* this development occurs. Piaget believed that in this first stage of cognitive development, the acquisition of all knowledge is facilitated by the child's sensorimotor experiences. Even those who have serious reservations about Piaget's theory concede that some of the child's knowledge in these early months of life is established by motor and sensory contact with her environment. These same people suggest, however, that some of the child's cognitive abilities, including object permanence and the ability to imitate, may be genetically determined, and that other abilities may be products of innate perceptual processing of auditory and visual information. That is, some of the knowledge the child demonstrates during the first year, and even the first half year, comes through watching and listening, not through direct physical contact with the things in her world.

Some critics believe that recent research findings suggest that cognitive development does not progress in the fairly rigid, step-by-step manner implied by Piaget's stages. According to Piaget's theory, a range of cognitive abilities develop together within each substage of the sensorimotor period, and they undergo comparable changes within each succeeding stage. The research evidence suggests that the specific cognitive abilities of a given child might be at different levels of maturity at the same time, and that when there is a change in one ability, there will not necessarily be a directly correlated change in another. Cognitive development, these critics argue, is variable because it depends on biological maturation interacting with environmental experiences. The most extreme of these critics believe we should completely dismiss the notion of stages in our understanding of cognitive development. They believe that the bases of cognitive abilities are constant at all ages and that, over time, each child gradually figures out how to apply each ability to the completion of thought-related tasks (Gelman & Baillargeon, 1983). Others take a more moderate view. They believe that Piaget's stage concept, with appropriate modifications, remains viable. Flavell (1985), for example, has difficulty accepting the idea that cognition and its development is as widely variable as some have suggested. He believes that the varying cognitive abilities all theorists and researchers recognize in developing children must somehow be tied together in a coherent manner. These connections among cognitive abilities, in combination with maturational changes, suggest to Flavell that there must be some stage foundation to cognitive development.

So, where does this leave us? There is little doubt, even among the most ardent critics of Piaget's theory, that Piaget has appropriately identified the cognitive abilities the child acquires, and there is consensus that Piaget's general time frame for the maturity of cognitive abilities is, for the most part, on target. It is clear that some of Piaget's estimates about when certain cognitive abilities first appear were not correct. Children show the first signs of certain cognitive abilities much earlier than Piaget predicted. It also seems fair to conclude, based on recent research evidence, that early knowledge is not the product of sensorimotor experience only, that some cognitive abilities may be genetically predetermined, and that others may be influenced at least as much by innate perceptual abilities and experiences as by direct environmental contact. On the issue of stages, legitimate debate persists. It would not be unreasonable to assume, however, that when the dust from this particular battle settles, we will have concluded that some semblance of a stage model is still useful in understanding cognitive development, even though any future stage model will almost certainly accommodate wide individual variations.

The Sensorimotor Stage and Language: A Summary

In closing this section on Piaget's theory of cognitive development, it will be useful to return to our primary focus, language. Even though, as we noted earlier, Piaget did not specifically theorize about language development, he and others who have endorsed his theory have related aspects of cognitive development, as Piaget has described it, to language. Table 3.3 contains a brief summary of key aspects of cognitive development that are related, or appear to be related, to language development. In processing this information, keep in mind that *relationship* does not necessarily mean *cause–effect*. In fact, most of the research data do not suggest that the connections between cognitive and language factors are more than correlational relationships.

Table 3.3 Sensorimotor and Language Events: A Summary

Sensorimotor Concept/Behavior	Language Behavior
Object permanence	1. Object permanence appears to be related to early semantic functions, including nonexistence, disappearance, and recurrence. 2. Brown (1973) suggests that the understanding of object permanence reflected in substage 4 may be adequate for the acquisition of the child's first productive words.
Causality	1. An understanding of causality is a cognitive prerequisite for communication (Bates & Snyder, 1987; Greenwald & Leonard, 1979; Snyder, 1978). 2. There appears to be a significant relationship between causality and the child's ability to understand verbs and semantic relations (Miller, Chapman, Branston, & Reichle, 1980).
Means–ends	1. An understanding of means–ends is critical to language development. 2. There is a significant correlation between an understanding of mean–ends and language development during the early portion of substage 4 (Bates et al., 1975, 1979; Bates, Benigni, Bretherton, Camaioni, & Volterra, 1977). This cognitive ability is particularly important to the development of communicative intentionality. 3. The understanding of means–ends reflected in substage 6 appears to be significantly related to the emergence of two-word utterances (Zachary, 1978).
Imitation	1. Imitation is significantly correlated with gestural development at nine to ten months. 2. Deferred imitation is significantly correlated with naming and with recognitory gestures (i.e., gestures that represent the functions or uses of objects) (Bates & Snyder, 1987). 3. When the child produces deferred imitation, we can assume that she has a true understanding of symbolic function because in deferred imitation, the referent for the imitation need not be present.
Play	1. There is a significant correlation between object play and language at ten to thirteen months (Bates et al., 1979; James, 1980). 2. Children who show a propensity for using a variety of schemes for objects in their early play experiences tend to progress more dramatically in language development than children who are more limited in their use of object schemes (Bates et al., 1975; Greenwald & Leonard, 1979; Sugarman, 1978). 3. A child will produce meaningful words as symbols for people, things, and events before he has demonstrated complete competence in symbolic play.

Nevertheless, it is intriguing to think about what these relationships might mean relative to both cognitive and language functions.

Vygotsky's Theory of Cognitive Development: A Sociocultural Perspective

The question we posed at the beginning of this chapter has significant relevance in relation to Vygotsky's theory of cognitive development: *Does thought shape language, or does language shape thought?* Hold that question in mind as this section unfolds, and try to determine how Lev Vygotsky would answer it.

Like Piaget, Vygotsky believed that the child is an active agent in her quest for knowledge. Beyond this general agreement, however, emerges a striking difference in the views of the two men. Whereas Piaget believed that the child operates independently, especially during the early stages of cognitive development, Vygotsky was convinced that the child's cognitive development is heavily influenced by her environment and by her culture from the very beginning of knowledge acquisition. In fact, Vygotsky believed that the developing child interacts with her environment in order to develop cognitive abilities that will allow her to adapt to her culture. In other words, during the course of intellectual development, there is a synergistic relationship between what the child brings to the cognitive table in terms of innate abilities and self-directed exploration and what her environment and culture bring to the table.

Vygotsky's views about cognitive development were not merely the result of academic musing but were forged in his own life experiences. We will best understand the theory, therefore, if we take a brief look at the man. In an interesting coincidence, the two men who have exercised the most profound influences on our understanding of cognitive development, Jean Piaget and Lev Vygotsky, were born in the same year, 1896. Tragically, Vygotsky's life was cut short at thirty-seven years by tuberculosis. The brief professional life he had was exceptionally productive, but he did not have the same long-term opportunity for reflection that Piaget had. For that reason, his theory is not as fully developed and not as detailed as Piaget's theory.

Vygotsky's own boyhood experiences related to learning shaped his views of cognitive development. As a youngster, he did not attend a formal school. He was taught at home by a tutor who believed that education involves more than simply filling an empty intellectual vessel. The tutor challenged the young Russian boy to be fully engaged in the process of learning, to answer and pose questions, to process answers, to think about how one piece of knowledge is integrated with established knowledge, to consider how one question leads to another. His was a truly interactive learning experience, and he came away from this personal experience believing that knowledge acquisition and intellectual development must necessarily proceed in this interactive manner.

Vygotsky's later educational experiences resulted in another critical difference between his views about cognitive development and Piaget's. Piaget, you will recall, did not give language any unique status in the process of cognitive development. He viewed language as simply one of a number of symbolic abilities the child acquires over the course of intellectual development. Vygotsky always viewed language as a key player in cognitive development, a perspective that was undoubtedly enhanced by his academic interest in literature, his major field of study at the University of Moscow. It is not surprising that when he shifted his attention to the study of cognitive development, he retained a focus on language.

One might well ask why there is so much interest in Vygotsky's views about cognitive development today. After all, this man's views about cognition were published more than seventy years ago. According to Wertsch and Tulviste (1992), the present interest in Vygotsky's theory can be traced to his belief that the child is not an independently operating agent, that the child's cognitive development is the product of an interaction between the child's innate abilities and his social experiences. It is noteworthy that Vygotsky's view of intellectual development is generally consonant with the dominant view of language development today, the social interactionist view. The marriage between a sociocultural view of cognition and a social interactionist view of language is a natural and eminently logical phenomenon.

Even though some people might be tempted to park Vygotsky at the nurture end of the nature-versus-nurture continuum, that would be an oversimplification of his views about development. Vygotsky begins, in fact, with a nature base. He believes that human children are born with fundamental cognitive and perceptual abilities, including capacities for memory and attending, abilities that human beings share with other animals. During the first two years of the human child's life, these abilities develop and mature according to a mostly biological calendar and as a result of the child's primitive contacts with his environment. The nature of cognitive development changes radically, however, as soon as the child can mentally represent the environmental phenomena he is experiencing. This mental representation includes, as a primary component, language.

At this point, armed with naturally developing cognitive and perceptual abilities and with emerging language skills, the child is able to engage in the social dialogues that are so inextricably connected to cultural activities. The groundwork is now laid for the component of Vygotsky's theory of cognitive development most closely associated with his name, *private speech*. When the young child begins to talk to herself, she crosses an important threshold in her cognitive development. From this point forward, and as a direct result of the power of language, the child's mental abilities will be shaped into the higher-order cognitive processes of an intelligence that clearly separates human beings from animals with lesser cognitive capacities. That is, the child uses language to direct her actions and to learn how to get things done (Wertsch & Tulviste, 1992).

Before we take a closer look at private speech and other critical elements of Vygotsky's theory, there is another basic difference between Piaget and Vygotsky that must be stressed. Piaget, as we have noted at a number of junctures in this chapter, believed that cognitive development proceeds in a predictable stage-by-stage manner. Vygotsky's view was that cognitive development does not proceed through exactly the same progressive sequence for all children. He argued that while each child experiences progressive changes in the way she thinks and behaves as a cognitive creature, the progression is continuous rather than stage by stage. More important, each child's cognitive development is shaped by the influences of the important adults and peers in the social environment and by the experiences unique to her culture.

While Vygotsky and Piaget would agree that there are systematic changes in cognitive development, Vygotsky would argue that these systematic changes vary widely across cultures because the nature of social interactions between children and the important people in their lives varies widely by culture. The tasks around which learning occurs differ from culture to culture. In some cultures, for example, girls are expected to perform domestic tasks at a young age. In other cultures, boys are expected to learn how to hunt and fish. In our culture, children are free of these kinds of responsibilities and are encouraged to play and "have fun." It is not difficult to imagine significant differences in the kinds of interactions that will occur between adults and children in each of these cultural situations. If little girls are expected to perform domestic tasks at an early age, they will be taught these skills by their primary caregivers and other significant adults. These lessons will involve communicative exchanges unique to the tasks being taught. Learning the skills inherent to the tasks will involve unique problem-solving challenges. Little boys who must learn how to hunt, fish, and forage will have radically different interactions with their caregivers than little boys whose caregivers teach them how to play baseball and fly kites. Children who live in cultures that place a premium on written language will face different cognitive challenges and will experience different social and communicative interactions with their significant others than children who live in cultures that depend mostly or solely on spoken language. A list of possible major cultural differences that might affect the way children acquire knowledge relative to cultural expectations and to the social/communicative interactions that facilitate the acquisition of knowledge would be impressive in its length and breadth.

Vygotsky's point is that cognitive development does not occur in isolation, but is a function of a person's social and cultural environment. That there are cross-cultural differences in the nature of social/communicative exchanges between young children and adults has been demonstrated by research that lends support to Vygotsky's argument (Bakeman, Adamson, Konner, & Barr, 1990; Saxe, 1988; Childs & Greenfield, 1982; Draper & Cashdan, 1988). We will now turn our attention to some of the critical elements in Vygotsky's theory, beginning with private speech.

Private Speech

Anyone who has watched young children play has heard private speech. A preschool child who is trying to construct a building out of blocks might say to himself, "This piece is too big. It sticks out. I need a smaller one." A child with a fistful of crayons and a coloring book might mutter to herself, "What color should the house be? I think

I'll make it purple. No, that's not right. Houses aren't purple. It should be white. Where's the white crayon?" Yet another child, trying to put plastic pieces of varying geometric shapes into a box with holes corresponding to these shapes, might be heard to say to herself, "This one is round, so it won't fit here, but it will fit here. Whoops, it didn't fit because it's too big. I need to find the small round one. There it is!"

What is all this self-talking about? The answer to that question depends on the expert to whom it is addressed. Piaget referred to this self-directed talk as *egocentric speech,* which he believed is nonsocial and relatively purposeless. It is speech produced by the individual child for the individual child who cannot mentally represent the viewpoints of other people. Based on what we have already established about Vygotsky's theory, you would expect a very different response from his perspective, and your expectation will be realized. Vygotsky (1986) believed that when children speak to themselves, they are guiding themselves through their actions. Especially early in their lives, children use self-directed speech, or private speech, literally to help themselves think through problems and tasks, to help themselves choose actions that are most appropriate to doing whatever it is they are trying to do. Private speech is a first step toward more elaborate cognitive skills. It helps the child learn how to pay attention, how to memorize and recall bits of information from memory, how to formulate and execute plans in solving problems, and, in a very real sense, how to think, ponder, or muse. As the child gets older, the nature of self-directed talking changes. In the beginning, the child talks out loud. As she gets older, she might whisper or mutter under her breath. Eventually, her private speech will be truly private. It will be silent and internalized. In short, it will become exactly the kind of private speech you use every day to think through your problems, to choose plans of actions for solving your problems, to reflect on the meaning of life and the futility of the Chicago Cubs.

The weight of the research evidence relative to self-directed talking comes down heavily on the side of Vygotsky. For that reason, most people who refer to self-directed talking today refer to it as *private speech* and no longer as *egocentric speech.* The most telling evidence supporting Vygotsky's view about private speech shows that children are more likely to talk to themselves when they are engaged in difficult tasks, when they are struggling with tasks and making mistakes, or when they are unsure about what they should do next (Berk, 1992). The research also confirms that Vygotsky was correct about the changes that occur to private speech as children mature. That is, it becomes less overt and more private until it becomes essentially speech in thought form (Berk & Landau, 1993; Frauenglass & Diaz, 1985). From a cognitive development point of view, Vygotsky's most crucial assertion is that private speech provides a foundation for higher-order cognitive functions. When the child engages in make-believe play, for example, private speech is a critical element of that activity. The co-existence of these two activities suggests that private speech helps the child place the control of action within the constraints of thought (Krafft & Berk, 1998). Research indicates that children who are uninhibited self-talkers when they are confronted with challenging tasks are more attentive, more fully engaged, and more likely to complete tasks successfully than children who are more reticent self-talkers

(Behrend, Rosengren, and Perlmutter, 1992; Bivens & Berk, 1990). There is also evidence that preschool children who participate in elaborate sociodramatic play, an activity that depends heavily on private speech, make more rapid progress in learning to follow classroom rules than children who are less inclined to participate in this kind of activity (Elias & Berk, 2002).

Social Keys to Cognitive Development

Keep in mind that Vygotsky believed that the establishment of higher-order cognitive functions begins in children's social interactions with the important people in their environment, interactions that reflect the culture of which they are members. This means that, from Vygotsky's point of view, we cannot talk about cognitive development without taking these social interactions into account. Children learn how to do things, and they learn how to process their thoughts in ways that appropriately reflect the culture in which they live, by interacting with adults who already know how things should be done and how to think in ways that are culturally acceptable. The child might be able to handle some tasks with which she is confronted without any direct intervention or assistance. That is, she will figure some things out, just as Piaget suggested, by independent discovery. There are many other tasks, however, that the child cannot manage on her own. She needs help from people who have greater knowledge, experience, and skill than she possesses. These tasks fall into what is called the *zone of proximal development.* Within this zone are those tasks with which the child needs help, and the help typically comes in the form of language. As a child and adult work together to learn a skill or solve a task problem, they talk to one another. The child retains language from these exchanges that she incorporates into her private speech. At some later time, she will use this private speech, now enhanced by the language she has garnered from these dialogues, to solve problems on her own.

If he had lived longer and continued to revise and elaborate his theory, Vygotsky would have probably tried to identify the features of adult–child dialogues that would most effectively facilitate the development of the child's cognitive abilities. In the absence of direction from Vygotsky himself on this subject, researchers have identified at least two attributes of these dialogues they believe are crucial in transferring the adult's cognitive competence to the child's cognitive development. The first of these attributes is *intersubjectivity.* An interaction is characterized by intersubjectivity if two people working together on a common task with different levels of understanding about how the task can or should be accomplished manage to merge what they know into a shared understanding as the task is completed. In this kind of interaction, each partner accommodates the viewpoint and competence of the other partner. An adult-to-adult dialogue characterized by intersubjectivity might include comments such as these: "What I hear you saying is . . ." or "I think I understand what you are saying . . . , but have you considered . . . ?" Each adult partner tries to understand the other partner's perspective, tries to gauge the other partner's knowledge base, tries to take from that knowledge base what she does not understand, and tries to impart knowledge he has that his partner might lack. This kind of dialogue demonstrates mutual respect and a shared determination to solve a problem for which the partners feel a united ownership. In an interaction shared by an adult and a child, the adult will convey what she knows to the child in a manner that fits what the child already knows and that does not exceed the child's ability to understand. You will recognize that this is exactly what occurs in any good teaching–learning situation even when the teacher and learner are both adults. That is, the teacher conveys her knowledge to the student by drawing on what the student already knows, by taking into account the student's abilities to understand, and by challenging the student to expand his own knowledge. In an interaction characterized by intersubjectivity, therefore, the child is challenged by the adult's dialogue and demonstrations to extend his understanding so that he develops a more mature, adultlike strategy for completing the targeted task (Rogoff, 1990).

The second attribute that characterizes facilitating dialogues is *scaffolding* (Bruner, 1983; Wood, 1989). To understand this feature of dialogues, we should first consider the literal meaning of the word *scaffold* and consider how scaffolds are used in real life. According to ***www.Dictionary.com,*** a *scaffold* is "a temporary platform, either supported from below or suspended from above, on which workers sit or stand when performing tasks at heights above the ground." We have all seen painters and window washers on scaffolds. At one time, scaffolds were no more than planks of wood attached to ropes. Today they are more sturdy mechanisms made of steel and protected by backup safety systems to guard against mechanical failures, but the general idea of a scaffold has not changed. When the window washer completes the windows on the third floor of a building, the scaffold is raised to the fourth floor, and it continues to be raised until all the windows on all the floors are squeaky clean.

How does scaffolding relate to cognitive development and to the dialogues and interactions that facilitate cognitive development? Just as a real-life scaffold is adjusted to the height necessary for the completion of a task such as washing windows, adults can provide scaffolds for the child when she is trying to reach new heights of cognitive competence. If the child has little idea about how to accomplish a targeted task, adults will set the scaffold low in the sense that they provide direct instruction. At this level, adults might try to segment the task into smaller tasks, building on what the child does know and can do, and then helping her master the next level, and then the next, until she can compete the whole task. When we teach children to write, for example, we do not expect the child to move from no writing skill to adult mastery in one step. We begin by asking the child to draw vertical lines, horizontal lines, and circles, skills she already has or that she can easily master. We scaffold the skills upward from the easiest and most basic of drawing skills to increasingly more elaborate writing skills until the child is actually producing written letters. As the child's cognitive competence increases, her need for direct support decreases. The adult who is a skillful scaffolder will gradually withdraw cognitive supports as the child gradually demonstrates less need for them, but the same sensitive scaffolder will be prepared to introduce the supports again if the child's independent efforts are producing more

Table 3.4 Key Features of Vygotsky's Theory

- Children are active participants in their quest for knowledge.
- Cognitive development is heavily influenced by the environment and culture.
- Language is a key player in cognitive development.
- Children use *private speech* to guide themselves through their actions.
- Children are born with basic cognitive and perceptual abilities.
- Children's cognitive abilities during the first two years of life develop and mature according to a biological calendar.
- At about two years, cognition and language influence each other.
- Children's ability to represent their environment mentally, including their use of language, facilitates cognitive development.
- Cognitive development does *not* proceed through exactly the same sequence for all children.

frustration and failure than success. The general rule in effective scaffolding, therefore, is to adjust support so that it meets the changing cognitive needs of the child.

Does effective scaffolding make a difference? There is research evidence that indicates it does. In studies focusing on the possible benefits of this strategy, some mothers used scaffolding more effectively than others in the process of teaching their children how to solve a particularly difficult puzzle. The children of the more effective scaffolders used more private speech and were more successful in independently solving a similar puzzle than the children of mothers who were less skillful in the use of scaffolding (Behrend, Rosengren, & Perlmutter, 1992; Berk & Spuhl, 1992.)

During his tragically brief life, Vygotsky gave us much to think about relative to cognition, cognitive development, and the synergistic relationship between cognition and language (see Table 3.4). Researchers continue to test the principles and concepts of his theory, and, so far at least, his views that cognitive development occurs within the larger context of social and cultural experiences and that language directs cognition as much as cognition directs language are holding up well to empirical scrutiny.

The Perceptual Groundwork for Communication

Before we proceed to a detailed description of speech and language development in the next three chapters, we must more fully address the perceptual preparation for communication, a topic briefly introduced when we discussed the principle of distancing earlier in this chapter. **Perception,** you may remember, refers to the processes by which a person selects, organizes, integrates, and interprets the sensory stimuli he receives. Since children must somehow make sense of the sensory information they receive related to communication in general and speech specifically before they can create their own communicative output, we should know something about what they receive and what catches their attention during the preparation period. What follows then is a brief summary of what we believe are children's earliest perceptual abilities as they pertain to communication.

The Relationship between Cognition and Perception

It should be fairly obvious that perception cannot be completely separated from cognition. To understand, think, solve problems, and engage in all other activities associated with cognition, we must be able to sort through the stimuli our senses are receiving, recognize important stimuli, ignore unimportant ones, and then categorize, integrate, and interpret the stimuli we have selected. The further into perception we proceed, the closer to cognition we get, until the line between them becomes effectively blurred to the point of virtual elimination.

Stern (1977) makes a useful distinction between **perceptual stimulation** and **cognitive stimulation.** As a result of perceptual or sensory stimulation, a child recognizes that stimuli are present and reacts to the major characteristics of the stimuli. If they are auditory stimuli, for example, he reacts to the loudness and pitch changes of the sounds he is receiving. If they are visual, he reacts to things such as size and shape. This level of perception develops early. As the child develops intellectually, he shows evidence of cognitive stimulation, which means he not only recognizes stimuli by their sensory characteristics but also understands what they mean and how they compare to other stimuli he has received. He understands, for example, the difference between the ringing of the doorbell and the ringing of the telephone. When the doorbell rings, he runs to the door because he knows someone will be there. When the telephone rings, he picks up the receiver because he knows someone will answer. He combines his ability to make discriminations among similar and dissimilar bits of sensory information with his ability to make mental judgments about what this information means. This complex marriage of perception and cognition continues throughout the child's development years and beyond. In fact, as long as a person can receive new information, process it, and think about it, the marriage thrives.

Visual Perception

You might wonder what visual perception has to do with language and especially with speech. Actually, what the child sees can be very important in the language acquisition process. Sachs (1989) contends that visual and tactile stimuli "play a great role in establishing the bond between adult and child" (p. 38). This in no way minimizes the importance of auditory stimulation, but it does suggest that what the child sees helps to direct and fix her attention. Presumably, once the speaker has gained the child's attention by whatever visual or tactile stimuli are required, the child will gain more from the auditory stimuli produced by the speaker. Even though we have no proof that this connection of sensory modalities is necessary for speech development, it is probably more than coincidental that infants are interested in the kinds of visual stimuli that are characteristic of early child–adult interactions.

Vision is the first sensory system the child controls (Tiegerman, 1989). Within hours after birth, the infant can follow movement visually (Greenman, 1963) and is able to focus on a target seven and a half inches removed, the distance at which vision achieves its optimal focus (Owens, 2001, p. 160). This is potentially significant because when the child is being fed, his mother's eyes are almost exactly eight inches away, and his mother watches him almost constantly during feeding (Stern, 1977) while he returns the visual favor. It is tempting to conclude, as some observers have, that the child is genetically preprogrammed for this visual coupling, which, it is further assumed, leads to bonding between the child and mother.

By the time the child is three months old, she can control eye movements sufficiently to determine the visual information she chooses to receive. She looks at things and people she finds interesting, and she turns away when she is no longer interested. The infant prefers objects of contrasting colors, and she likes things that move (Haith, 1976). She is attracted to objects with designs of varying angles and curves, and visually complex objects that reflect light variably (Fantz, 1964; Freedman, 1964; Haaf & Bell, 1967). What makes this fascinating is that the infant shows strong interest in the human face, an object that meets all these criteria for preference and interest. The face can consist of many colors when you include all the parts: hair, eyes, eyebrows, lashes, lips, and cheeks. The face is capable of almost infinite movement and has many angles and curves that reflect and shade light. Again, it is tempting to conclude that the child is born with visual interests that perfectly match the facial characteristics of her primary object of attention and affection, the caregiver.

Much attention has been paid by researchers and theorists to the child's interest in the human face in general, the caregiver's face in particular, and to the eye contact or gaze between child and caregiver. There has been much speculation about what all this might suggest about bonding in the child–caregiver relationship. Certainly no one questions the newborn's preoccupation with looking at his caregiver's face. So fixed is he on looking at the caregiver's face in the first few weeks of his life that it is difficult to direct his visual attention anywhere else. By the time he is just two weeks old, he may be able to distinguish, on the basis of face and voice, his caregiver from other people (Bower, 1977). When he is three weeks old, he will respond to his caregiver's face and other human faces by smiling (Trevarthen, 1979). By the time he is three months old, the infant and his caregiver exchange gazes in a manner that suggests adultlike conversational turn taking (Jaffe, Stern, & Perry, 1973). At the very least, this is intriguing stuff. At most, contingent on more research that would allow for more confident conclusions, it might suggest that the child is genetically tuned to certain visual stimuli that are important in capturing his attention and in helping to establish a communicative relationship with his caregiver, a relationship many social interactionist theorists believe is important, if not vital, to normal communication development.

Auditory Perception

Just as children seem to have a special interest in the visual characteristics of the human face, they seem to be especially attracted to the human voice and speech. It is important to establish, however, that there are characteristics of sounds in general that appeal to infants, characteristics found in human speech. This could mean that children are interested in these characteristics because they are born with speech perceptual abilities and find these sound characteristics interesting whether they occur in speech or nonspeech sounds. It could mean that children are born with an auditory system designed to make discriminations among sounds we believe they find interesting and not designed to make discriminations among sounds we assume they are ignoring. It could, of course, be only coincidental that children react to sound features that happen to be characteristic of human speech. Much more research needs to be conducted before we know *why* the children react as they do to specified features of sound. In the meantime, we can account for at least some of *what* they seem to find appealing in the sounds they hear.

It would seem important to first assess the very young infant's ability to determine the direction from which a sound is coming. An early study by Wertheimer (1961) indicated that a child just after birth moved his eyes in the direction of clicking sounds, but other studies since have not confirmed this finding. A more reasonable suggestion of the localization of sound in young infants is turning the head, a behavior studied by Muir and Field (1979). Using head turning as a criterion for localizing sound, they found that infants ranging in age from two to seven days turned in the direction of a rattling noise about three-fourths of the time. This consistency allows us to conclude that newborns can determine at least the general direction of sound sources.

From the time the child is born, perhaps even while he is still in the uterus, he can make many kinds of auditory discriminations. Some newborn children, for example, can discriminate between a pure tone at four hundred Hertz and another at one thousand Hertz (Bridger, 1961), and there is evidence that they seem to make their best discriminations among frequencies characteristic of human speech (Eisenberg, 1976).

Newborns can make gross discriminations about the loudness levels of sounds. When they listen to white noise (a mixture of a wide range of frequencies) that is varied in loudness, there are noticeable changes in heart rate and in the startle reflex (Bench, 1969). Similar changes in behavior occur when children hear pure tones varied by loudness (Bartoshuk, 1964).

Although it is important to remember that we are dealing with only the broadest judgments of differences, some evidence suggests that infants respond differentially to sounds of varying durations (Clifton, Graham, & Hatton, 1968; Ling, 1972). In reference to the Ling study, Reich (1986) cautions that it "does not demonstrate that the infant can detect these differences, only that it reacts more to signals of longer duration" (p. 15). At the least, this research indicates that infants are aware of when sounds begin and end and how long they are sustained, and it is probable that infants are able to make some discriminations concerning durations.

An Early Interest in the Human Voice and Speech

One of the most exciting general findings of the research related to the early perceptual abilities of children is that infants show a greater interest in human speech than other noises (Eisenberg, 1976; Jensen, Williams, & Bzoch, 1975). There is evidence that a child may prefer the acoustic characteristics of a speech passage his mother recited while she was pregnant over the acoustic characteristics of something she did not read (DeCasper & Spence, 1986), and there is evidence that a child as young as three days recognizes his mother's voice and discriminates it from the voices of other mothers (DeCasper & Fifer, 1980). All of this can be interpreted to mean that, just as children are born with basic biological abilities to produce speech and language, they are born with biological perceptual abilities to receive and interpret speech and language. Whether or not a conclusion as sweeping as this is warranted, we can conclude that a newborn infant is able to distinguish between speech and nonspeech sounds, that he seems to prefer speech, that he recognizes his mother's voice very early, and that he seems to be aware of differences between sounds to which he was exposed while in the uterus and sounds to which he was not exposed. These are significant perceptual abilities.

As impressive as the infant's general speech discrimination is, it is perhaps even more impressive that as early as one month, a child can discriminate among speech sounds. One of the methods used to assess this ability in infants is known as *non-nutritive sucking* or *high-amplitude sucking* and was developed at Brown University (Eimas, Siqueland, Jusczyk, & Vigorito, 1971). In this procedure, the infant sucks on a specially designed pacifier connected to a sound generator. When she sucks on the pacifier with enough vigor, she hears a predetermined sound. Since the only thing that changes in this exercise is the sound produced by the sucking, it is reasonable to assume that, if the infant does not recognize the difference between the first sound and the second, there will be no change in the rate of sucking, but this is not what happens. When Eimas et al. (1971) presented "ba," the one-month-old infant sucked vigorously and quickly, but after a few minutes lost interest and decreased the rate of sucking. When a new sound, "pa," was introduced, the infant increased the rate of sucking. A number of studies reviewed by Aslin, Pisoni, and Jusczyk (1983) have shown the same reaction with a variety of speech sounds.

Since this ability is demonstrated at such a young age, it appears to be an innate ability rather than environmental. In an attempt to answer this particular nature–nurture question, Trehub (1976) tested the ability of Canadian infants and English-speaking adults to discriminate between two Czech sounds. Although the infants discriminated between the Czech sounds as well as between English sounds such as "p" and "b," the adults had great difficulty with the Czech sounds. Trehub concluded that children are born with the ability to discriminate among sounds found in all languages. As speakers become more immersed in their own languages, they lose some of this discriminative ability.

Taking the question to the next logical level, Werker and Tees (1984) tried to determine how quickly the infant loses this open-ended ability to discriminate speech sounds. They presented non-English sounds to English-speaking children ranging in age from six months to twelve months. Infants between six and eight months had little difficulty making the necessary discriminations. Those between eight and ten months had more difficulty, and those between ten and twelve months had the most difficulty. It appears then that the ability to discriminate a wide range of sounds representing many languages declines early in the child's life. Werker and Tees suggest that it is probably not coincidental that children's discrimination abilities become more narrow as they are acquiring their own sound system and language. Environment does play a role in shaping discrimination abilities, therefore, but rather than expanding these abilities, children's environmental experiences make their discriminations more selective, more consistent with the speech sounds native to their language.

I'm Ready! Let's Talk!

There is much we still do not know about the child's preparation for language, but it should be obvious that the child does not just sit in his crib waiting for that thrilling moment when he begins to speak. From the time the child is born, even before he is born, he is receiving sensory information about his world. From the moment of his birth, he processes all of this data in attempts to understand the nature of objects, people, and sounds. From the earliest moments of his life, he can make distinctions among things he sees and things he hears, and many of these distinctions seem to be relevant to his future social and communicative development. Over the first two years of his life, he progresses from an almost completely reflexive and sensory creature to a person who is able to think and solve problems. He progresses from an intellectual view of the world that is strictly *reality based* and hands-on, to a view that allows for *mental representation* of all that is real and even some that is not. When the child is able to capture the world in his brain and in his thought processes, when he is able to transform things, people, places, events, and actions into abstract, representational forms, he is ready for language. Readiness does not come in one magic moment, of course, and language does not spill out of the child in a complete package. Language, like the cognitive and perceptual abilities on which it is based, emerges in a progressive manner, in steps and stages that are as interlocking and integrated as are the stages of cognitive development. Even in this chapter, which has focused on the preparation for speech and language, we have seen substantial evidence of communicative ability and output. In the next three chapters we will look more closely at speech and language development, a progression that amounts to an explosion in the preschool years but slows down and becomes more evolutionary in nature as the child moves toward adolescence.

As we close this chapter and look ahead to a detailed examination of language development, we should emphasize that while cognitive development and language development are inextricably connected, and while there are clearly cause–effect relationships between cognition and language use, they do not develop in a simplistic parallel manner. The child is clearly a thinker before she is a speaker. She conceptualizes before she can produce the words that represent the concepts she understands. She can link thoughts before she can she can produce grammatically complete utterances that express those cognitive linkages. The lag between cognitive development and the emergence of correlative language forms was identified quite accurately in an October 2004 installment of the syndicated comic strip, *Hi and Lois*, written by Greg and Brian Walker and drawn by Chance Browne. In the first panel of this installment, Lois and a friend are watching Lois' little girl, Trixie, interact with another little girl. Trixie is watching in silence as the other little girl coos and gestures. Lois' friend says, "Cute! She's trying to talk to Trixie." Lois says, "I wonder why Trixie's not responding." In the second panel, the cooing little girl continues her efforts while we read Trixie's thoughts: "I refuse to engage in meaningless babble until my verbal skills catch up to my cognitive abilities." Trixie would get some arguments from language people about the idea that babbling is *meaningless,* but she is right on target about the delay between thinking and talking. In the chapters that follow, we will take a close look at the developmental process by which the gap between cognition and language is closed, a process that results in such a thorough integration of cognition and language that in mature communication, the line that separates what we think and what we say is nearly nonexistent.

Review Questions

1. What does common sense suggest about the relationship between language and thought?
2. Define and provide examples for the following concepts included in Piaget's theory of cognitive development: schema, assimilation, accommodation, and equilibrium.
3. Identify and briefly describe each of Piaget's four stages of intellectual development from birth through adolescence.
4. What is the principle of distancing? What does this principle contribute to our understanding of cognitive and language development?
5. Define each of the following key concepts and behaviors as the primary players in the sensorimotor stage of cognitive development: object permanence, causality, means–ends, imitation, play, and communication.
6. Six substages comprise Piaget's sensorimotor stage of intellectual development. Identify what you believe are the most important developmental changes in each substage, and justify your selections.
7. How are the cognitive theories of Piaget and Vygotsky similar? What are their major differences?
8. What does recent research suggest about Piaget's predictions regarding the emergence of *object permanence?*

Why is there such a disparity between what Piaget predicted and what empirical evidence seems to suggest about the emergence of this cognitive ability?

9. What does the evidence suggesting that *mental representation* occurs earlier than Piaget predicted suggest about the explanation of early cognitive abilities solely within the context of sensorimotor experiences?
10. Why do some critics of Piaget's theory believe that the stage concept of cognitive development is no longer viable? Why do others believe that the stage concept, in some form, still has value in understanding how intellectual development occurs?
11. How did Vygotsky's own life experiences shape his views about cognitive development?
12. Why is Vygotsky's theory referred to as a *sociocultural* theory of cognitive development?
13. Differentiate Vygotsky's *private speech* from Piaget's *egocentric speech.* Why is *private speech* the preferred label for self-directed talk today?
14. What is meant by the *zone of proximal development?*
15. Identify and describe the two attributes of adult–child dialogues that presumably facilitate cognitive development.

16. How are cognition and perception related to one another?
17. How is visual perception related to speech and language development?
18. What auditory perceptual abilities does the newborn child have that

seem to be related to early communication development?
19. Summarize what is known about the infant's interest in the human voice and speech.

References and Suggested Readings

Anisfeld, M. (1984). *Language development from birth to three.* Hillsdale, NJ: Erlbaum.

Aslin, R., Pisoni, D., & Jusczyk, P. (1983). Auditory development and speech perception in infancy. In M. Haith & J. Campos (Eds.), *Handbook of child psychology: Vol. 2. Infancy and developmental psychobiology.* New York: Wiley.

Baillargeon, R. (1987). Object permanence in 3.5- and 4.5-month-old infants. *Developmental Psychology, 23,* 655–664.

Baillargeon, R., & DeVos, J. (1991). Object permanence in young infants: Further evidence. *Child Development, 62,* 1227–1246.

Baillargeon, R., DeVos, J., & Graber, M. (1989). Location memory in 8-month-old infants in a non-search AB task: Further evidence. *Cognitive Development, 4,* 345–367.

Baillargeon, R., Graber, M., DeVos, J., & Black, J. (1990). Why do young infants fail to search for hidden objects? *Cognition, 36,* 255–284.

Bakeman, R., Adamson, L., Konner, M., & Barr, R. (1990). !Kung infancy: The social context of object exploration. *Child Development, 61,* 794–809.

Barr, R., & Hayne, H. (1999). Developmental changes in imitation from television during infancy. *Child Development, 70,* 1067–1081.

Bartoshuk, A. (1964). Human neonatal cardiac responses to sound: A

power function. *Psychodynamic Science, 1,* 151–152.

Bates, E., Benigni, L., Bretherton, I., Camaioni, L., & Volterra, V. (1977). From gesture to the first word: On cognitive and social prerequisites. In M. Lewis & L. Rosenblum (Eds.), *Interaction, conversation, and the development of language.* New York: Wiley.

Bates, E., Benigni, L., Bretherton, I., Camaioni, L., & Volterra, V. (1979). *The emergence of symbols: Cognition and communication in infancy.* New York: Academic Press.

Bates, E., Bretherton, I., Snyder, L., Shore, C., & Volterra, V. (1980). Vocal and gestural symbols at 13 months. *Merrill-Palmer Quarterly, 26,* 407–423.

Bates, E., Camaioni, L., & Volterra, V. (1975). The acquisition of performatives prior to speech. *Merrill-Palmer Quarterly, 21,* 205–224.

Bates, E., & Snyder, L., (1987). The cognitive hypothesis in language development. In I. Uzgiris & J. Hunt (Eds.), *Infant performance and experience: New findings with the ordinal scale.* Urbana: University of Illinois Press.

Behrend, D., Rosengren, K., & Perlmutter, M. (1992). The relation between private speech and parental interactive style. In R. Diaz & L. Berk (Eds.), *Private speech: From social interaction to self-regulation.* Hillsdale, NJ: Erlbaum.

Bench, J. (1969). Audio-frequency and audio-intensity discrimination in the human neonate. *International Audiology, 8,* 615–625.

Berk, L. (1992). Children's private speech: An overview of theory and the status of research. In R. Diaz & L. Berk (Eds.), *Private speech: From social interaction to self-regulation.* Hillsdale, NJ: Erlbaum.

Berk, L. (1994). *Child development* (3rd ed.). Needham Heights, MA: Allyn & Bacon.

Berk, L. (2003). *Child development* (6th ed.). Boston: Allyn & Bacon.

Berk, L., & Landau, S. (1993). Private speech of learning disabled and normally achieving children in classroom academic and laboratory contexts. *Child Development, 64,* 556–571.

Berk, L., & Spuhl, S. (1995). Maternal interaction, private speech, and task performance in preschool children. *Early Childhood Research Quarterly, 10,* 145–169.

Bivens, J., & Berk, L. (1990). A longitudinal study of the development of elementary school children's private speech. *Merrill-Palmer Quarterly, 36,* 443–463.

Bloom, K., & Lo, E. (1990). Adult perceptions of vocalizing infants. *Infant Behavior and Development, 13,* 209–213.

Borden, G., & Harris, K. (1984) *Speech science primer: Physiology, acoustics, and perception of speech* (2nd ed.). Baltimore: Williams & Wilkins.

Bower, T. (1977). *The perceptual world of the child.* Cambridge, MA: Harvard University Press.

Bridger, W. (1961). Sensory habituation and discrimination in the human neonate. *American Journal of Psychiatry, 117,* 991–996.

Brockman, L., Morgan, G., & Harmon, R. (1988). Mastery motivation and developmental delay. In T. Wachs & R. Sheehan (Eds.), *Assessment of young developmentally disabled children.* New York: Plenum.

Brown, R. (1973). *A first language: The early stages.* Cambridge, MA: Harvard University Press.

Bruner, J. (1983). *Child's talk: Learning to use language.* Oxford: Oxford University Press.

Bryen, D. (1982). *Inquiries into child language.* Boston: Allyn & Bacon.

Childs, C., & Greenfield, P. M. (1982). Informal modes of learning and teaching: The case of Zinacanteco weaving. In N. Warren (Ed.), *Advances in cross-cultural psychology* (Vol. 2). London: Academic Press.

Clifton, R., Graham, R., & Hatton, H. (1968). Newborn heart-rate response and response habituation as a function of stimulus duration. *Journal of Experimental Child Psychology, 6,* 265–278.

Cole, M., John-Steiner, V., Scribner, S., & Souberman, M. (Eds.). (1978). *Mind in society: The development of higher psychological processes.* Cambridge, MA: Harvard University Press.

DeCasper, A., & Fifer, W. (1980). Of human bonding: Newborns prefer their mothers' voices. *Science, 208,* 1174–1176.

DeCasper, A., & Spence, M. (1986). Prenatal maternal speech influences newborns' perception of speech sounds. *Infant Behavior and Development, 9,* 133–150.

D'Odorico, L. (1984). Nonsegmental features in prelinguistic communications: An analysis of some types of infant cry and noncry vocalizations. *Journal of Child Language, 11,* 17–27.

Draper, P., & Cashdan, E. (1988). Technological change and child behavior among the !Kung. *Ethnology, 27,* 339–365.

Dunst, C. (1980). *Clinical and educational manual for use with the Uzgiris and Hunt scales of infant psychological development.* Baltimore: University Park Press.

Elias, C., & Berk, L. (2002). Self-regulation in young children: Is there a role for sociodramatic play? *Early Childhood Research Quarterly, 17,* 1–17.

Eilers, R., & Oller, K. (1983). Speech perception in infancy. In E. Lasky & J. Katz (Eds.), *Central auditory processing disorders: Problems of speech, language, and learning.* Austin, TX: PRO-ED.

Eimas, P., Siqueland, E., Jusczyk, P., & Vigorito, J. (1971). Speech perception in infants. *Science, 171,* 303–306.

Eisenberg, R. (1976). *Auditory competence in early life: The roots of communicative-behavior.* Baltimore: University Park Press.

Fantz, R. (1964). Visual experience in infants: Decreased attention to familiar patterns relative to novel ones. *Science, 146,* 668–670.

Flavell, J. (1977). *Concept development.* Upper Saddle River, NJ: Prentice Hall.

Flavell, J. H. (1985). *Cognitive development* (2nd ed.). Upper Saddle River, NJ: Prentice Hall.

Frauenglass, M., & Diaz, R. (1985). Self-regulatory functions of children's private speech: A critical analysis of recent challenges to Vygotsky's theory. *Developmental Psychology, 21,* 357–364.

Freedman, D. (1964). Smiling in blind infants and the issue of innate vs. acquired. *Journal of Child Psychology and Psychiatry, 5,* 171–184.

Gelman, R., & Baillargeon, R. (1983). A review of some Piagetian concepts. In P. H. Mussen (Ed.), *Handbook of child psychology: Volume 3. Cognitive development* (4th ed.). New York: Wiley.

Göncü, A. (1993). Development of intersubjectivity in the dyadic play of preschoolers. *Early Childhood Research Quarterly, 8,* 99–116.

Gopnik, A., & Meltzoff, A. (1987). The development of categorization in the second year and its relation to other cognitive and linguistic developments. *Child Development, 58,* 1523–1531.

Greenman, G. (1963). Visual behavior of newborn infants. In A. Solnit & S. Provence (Eds.), *Modern perspectives in child development.* New York: Hallmark.

Greenwald, C., & Leonard, L. (1979). Communicative and sensorimotor development in Down's syndrome children. *American Journal of Mental Deficiency, 84,* 296–303.

Haaf, R., & Bell, R. (1967). A facial dimension in visual discrimination by human infants. *Child Development, 38,* 893–899.

Haight, W., & Miller, P. (1993). *Pretending at home: Early development in a sociocultural context.* Albany, NY: SUNY Press.

Haith, M. (1976, July). *Organization of visual behavior at birth.* Paper presented at the 21st International Congress of Psychology, Paris, France.

Hayne, H., Boniface, J., & Barr, R. (2000). The development of declarative memory in human infants: Age-related changes in deferred imitation. *Behavioral Neuroscience, 114,* 77–83.

Hayne, H., Rovee-Collier, C., & Perris, E. (1987). Categorization and memory retrieval by three-month-olds. *Child Development, 58,* 750–767.

Jaffe, J., Stern, D., & Perry, C. (1973). "Conversational" coupling of gaze behavior in prelinguistic human development. *Journal of Psycholinguistic Research, 2,* 321–330.

James, S. (1980). *Language and sensorimotor cognitive development in the young child.* Paper presented at the annual convention of the New York Speech–Language–Hearing Association.

James, S. (1990). *Normal language acquisition.* Austin, TX: PRO-ED.

Jensen, P., Williams, W., & Bzoch, K. (1975, November). *Preference of young infants for speech vs. nonspeech stimuli.* Paper presented to the annual American Speech and Hearing Association convention, Washington, D.C.

Johnston, E., & Johnston, A. (1984). *The Piagetian language nursery: An intensive group language intervention program for preschoolers.* Rockville, MD: Aspen.

Kelly, C., & Dale, P. (1989). Cognitive skills associated with the onset of multiword utterances. *Journal of Speech and Hearing Research, 32,* 645–656.

Klein, P., & Meltzoff, A. (1999). Long-term memory, forgetting, and deferred imitation in 12-month-old infants. *Developmental Science, 2,* 102–113.

Krafft, K., & Berk, L. (1998). Private speech in two preschools: Significance of open-ended activities and make-believe play for verbal self-regulation. *Early Childhood Research Quarterly, 13,* 637–658.

Lillard, A. (2001). Pretending, understanding pretense, and understand-ing minds. In. S. Reifel (Ed.), *Theory in context and out: Play and culture studies, Vol. 3* (pp. 233–254). Westport, CT: Ablex.

Ling, D. (1972). Acoustic stimulus duration in relation to behavioral responses of newborn infants. *Journal of Speech and Hearing Research, 15,* 567–571.

Mandler, J. (1992a). The foundations of conceptual thought in infancy. *Cognitive Development, 7,* 273–285.

Mandler, J. (1992b). How to build a baby: II. Conceptual primitives. *Psychological Review, 99,* 587–604.

McCormick, L. (1990). Bases for language and communication development. In L. McCormick & R. Schiefelbusch (Eds.), *Early language intervention: An introduction* (2nd ed.). Upper Saddle River, NJ: Prentice Hall.

McCune, L. (1993). The development of play as the development of consciousness. In M. H. Bornstein & A. O'Reilly (Eds.), *New directions for child development* (No. 59, pp. 67–79). San Francisco: Jossey-Bass.

Meltzoff, A. (1988a). Imitation of televised models by infants. *Child Development, 59,* 1221–1229.

Meltzoff, A. (1988b). Infant imitation after a 1-week delay: Long-term memory for novel acts and multiple stimuli. *Developmental Psychology, 24,* 470–476.

Meltzoff, A., & Moore, M. (1999). Persons and representations: Why infant imitation is important for theories of human development. In J. Nadel & G. Butterworth (Eds.), *Imitation in infancy* (pp. 9–35). Cambridge: Cambridge University Press.

Miller, J., Chapman, R., Branston, M., and Reichle, J. (1980). Language comprehension in sensorimotor stages 5 and 6. *Journal of Speech and Hearing Research, 4,* 1–12.

Moerk, E. (1977). *Pragmatic and semantic aspects of early language development.* Baltimore: University Park Press.

Moore, K., & Meltzoff, A. (1978). Object permanence, imitation, and language development in infancy: Toward a neo-Piagetian perspective on communicative development. In F. Minifie & L. Lloyd (Eds.), *Communicative and cognitive abilities—Early behavioral assessment.* Baltimore: University Park Press.

Muir, D., & Field, J. (1979). Newborn infants orient to sounds. *Child Development, 50,* 431–436.

Muma, J. (1978). *Language handbook.* Upper Saddle River, NJ: Prentice Hall.

Oakes, L., Madole, K., & Cohen, L. (1991). Infants' object examining: Habituation and categorization. *Cognitive Development, 6,* 377–392.

O'Reilly, A. (1995). Using representations: Comprehension and production of actions with imagined objects. *Child Development, 66,* 999–1010.

Owens, R. (2001). *Language development: An introduction* (5th ed.), Boston: Allyn & Bacon.

Owens, R. (2005). *Language development, An introduction* (6th ed.). Boston: Allyn & Bacon.

Piaget, J. (1952). *Origins of intelligence in children.* New York: International Universities Press.

Piaget, J. (1954). *The construction of reality in the child.* New York: Basic Books.

Piaget, J. (1963). *The origins of intelligence in children.* New York: Norton.

Reed, V. (1986). Bases of language functioning. In V. Reed (Ed.), *An introduction to children with language disorders.* New York: Macmillan.

Rees, N. (1975). Imitation and language development: Issues and clinical implications. *Journal of Speech and Hearing Disorders, 40,* 339–350.

Reich, P. (1986). *Language development.* Upper Saddle River, NJ: Prentice Hall.

Rice, M. (1983). Contemporary accounts of the cognitive/language relationship: Implications for speech–language clinicians. *Journal of Speech and Hearing Disorders, 48,* 347–359.

Roberts, K. (1988). Retrieval of a basic-level category in prelinguistic infants. *Developmental Psychology, 24,* 21–27.

Rogoff, B. (1990). *Apprenticeship in thinking.* New York: Oxford University Press.

Sachs, J. (1989). Communication development in infancy. In J. Berko-Gleason (Ed.), *The development of language.* Upper Saddle River, NJ: Merrill/Prentice Hall.

Saxe, G. G. (1988). Candy selling and math learning. *Educational Researcher, 17,* 14–21.

Sherman, T. (1985). Categorization skills in infants. *Child Development, 56,* 1561–1573.

Snyder, L. (1978). Communicative and cognitive abilities and disabilities in the sensorimotor period. *Merrill-Palmer Quarterly, 24,* 161–180.

Stark, R. (1979). Prespeech segmental feature development. In P. Fletcher & M. Garman (Eds.), *Language acquisition.* New York: Cambridge University Press.

Stern, D. (1977). *The first relationship.* Cambridge, MA: Harvard University Press.

Sugarman, S. (1978). A description of communicative development in the prelanguage child. In I. Markova (Ed.), *The social context of language.* New York: Wiley.

Tiegerman, E. (1989). The cognitive bases in language development. In D. Berstein & E. Tiegerman (Eds.), *Language and communication disorders in children* (2nd ed.). Upper Saddle River, NJ: Merrill/Prentice Hall.

Tomasello, M., Striano, T., & Rochat, P. (1999). Do young children use objects as symbols? *British Journal of Developmental Psychology, 17,* 563–584.

Trehub, S. (1976). The discrimination of foreign speech contrasts by infants and children. *Child Development, 47,* 466–472.

Trevarthen, C. (1979). Communication and cooperation in early infancy: A description of primary intersubjectivity. In M. Bullowa (Ed.), *Before speech*. New York: Cambridge University Press.

Vygotsky, L. (1986). *Thought and language* (A. Kozuhn, Trans.). Cambridge, MA: MIT Press. (Original work published 1934)

Wadsworth, B. (1971). *Piaget's theory of cognitive development*. New York: McKay.

Werker, J., & Tees, R. (1984). Cross-language speech perception: Evidence for perceptual reorganization during the first year of life. *Infant Behavior and Development, 7,* 49–64.

Wertheimer, M. (1961). Psychomotor coordination of auditory and visual space at birth. *Science, 134,* 1692.

Wertsch, J., & Tulviste, P. (1992). L. S. Vygotsky and contemporary developmental psychology. *Developmental Psychology, 28,* 548–557.

Westby, C. (1980). Assessment of cognitive and language abilities through play. *Language, Speech, and Hearing Services in Schools, 11,* 154–168.

Wood, D. (1989). Social interaction as tutoring. In M. Bornstein & J. Bruner (Eds.), *Interaction in human development*. Hillsdale, NJ: Erlbaum.

Zachary, W. (1978). Ordinality and interdependence of representation and language development in infants. *Child Development, 49,* 681–687.

4

In the Beginning: Communication Development from Birth to Two Years

CHAPTER OBJECTIVES

Three chapters trace language development from birth through the school-age years. In this chapter, we consider language development from birth through two years. We emphasize that the child is a communicator from the beginning of her life, and the changes in her communication system over the first two years are dramatic. She begins by crying, and by the time she is two years old, she has already been talking for a year.

As a framework for our discussion of language acquisition in this chapter and the next, we use a stage view of development. Although we focus primarily on speech and language *production*, we also consider the vital role of *comprehension* in communication development. Specifically, this chapter is designed to facilitate understanding of the following topics:

- The *receptive* component of the infant's communication system, including the early discrimination abilities that appear to be linked in a preparatory sense to speech production

- Infant–adult interactions that create a communication environment conducive to speech and language development
- Speech production during infancy from first cries to first words
- The stage concept of language acquisition, including the strengths and potential dangers in this view of human development
- *Morphology, morphemes,* and *mean length of utterance (MLU)*

- *Stage 1* (twelve to twenty-six months) of language development, with special attention to the classification and functions of first words, early conversational skills, and the emergence of word combinations
- The relationship between comprehension and production in an emerging communication system
- The role of the caregiver in stage 1 of language development

---

To the casual observer, the child's first year of life is fairly uneventful. It seems to be a succession of days marked by sleeping, eating, spitting up, crying, and soiling diapers. The more educated observer understands that much more is going on than this. The child comes into the world genetically programmed to become a whole person, a thinking, acting, reacting, speaking human being, and he does not wait until his first birthday to begin his growth into personhood. He is born with an enormous intellectual capacity that begins to develop immediately. He has fairly sophisticated perceptual abilities that he uses within the first hours and days of his life. Much of his first year is devoted to making contact with his world, first through his senses. He absorbs the sights, sounds, and textures of this new environment into which he has been hurled. He makes immediate connections to those people who will be most important in his early development. In the beginning, he does not understand his relationship to the people and things in his environment, but in a very real sense he *relates* to these people and things by looking at them, listening to them, by grasping them, and putting them into his mouth. The newborn child is not a mass of tissue simply waiting to be molded. During the first year of his life, he is a vital, active, exploring, thinking creature, and from the very beginning he is a **communicator.**

From the Beginning, the Infant Communicates

Before the child develops language, she communicates. Before she sends *intentional* messages, she communicates. As noted in the opening chapter of this book, human beings communicate even when they do not intend to communicate. We cannot help ourselves! When the newborn infant cries, she is sending a message. It is not always a clear message, and she does not send it with any sense of purpose, but those within hearing distance receive something they perceive as a message. A listener will likely interpret this reflexive cry to mean, "I am hungry," "I am sleepy," or "I am in pain." When the child responds to stimuli with the startle reflex by kicking her legs and pumping her arms, the observer interprets the action to mean, "I'm excited," or "I'm frightened." When the child smiles, the listener senses that the child is communicating something like "I see you. You're really special to me, and I love you." There are no boundaries when these signals, most of which are reflexive responses to specific stimuli, are interpreted by people who are anxious to connect to the child. Some adults even attach messages to noises such as sucking, gurgling, and burping—"Oh, he's telling us he's hungry," or "She really enjoyed those strained peas!"

The preceding chapter traced cognitive development over the first two years, and explored the perceptual abilities the child has from the earliest days of his life. The infant uses his perceptual abilities to receive and process sensory data. As he uses this information to develop an understanding of objects, cause–effect, and means–ends, he moves closer to intentional communication. Before the first year ends, there is evidence of communicative intent. Over the next few years, the child becomes an amazingly sophisticated and effective communicator. This chapter and the next will trace the impressive progression in communicative ability and the emergence of language that characterize the child's development through the preschool years. Begin by taking a closer look at communication development during infancy.

I May Be Naked, But I Have All My Parts and They Work!

As you study the development of communication in general and language specifically, keep in mind that the child is born with all the anatomical equipment she needs for receiving and producing speech and language. Even though growth and neuromuscular maturation must occur before these structures are used with intricate skill, the child uses all of her communication equipment from the beginning. She uses her ears to hear. She uses her larynx first to make crying noises and within just a few weeks to make sounds of pleasure as well. The adjustments she makes with her articulators during the first year are mostly random and meaningless, but within just a few months she is making vowel-like adjustments in the speech mechanism, and by the end of the first year, she is making the kinds of movements and contacts that are necessary to produce consonants. The point is that human children are ready to talk, and they waste no time in preparing for that day when their communication strategy will include **language.**

Perhaps the most impressive part of the infant's communication system is the *receptive* component. He has very good hearing and is able to process the auditory stimuli he receives in ways that suggest a strong innate interest in speech. This is important because there seems little question that speech and language development depends on the ability to receive and process sensory data, especially auditory data. Owens (2001, p. 153) suggests that speech and language development depends on six perceptual abilities:

1. The ability to attend specifically to speech
2. The ability to discriminate speech sounds
3. The ability to remember a sequence of speech sounds in the correct order
4. The ability to discriminate between sequences of speech sounds

5. The ability to compare a sequence of speech sounds to a model that has been stored in memory
6. The ability to make discriminations among intonational patterns

These six abilities will provide a framework for a discussion of *speech perception*, an essential component in the process of language development. You may recognize that the first two of these abilities were discussed in the final section of the preceding chapter. The infant not only can make gross discriminations among sounds relative to the direction of the sound source, pitch, loudness, and duration but also seems to have a special and discriminatory interest in speech and the human voice. In addition, the child as young as one month can make discriminations among speech sounds. At first, this speech sound discrimination ability is fairly open-ended. That is, the six-month-old infant can discriminate among a wide range of sounds, but by the end of the first year, his discrimination skills are already becoming more focused on the speech sounds of his native language.

Remembering a Sequence of Sounds in the Correct Order

It will be immediately obvious to anyone who listens to young children that they do not begin to talk by producing speech sounds in isolation. From the beginning, a child produces sounds in sequences. The first sequences are very simple, of course, but she does link sounds together. It would seem logical, therefore, that in processing the speech she hears, the child would need to hear not only the specific sounds in the models presented to her but also the correct order of sounds as they are sequenced.

Since this is a matter of memory as much as perception, we need to know when the infant begins to develop a memory. There is evidence that the infant as young as one month can remember an object if it reappears within two and one-half seconds, and by the time he is four months old, he can remember the object after five to seven seconds (Owens, 2005, p. 74). Although this may not be impressive by adult standards, it does represent the beginning of the short-term memory that is essential in processing speech.

Discriminating between Sequences of Sounds

Imagine what it would be like to listen to speech and not know where words begin and end. What if you could not distinguish differences between sequences of sounds? It you have listened to a language you do not speak, you should be able to relate to this experience. Let's say you do not speak Japanese. When you listen to Japanese being spoken, you cannot tell which sequences of sounds are words. You cannot tell where sentences begin and end. You certainly cannot make any meaningful discriminations among the sequences of sounds you are hearing. It is reasonable to assume that the newborn child's experience with speech is very similar to this. She hears continuous strings of sounds with no idea about where the boundaries are and with no ability to make *meaningful* discriminations among strings of sounds in the sense that she associates the strings of sounds with specific people, things, events, or ideas. The ability to make this kind of discrimination must develop. When does it begin?

You learned in the preceding chapter that the infant as young as one month can discriminate among individual speech sounds (Aslin, Pisoni, & Jusczyk, 1983; Eimas, Siqueland, Jusczyk, & Vigorito, 1971). Additional evidence indicates that by the time the infant is six and one-half months old, she can discriminate differences in strings of syllables (Goodsitt, Morse, VerHoeve, & Cowan, 1984), although there is much not yet known about how the infant makes these discriminations. The point is that the infant possesses the ability to discriminate among sounds and among sequences of sounds within the first six or seven months of life. Because words are sequences of sounds, the ability to recognize differences among strings of sounds is crucial to the acquisition of language. And because some words are identical except for one sound, it is also essential that the language-acquiring child be able to recognize differences among individual speech sounds. By nine months, the child can make distinctions among the speech sounds specific to her language in the models presented to her, and she is on the threshold of being able to produce words that reflect her understanding of speech sound differences.

Comparing Sequences of Sounds to Stored Models

By the second half of the first year, the child is beginning to understand words. Consider what this means in terms of memory and sequences of sounds. When someone produces the right sequence of sounds, such as "mama," the child recognizes the sequence because it matches a combination of sounds she has stored in her memory, a combination she associates with a person or object in her environment. Recall that the sound sequence–meaning association may not be the same for the child as for an adult, but this does not minimize the significance of the association. The child at eight or nine months, for example, might understand the word *mama* to mean "any female person who's usually there when I want her." Within the next eight or nine months, through the cognitive processes of accommodation and assimilation, she will sort out female persons into narrower and more appropriate schemata. She will recognize other sequences of sounds that are used to refer to these schemata, sequences that will be stored in her progressively more powerful memory. Notice how cognitive development, memory, and perceptual abilities interact as the child takes the first steps in language acquisition. These interactions are absolutely essential and increasingly obvious as language development accelerates.

Discriminating Intonational Patterns

Have you ever thought about how much of the meaning in the messages you send and receive depends on variables of speech such as rate, rhythm, stress, and intonational patterns? Calculating an exact percentage is impossible because how much meaning is sent verbally and nonverbally depends on each utterance. In some communications, the words are of such great importance that other variables do not really matter. If a speaker is simply providing information, for example, nonverbal variables would not contribute much to the total meaning. In other situations, the word or words are almost superfluous. Imagine a situation in which you see a friend do something you think is a little suspicious. You look at her and say, "So?" It's difficult to imagine this scenario without imagining the intonational pattern that would be superimposed on the "So?"

Now think about how important these nonverbal variations are in communications with young children or even with the family dog. If you say to your dog, "I'm going to take you outside and beat you with a stick," but say it in a manner that suggests this is going to be a happy occasion, the dog will wag its tail and jump up and down in joyful anticipation. In much the same way, the infant responds more positively to speech with "happy" and "friendly" intonational patterns than to speech that sounds stern, angry, or threatening. You read in Chapter 3 that a newborn child can discriminate among pure tones (Bridger, 1961) and makes his best discriminations among frequencies characteristic of speech (Eisenberg, 1976). By the time he is six months old, the infant recognizes and even imitates intonational patterns (Kessen, Levine, & Wendrich, 1979). The melody of speech created by pitch changes and intonational patterns is an important element in creating and receiving messages from the earliest days of the child's communicative life, and it continues to be important as language emerges and communication becomes more sophisticated. In many cases, for children and adults, *what* is said may be less important in determining the ultimate meaning of a message than *how* the words are spoken. Depending on the intonational pattern used and other elements of speech such as loudness, rate, and stress, the sentence "Get out of here" might be interpreted as an urgent threat to one's health and safety, or it might be interpreted as a light-hearted "You're kidding me, aren't you?"

Creating a Communication Environment: Infant–Adult Interactions

Not only is the child ready and able to communicate from the beginning of his life, but those who take care of the child seem eager to communicate with him, often even before birth. We have all heard about parents who talk to their children in utero, read to them, or play music for them. These parents are so anxious to connect to their babies, they cannot wait for their births! They want to establish meaningful interpersonal relationships with these new humans, and they want to talk to them. Parents often attach messages to the movements of the child in the uterus, and after he is born, as we have already mentioned, they are likely to associate meaning with every noise the child makes, from cries to burps. It is not surprising, therefore, that parents and other adults do talk to babies.

The speech directed at infants, as you know from your own experiences, is not the same as speech directed at adults. In fact, we sometimes call the speech we use with infants "baby talk." We all recognize this kind of speech when we hear it, but have you ever considered what baby talk really is? Are certain characteristics of baby talk the same in all cultures? Does baby talk serve a purpose for the child or for the adult? Is baby talk an important, perhaps necessary, part of language acquisition?

Baby Talk, Motherese, Parentese, or Child-Directed Speech

When language experts say that parents refer to "baby talk," this does not mean language forms typically ascribed to the speech of young children, as in the utterance

"Doe to 'tore" for "Go to store." *Baby talk* refers to the special way parents talk to their children. Many language people believe that the unique characteristics of baby talk facilitate the acquisition of language. There is evidence, in fact, that the input provided in this kind of language enables deaf children to reach normal developmental milestones when they are presented from birth with sign language comparable in form to baby talk (Petitto, 1984, 1985a, 1985b, 1986, 1987, 1988; Pettito & Marentette, 1990, 1991).

Sachs (1989, p. 36), in summarizing some of the relevant research findings, has identified some of the unique characteristics of speech directed to babies. In talking to babies, for example, speakers place more emphasis on components of speech such as pitch, rate, loudness, stress, rhythm, and intonation than on the words themselves. Kaye (1980) notes that mothers use considerable repetition in their speech and that each successive utterance is semantically similar to the preceding utterance. Most early topics tend to focus on objects children can see and hear (Bruner, 1975; Phillips, 1973). When children reach the sixth month of life, their mothers tend to employ an informational style of talking, a style that is less centered on objects and more centered on their infants' surroundings and behaviors (Penman, Cross, Milgrom-Friedman, & Meares, 1983).

Although there may be exceptions, baby talk in most languages is produced at higher than normal pitch levels, and with intonational patterns that include greater extremes of high and low pitches than are typically used in adult-to-adult speech. These characteristics are so universal, one might believe they are the salient features in baby talk to which infants respond most positively, but that may not be the case. In one study, six-month-old babies were exposed to speech that had the stereotypical high pitch levels and exaggerated prosodic elements commonly associated with baby talk, but there was no apparent *joy* or *happiness* in these samples. The babies were also exposed to speech delivered in a typical adult-to-adult style but was expressed in an obviously *joyful* manner. These babies preferred speech that was joyful or happy, even if it lacked the characteristics of pitch and highly variable intonational patterns associated with baby talk (Singh, Morgan, & Best, 2002). One specific characteristic of baby talk that seems to transcend speech is rhythm. The rhythm of speech directed to babies is more regular than adult speech, resulting in what some researchers describe as a *singsong cadence*. What is most interesting, however, and probably not coincidental, is that mothers who sign to their deaf children incorporate rhythms with their hands that are remarkably similar to the rhythms underlying the speech directed to hearing children (Fernald, 1994). There are, of course, many characteristics of speech directed to children that distinguish it from adult-to-adult speech, included those summarized in Table 4.1.

Based on what is known about the infant's perceptual abilities, the characteristics of talk directed to babies are not surprising. The child is able to make distinctions among pitch levels at an early age, and she prefers pitches in the speech range. There is also evidence that infants can make at least gross discriminations among loudness levels, sounds of varying durations, and different consonants in consonant–vowel–consonant (CVC) syllables (Moon, Bever, & Fifer, 1992). Note that infants not only prefer speech over other kinds of sounds but, according to

Table 4.1 Motherese (Child-Directed Speech) Characteristics

- Higher than normal overall pitch level
- More frequent use of pitch extremes—high and low
- More regular rhythm
- References to objects the child can see and/or hear
- Longer than normal pauses between segments
- Slower than normal rate
- Utterances that are shorter than normal in length
- Facial expressions are exaggerated
- Sentences are simple syntactic constructions
- More utterance repetitions
- Greater loudness variation

some research (Fernald, 1985; Sullivan & Horowitz, 1983), also prefer speech with baby talk characteristics to adult speech. One must be careful, however, about the conclusions drawn from these findings. It is possible that infants prefer baby talk because they are innately tuned to the characteristics of baby talk, but it is also possible that the preference is an environmental phenomenon that develops because infants associate baby talk with their caregivers. Why do adults use this kind of speech with babies? It is unlikely that parents make a conscious decision to use higher than normal pitches, widely varying intonation contours, and singsong cadences because they are familiar with the research literature that suggests these characteristics are appropriate for speech directed at babies. It may simply be that through trial and error, adults have learned that they are better able to gain the attention of an infant by using baby talk, and it would be difficult to argue against the idea that each generation "learns" how to use baby talk by observing members of the preceding generation communicating with babies.

Even if we cannot determine whether baby talk is the product of genetics or environment, we can appreciate its role in child–adult interactions. In Chapter 3, we indicated that the infant has an early and powerful interest in the caregiver's face. He has a similar interest in the caregiver's voice and speech. The caregiver quickly learns that she can use her face, voice, and speech to capture the infant's attention, and she learns the features of her child's communicative efforts that are most meaningful in their exchanges (Meadows, Elias, & Bain, 2000). On the basis of present knowledge, it might be a stretch to argue that this kind of contact is essential for speech and language development, but there seems little doubt that during special moments when the caregiver is attending carefully to all aspects of the child's reflexive and learned behaviors and when she gazes into the baby's attentive eyes and fills his discriminating ears with the lilting, soothing sounds of speech, an important bond is being formed, a bond that certainly has the potential to facilitate communication acquisition.

Working Together: A Mother–Child Partnership

An implication shared by words such as *communication* and *interaction* is that both partners are involved in the process—and that is one of the most important points to

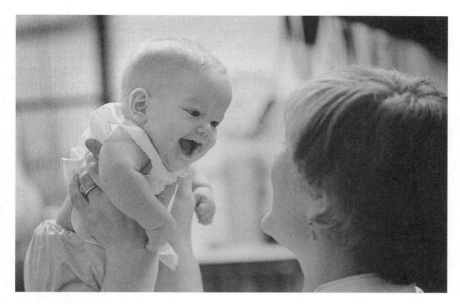

Infant–adult interaction, a precursor of communication.

be made about infant communication. It is noteworthy, for example, that in addition to their interest in baby talk or motherese, researchers have directed their attention to the *joint* nature of the interaction between caregiver and child and whether or not the sharing of communication in the earliest months of the child's life really matters. It does matter. There is evidence that when mothers encourage their infants to attend, the language development of those infants is enhanced (Karras, Braungart-Rieker, Mullins, & Lefever, 2002). When caregivers encourage their infants to pay attention to objects and when caregivers attach names to those objects, those children add words to their vocabularies more quickly than children whose caregivers are not as pro-active in establishing joint communications during infancy (Campbell & Namy, 2003). It is also important to note that the language advantages derived from interactive communications between caregivers and infants remain noticeable in children at one year, at eighteen months, and at thirty months (Rollins, 2003). Taken together, the research indicates that joint communication is important at the beginning, to establish a base for speech and language development, and the influences of those early interactions are felt throughout the acquisition period. Also, joint communication is not a one-dimensional phenomenon. The sense of *togetherness* suggested by the word *joint* is expressed in several ways.

Joint focus of attention, sometimes called *joint reference,* suggests that the caregiver and child are focusing on the same object or event at the same time. Owens (2005, pp. 173–174), notes that there are four phases in the development of establishing joint focus of attention (see Table 4.2). During phase 1, which extends from about four to six weeks, the caregiver might place an object where the child can see it, move it to

Table 4.2 Four Phases in the Development of Joint Reference

Phase	Approximate Age Range	Key Features
1	4–6 weeks	Caregiver places object where child can see it and calls attention to the object with a verbal stimulus such as "Look!"
	By 6 months	May recognize caregiver's pitch pattern as a signal to establish joint attention.
2	7 months	Child begins to demonstrate efforts to communicate intentionally; may create joint reference by pointing to an object of interest.
	By 8 months	Child may reach for an object and look to caregiver for a response.
3	8–12 months	Child uses combinations of gestures and vocalizations to indicate interest in objects.
4	12 months	Child exercises control over topic; produces names of objects and events.

make certain the child focuses on it, and say the child's name or something such as "Look!" to ensure that the child is paying attention. Even though these exchanges may initially be meaningless to the child, she will pay attention to the caregiver's utterances by three months; by six months, she may recognize that the caregiver's pitch pattern is a signal to establish joint attention (Ryan, 1974).

The child enters phase 2 at about seven months. At this point, the child begins to demonstrate an intention to communicate and may create joint referencing by pointing to an object or event of interest. By eight months, the child may reach for an object and look to her caregiver for a response. It is not difficult to imagine that in this scenario, the caregiver enthusiastically responds by handing the object to the child and providing her the kind of accolades we might expect from cheerleaders at a basketball game. Well, it might not be quite that dramatic, but there is no doubt that the caregiver will be pleased and proud, conveying that message to the child with considerable verve.

During phase 3, which ranges from about eight to twelve months of age, the child produces gestures, such as pointing, showing, and reaching, accompanied by vocalizations. When the caregiver observes the child using a gesture, she might seize the opportunity to ask the child about her intention, and she might incorporate the same gesture in her response.

When the child reaches her first birthday, she is entering the final phase of joint focus of attention. She can now name objects and events. She is beginning to exercise more control over the topics of her communicative exchanges with other people. As the child begins to take more initiative in these exchanges, her caregiver reduces the number of questions she asks her, and provides more labels for the objects and events on which the child is focusing her attention.

Constructing a conversation is another joint venture. Experts who focus on such matters believe that the physical and talking routines involved in infant–caregiver interactions make important contributions to the child's acquisition of conversational skills. The turn taking inherent in the daily routines associated with mealtime and taking a bath, for example, and the turn taking that is structured into playing games help form a framework in which the child can find where his behavior *fits* into a given communicative exchange. This framework is referred to as a *script* or *scaffold*. As the child repeatedly experiences these activities and the routines or scripts associated with them, his knowledge about the events themselves increases, and he develops a greater understanding about the kinds of communicative dialogues that are appropriate in varying circumstances. This is all part of learning what can and should be said and done in a range of situations that call for certain actions and certain kinds of talking. We all know that what might be appropriate in one circumstance is not appropriate in another, and we probably all know from personal experience that it takes some time to sort out what is proper and when it is proper. The sorting begins at a young age, and some folks never seem to get it quite right.

Snow (1977) has described the evolution of conversation between two mothers and their babies as they moved toward their second birthdays. When the children were about three months old, the communicative exchanges were very simple and were directed primarily by the children. When the children smiled or burped, for example, the mothers reacted with comments, sometimes in the form of questions. The mothers' utterances were short and simple, but there was no expectation on their parts that the babies understood the content. Even at this stage, however, the exchanges were conversation-like in the sense that each mother treated the behaviors of her child as though they were intentional messages. It was interesting that these mothers offered considerable courtesy in these "conversations." Whereas adults often make it difficult for one another to have their turns in conversation, these mothers tried to prompt responses from their babies, and they paused expectantly, waiting for responses. They made a clear attempt to encourage and allow the turn taking that characterizes real conversation, even though these children were not processing words as linguistic units.

As their children matured, the mothers in Snow's study developed greater expectations and made greater demands. Midway through the first year, the mothers were more selective in their responses to the noises their babies were making. They no longer treated bodily noises such as burps as equal to vocalized sounds such as cooing and babbling. The mothers tried to build conversations based on vocalized sounds and essentially ignored other noises. To maintain conversational turn taking, the mothers often imitated their babies' utterances. When the children responded by repeating their original vocalizations, these utterances were treated like appropriate turns in the conversations.

By the time the children in Snow's study reached the end of their first year, the communicative stakes had been raised considerably. There was an even stronger emphasis on speechlike behaviors in terms of what was judged to be conversationally acceptable, and the mothers often interpreted their babies' utterances as real words, even when they probably were not. Since children begin to produce true words at about twelve months and begin to combine words into multiple-word utterances by about eighteen months, conversation becomes much more adult-like as the second year unfolds.

We have yet to answer the most important question posed in the opening of this section. Is speech directed to the infant an important or necessary component of speech and language acquisition? No one has offered evidence that normal children who receive little speech from their caregivers *cannot* develop normal speech and language. On the other hand, evidence indicates that communicative stimulation from caregivers is helpful. One study directly applicable to this question was conducted by Clarke-Stewart (1973), who found that a child's language competence is correlated with the amount of speech and language stimulation the child receives from the caregiver. It is interesting that Clarke-Stewart observed that the caregiver's speech to others, speech to which the child is also exposed, does not have an influence on the child's language competence. This suggests that it is not the total quantity of speech to which a child is exposed that has an impact on communicative development, but the amount of speech that is intended specifically for the child. After reviewing the Clarke-Stewart study and related research, Sachs (1989) reached this conclusion about the importance of baby talk in the acquisition process: "It would seem that baby talk, the way adults communicate with infants, is not simply a culturally transmitted, functionless style but rather a well-founded mode of speech that helps develop communication abilities in the child" (p. 40).

Speech Production in Infancy: From Cries to Words

To this point, we have emphasized the importance of *reception* in the infant's earliest communication experiences, and we have addressed the issue of infant–caregiver interaction. If you think about speech production in the context of an input–output model, we have concentrated so far on the *input* portion of the model. Caregivers provide the speech and language stimuli that the infant feeds into his linguistic processor. The input portion is more complicated than simple absorption, however, because the infant does not simply *receive* information. He *interacts* with the sender, and, as we have just noted, there is evidence that linguistic information specifically directed to the child is more meaningful and more important than linguistic information directed to other people in the child's presence.

The output portion of communication does not begin with speech but with nonlinguistic behaviors. As the child matures intellectually, perceptually, and neuromuscularly, he is able to use the linguistic information he receives from his caregivers and others to make his communications more specific, more intentional, and more language-like. The beginning of the child's communicative output is very simple, sometimes very loud, and it sometimes interferes with a peaceful night's sleep. He cries!

Reflexive Cries and Other Biological Noises

The first sounds the infant makes, including her first cries, are **reflexive,** which means **unlearned.** In addition to crying, she will also burp, sneeze, and cough. These noises are sometimes called **vegetative** sounds to indicate that they are natural sounds made by a passive but living organism. The infant's first cries have often been described as "undifferentiated," which immediately after birth is undoubtedly true, but by the end of the first month, the infant's caregiver can usually differentiate among several basic cries (Wolff, 1969). When the child is hungry, she produces a repeating pattern of loud cry, silence, inhalation, and a resting period often accompanied by sucking noises. When she is in pain, she produces a cry best described as long, loud, and piercing. This cry may be followed by a silence during which she seems to be holding her breath. She may then produce a few whimpers before shrieking again. When the infant is in pain, she might also clench her fists and contort her face with tightened muscles and a frown. She is not a pretty sight, and the sounds of her anguish are often unmistakable. The infant's anger cry is similar in many respects to the pain cry, but when crying in anger, she moves a greater volume of air, and most listeners have no difficulty recognizing the underlying message of vexation and irritation.

Sounds of Comfort and Pleasure

By the time the infant is two months old, caregivers notice that crying behaviors are decreasing in frequency, but the cries become more varied and differentiated. According to D'Odorico (1984), the infant at four months is producing distinctive cries to signal discomfort, call, and request. The cries of discomfort would include the cries of pain and probably some of the cries of anger described earlier. At this stage, the child will cry to call someone, as in "Hey, somebody get in here quick!" He will also cry to make a request, as in "I'm hungry, and I'll thank you to give me a bottle."

The most positive change occurring at this time is the emergence of sounds communicating pleasure and comfort. By two months, the infant is **cooing.** Cooing is usually understood as the production of vowel-like sounds, but there may also be brief consonant-like sounds resembling "k" or "g." Although these sounds are sometimes produced by the infant when he is alone, they are often elicited when the caregiver talks to the infant or smiles during gaze coupling. In a typical exchange, the caregiver smiles and says something such as, "Aren't you a sweetheart." The infant responds with "O-o-o-o-u-u-u-u," and the caregiver imitates the coo. This cooing–imitation–cooing exchange can sometimes continue for fifteen minutes or longer, and most adults find it as delightful a communicative experience as the infant. The child at four months is not only cooing but laughing (Stark, 1979), and the laughter is at times sustained long enough that there is no question about the nature of the behavior. It may be difficult to determine what the child perceives as the punch line, but he finds something worthy of laughter.

Introductory or Transitional Babbling

According to Stark (1979) and Sachs (1989), "true" babbling does not begin until the child is six months or older. Beginning at about five months, however, the infant is producing vocalizations that seem to bridge cooing and true babbling. These are single-syllable productions consisting of vowel- and consonant-like sounds, and we can think of them as transitional behaviors that extend beyond cooing and prepare the way for babbling. Stark refers to these sequences as "marginal babbling."

True Babbling

We traditionally use the term **babbling** to describe repeated consonant–vowel sylla-bles, such as "mamama" or "nanana," productions that tend to appear at about six or seven months. The more specific term for this kind of production is **reduplicated babbling.** According to Stark, Bernstein, and Demorest (1993), reduplicated babbling occurs most often when the infant is investigating the environment or holding an ob-ject. The consonants most frequently incorporated into these utterances are produced at the front of the mouth—for example, *m, p, b, t, d,* and *n.* Some of the intonational contours the infant produced during cooing have disappeared (Stark, 1979), but the production of consonants suggests an increasing maturity in the child's control of the speech mechanism.

Whereas cooing is often elicited by social interaction between the infant and the caregiver, the infant will often babble most when she is by herself (Nakazima, 1975; Stark, 1981). Many researchers and writers have observed that during babbling, the in-fant produces a wide variety of sounds, many of which are not included in the sound system of her native language. Ferguson (1978) suggests that the sounds the child produces are largely the product of the limitations of her speech mechanism. As the structures of speech mature physiologically and as the infant becomes more absorbed in the sounds of her own language, her babbling more closely resembles her native language (Rees, 1972).

In addition to babbling, the infant between eight and twelve months produces an interesting behavior called **echolalia.** Echolalia is the immediate, parrotlike imitation of sounds, syllables, or words produced by someone else. The term *parrotlike* suggests that the infant does not understand what he is saying even though his imitations may be fairly accurate. If for no other reason, this behavior is important because it repre-sents a change in the nature of imitation in speech and language development. In the cooing stage, communication is maintained when the caregiver imitates the infant. In echolalia, the infant imitates the caregiver. In the months and years to come, the child's imitations of the speech models he hears become increasingly important in terms of acquiring the sound system, vocabulary, and structure of his language.

During true babbling, the infant's productions become more heavily dependent on self-hearing. For this reason, infants who are deaf sound very much like hearing children until they reach this point. Deaf infants cry, laugh, coo, and produce some marginal babbling, but when hearing infants begin to produce true babbling, deaf in-fants begin to restrict their output and use fewer consonant sounds than hearing in-fants at about eight months of age (Oller, Eilers, Bull, & Carney, 1985; Stoel-Gammon & Otomo, 1986).

Variegated Babbling and Jargon

Beginning at about nine months and continuing through eighteen months, the nature of babbling changes in the sense that it becomes more varied within a single utterance. Instead of simply repeating the same syllable as she did in the earlier stage, the child now produces successive syllables that differ from one another, as in "madagaba."

This more advanced babbling is known as *variegated* babbling. Stark (1986) found that some variegated babbling productions are consonant–vowel–consonant (CVC) combinations, in which the consonant is replicated, and vowel–consonant–vowel (VCV) combinations, in which the vowel is replicated. That is, the child might say "Gug" (CVC) or "Ugu" (VCV). As the name suggests, variegated babbling is characterized by a wider range of sounds, especially consonants, than reduplicated babbling. It should be noted that not all researchers are convinced that the variegated babbling period necessarily follows the reduplicated babbling period (Mitchell & Kent, 1990), but there is a certain logical appeal to the progression.

The seven- or eight-month-old infant attends to the intonational contours of adult speech. It makes sense then that, as he continues to experiment with sounds and sound combinations, he begins to incorporate intonational contours into his vocalizations, producing what is called *jargon* babbling. Jargon babbling productions are distinguished by melodic patterns. In fact, this form of babbling has many of the characteristics of real speech. If you attend just to the melody of jargon babbling utterances, they sound adult-like. The child produces the rhythm, stresses, rate variations, and intonational contours of his language, even though he produces few, if any, meaningful words.

Jargon babbling is to speech as humming or "la-la-la"ing is to singing when we do not know or cannot remember the lyrics. When the child produces these vocalizations, adult listeners hear what they believe are questions, commands, expressions of joy, statements of concern, and virtually every kind of communication imaginable. The son of a friend in graduate school was particularly proficient in jargon babbling. His father was a great storyteller. The son would "tell stories" in jargon babbling, some "funny" as evidenced by his laughter and some "serious" as reflected by the tone of his voice and the look on his face, using the same speech melodies as his father used. These vocalizations were delightfully entertaining, and, if the truth be told, many of the son's stories were better than the father's!

Although jargon babbling is interesting and clearly indicates that the child is paying attention to and imitating the melodic characteristics of adult speech, it is not language. Early in this same nine to eighteen month period, however, evidence suggests that the child is moving from prelinguistic communication to language. The child will not produce her first conventional words until she is about twelve months, but by the time she is nine or ten months old, she may be producing what are called **vocables, phonetically consistent forms, performatives,** or **protowords.** All of these terms refer to productions, unique to a given child, that are consistent patterns of sounds used in reference to particular things or situations. The son of von Raffler-Engle (1973), for example, produced the sound "e-e-e" to signal that he wanted an object, and he produced "u-u-u" to signal disapproval. These are not words, of course, but they represent an important transition from vocal play and babbling, vocalizations that are random and devoid of specific meaning, to productions that are purposive, consistent, and meaningful. Carter's (1975) analysis of vocables in one child suggests there may be a fairly direct connection between some vocables and corresponding true words. She found, for example, that vocables beginning with *m,* accompanied by a gesture to indicate "I want," gradually evolved into the words *more, my,* and *mine.* Some evidence suggests that vocables are present in children's productions, no matter which language they are acquiring (Blake & deBoysson-Bardies, 1992). See Table 4.3 for a summary of prevocalizations.

The Development of Communication Functions: Using Communication to Get Things Done

Although it is true that human beings talk even when they have nothing to say and even when no one, perhaps even the speaker, is listening, humans usually communicate for a purpose. We use speech intentionally to accomplish specific goals. We use speech to inform, to persuade, to direct, to flatter, to manipulate, to request, to express, to argue, to impress, to complain, and so on. The study of the functions, purposes, or intents of communication is called **pragmatics.** The term makes sense. *Pragmatic* means "practical," and pragmatics is the study of the practical aspects of communication. Do infants show an awareness of pragmatics or communicative function before they begin to produce language? Of course they do. In this section, we will briefly examine the stages of communicative function development in children.

As noted in Chapter 2, the pragmatics revolution stimulated interest in the functions served by communicative efforts. The work of Austin (1962) and Searle (1969), which focused on adult speech, suggests that there are three components to all speech acts: (1) *perlocutions,* which are concerned with how listeners interpret speech acts, (2) *illocutions,* which involve the intentions expressed by the speaker, and (3) *locutions,*

Table 4.3 Typical Development of Prelinguistic Vocalizations

Approximate Age Range	Vocalizations
0–1 month	• Reflexive cries, vegetative sounds
1–4 months	• Cooing (vowel-like sounds), differentiated crying (hunger, pain, etc.)
4–6 months	• Transitional or marginal babbling: single-syllable productions of vowel- and consonant-like sounds
6–8 months	• Reduplicated babbling (productions of the same syllable—e.g., "bababa")
8–12 months	• Echolalia (imitation of sounds and syllables—continues beyond 12 months)
	• Variegated babbling (changes in consonant–vowel combinations—e.g., "dadu")
	• Jargon babbling (intonational changes added to syllable productions to give impression of sentencelike behavior)
	• Vocables or protowords (productions unique to each child)

which include the meanings of utterances (see Figure 4.1). Bates, Camaioni, and Volterra (1975) borrowed these terms from Searle and applied them to the developing communication functions of children.

We will consider three stages of communication function development based on Searle's terms. To fully appreciate what happens in this development, understand that the child is developing the ability to produce goal-directed, intentional communication behaviors. The child is able to do this only to the extent that he takes into consideration the persons with whom he is communicating, and only to the extent that he is able to formulate messages for people other than himself.

How do children learn to use communication intentionally? Although there is probably not a clear and definitive answer to that question, you should not find it difficult to speculate about how communicative intent evolves. In the preceding chapter, we traced cognitive development through infancy. It should come as no surprise that there is a relationship between cognitive development and the developmental stages of early communication functions.

The *perlocutionary stage* of development extends from birth to approximately eight months of age. At the beginning of this stage, the infant is producing only reflexive cries. By the end of this stage, she is producing the goal-directed behaviors described in substage 3 of Piaget's sensorimotor period. By the end of the perlocutionary stage, the infant is using gestures to indicate that she recognizes the functions of common objects. She might lift a glass to her lips, for example, or put a spoon into her mouth. The production of these gestures demonstrates that the infant is organizing her world into conceptual categories. These early gestures have been called *recognitory* because they reflect the infant's ability to "recognize," albeit in a primitive way, the functionality of objects (Bates, Bretherton, Shore, & McNew, 1983).

The *illocutionary stage* extends from eight to twelve months of age. During this stage, the infant uses gestures or vocalizations to signal **intentionality.** By using a variety of gestures including pointing, showing, and requesting, the infant can convey

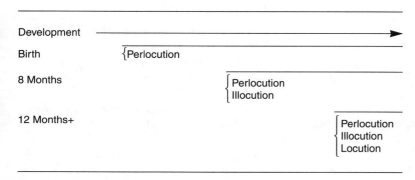

FIGURE 4.1 Development of the Three Stages of a Speech Act

Adapted from: McLaughlin, S. (1998), *Introduction to language development,* Singular Publishing Group, San Diego, CA.

differentiated intentions. At the same time, the infant might use vocables, those phonetically consistent forms of vocalization we referred to earlier, to express a range of specific and recognizable communicative functions.

Halliday (1975) concluded that his son, Nigel, between the ages of nine and sixteen months, produced a number of nonlinguistic utterances or vocables to convey meanings with four identifiable communicative intents. Nigel communicated to satisfy needs and wants, to control the behavior of others, to interact with others, and to express an emotion or interest (see Table 4.4).

Bates (1979) uses the term ***protodeclarative*** to describe the communicative gestures that are used to point out objects or events to which the child and adult attend together. The child might point to a cow, for example, not to request the cow or to ask about the cow but simply to say, "Hey, Mom, look at that big thing standing over there with a multifingered bubble on its belly!" Bates uses the term ***protoimperative*** in reference to gestures used by the infant to control or manipulate the behaviors of others. The child might point to an object to indicate that he wants the object. He might use a similar gesture to indicate that he wants a light turned off or on. He might shake his head vigorously and produce a different kind of vocalization to indicate that he does not want to eat any more strained peas. These are all protoimperatives.

The *locutionary stage* is the final stage. The child, who is now beyond the first birthday, is producing her first meaningful words. Words and gestures are now combined to express the same basic meanings or intentions that were previously conveyed by gestures or vocalizations.

Like Halliday (1975), Bruner (1981) found infant communications that reflect an interest in establishing contact with others. Bruner refers to this communicative function or intent as **social interaction.** These communications include behaviors used to greet another person, to attract and maintain the attention of another person, and to

Table 4.4 Early Communicative Functions

Function (Definition)	Example
Instrumental[a] (to have needs and wants satisfied)	"Uh-uh-uh" while pointing at refrigerator to get food or drink
Regulatory (to control the behaviors of other people)	"Kuh-kuh" while moving the caregiver's hands together to suggest the continuation of patty-cake
Interactional (to establish or maintain interpersonal contact)	"Muh-muh" while holding the caregiver's face to maintain attention on an object of shared interest
Personal (to express an emotion, interest, or attitude)	"Ga-ga" in angry tones while playing with a toy the child cannot manipulate properly

[a]The italicized terms are used by Halliday (1975).

establish the shared attention of the child and another person. As we have already noted, adults and especially parents react to virtually all of a child's behaviors as though they are purposive and have communicative intent. Harding (1983a, 1983b) believes that infant–adult interactions may help the infant learn about the practical nature of communication. She suggests that when caregivers reinforce and expand on behaviors such as eye contact, gesturing, crying, babbling, and other vocalizations (interpreting them as communication), infants are better able to recognize such behaviors as intentional communications, and produce them more often. In summary, then, the infant most likely acquires the ability to use nonverbal behaviors and vocalized behaviors with specific communicative intents as a result of overall biological maturation, cognitive development, and her social interactions with caregivers.

The first year of life has not been passive. The child has matured considerably. His intellectual abilities have progressed rapidly. He has interacted with his world and caregivers with enthusiasm and unbridled curiosity. He has communicated unintentionally and intentionally, but all of this has been merely prologue for what is about to occur. He is now ready for the magic and wonder of true language. As his first year comes to an end, he is about to become a linguistic communicator, beginning with his first real words.

Beyond Infancy: The Emergence of Language

The issue of stages was briefly discussed in the context of cognitive development. Keep in mind that we trace the development of many behaviors through stages because stages provide a convenient framework for understanding the changes that occur during the development of a behavior or, in the case of language, an aggregate of behaviors.

Consider for a moment how stages of speech and language development might be compared to grade levels in the study of mathematics. The mathematic skills you acquire and practice in first grade are clearly different from the skills you acquire and learn in trigonometry and precalculus as a senior in high school, but you reach advanced mathematic skills by acquiring and building on knowledge and skills that are progressively more sophisticated and complex as you move through the grade levels of elementary, junior high, and senior high school math courses. You begin by learning what numbers are and what they represent. You learn to add and subtract, and then you learn to multiply and divide, and you understand that multiplication is an advanced version of addition, and division is an advanced version of subtraction. You continue to add layer upon layer of mathematic knowledge, but each layer rests on all the layers below. Learning mathematics, then, is really a continuous process that involves learning new concepts, reviewing old concepts, and applying old concepts in new ways. The stages of mathematic acquisition are represented by grade levels and course names, but grade levels and course names are merely conveniences to help us organize the process of learning and to categorize the basic skills that are acquired at certain junctures in the overall development of mathematic competence.

In very much the same way, human beings learn speech and language in a continuous, uninterrupted manner. As the child acquires new words and new language forms, he is constantly reviewing prior language knowledge, and he is using language he has already acquired in new ways. We consider speech and language development in stages because it is a useful and convenient way to organize our discussion and because stages help us to understand how, and to some extent, *when* changes occur in language acquisition.

The *order* in which changes occur is far more important than the *ages* we will attach to these changes. All children will go through these stages in the same order, and, as was true of Piaget's cognitive stages, children do not skip stages of language development. *When* children go through these stages, however, might differ considerably. The age ranges associated with the stages are broad enough that most children will fit, but you should be careful not to read too much into the fact that a given child is either "ahead" or "behind" the normal age range for a given language behavior.

The specific stage model we use in our discussion of speech and language acquisition was developed by Roger Brown (1973). Brown's stages are widely used by researchers and authors to describe *syntactic* or structural development in children, and Brown's conclusions relative to these stages have been supported by the research of deVilliers and deVilliers (1978). Brown traced the development of syntax through five major stages (see Table 4.5). We will describe these stages, but in addition to syntax, we will include information about *semantic* or meaning development and about *pragmatic* development.

Brown tracked syntactic development by measuring the *mean length of utterance* (MLU), a concept more fully explained in the next section. Although age is not as reliable a measure of syntactic development as MLU, Miller and Chapman (1981) found that age and MLU are positively related. Because most people think about development in terms of ages, approximate age ranges will be provided as we move through Brown's five stages (Bernstein, 1989, pp. 108–118; Owens, 2005, p. 294). The rest of

Table 4.5 Overview of Brown's (1973) Stages of Syntactic Development

Stage/Description	Age Range (months)	Mean Length of Utterance (MLU)
1. Semantic roles and grammatical relations	12–26	1.0–2.00
2. Grammatical morphemes and the modulation of meanings	27–30	2.0–2.50
3. Modalities of the simple sentence	31–34	2.5–3.00
4. Embedding of one sentence within another	35–40	3.0–3.75
5. Coordination of simple sentences and propositional relations	41–46	3.75–4.50

this chapter describes the first stage of language development. The remaining four stages are discussed in the following chapter.

Tracking Language Development: Morphemes and Mean Length of Utterance

Before you can understand mean length of utterance, you must understand the units that are being counted; this brings us to morphology. **Morphology** is concerned with words and their parts as units of meaning. A **morpheme** is the smallest meaningful unit of language. It might be tempting to think of a word as being the smallest meaningful unit of language. It is true that a word might be a single morpheme, but some words contain several morphemes. It might seem that a single sound such as "s" cannot be a meaning unit, but in some cases, a single sound is a morpheme. It might even seem logical that a morpheme is the same as a syllable, but that is not always true, either. Sometimes a syllable is a morpheme, but sometimes it takes two or more syllables in the right combination to make one morpheme.

Confused? The confusion is helpful if it helps create the correct mind-set about morphemes. Morphemes are **units of meaning.** Morphemes can be sounds, or syllables, or whole words. A sound or sequence of sounds might be morphemes in some contexts but not in others, and they might be different kinds of morphemes depending on the context. Now let's sort out the confusion by identifying the possibilities.

There are two kinds of morphemes: free and bound. A **free morpheme** can stand alone and be meaningful. The following are free morphemes: *dog, cat, house,* and *go.* A **bound morpheme** is a unit of meaning that must be attached to a free morpheme to be meaningful. The word *tie* is a free morpheme meaning *to bind.* Notice what happens if we add *un-* to *tie* to produce *untie.* That word now means *to remove the binding.* By itself, *un-* has no meaning, but when it is attached to certain free morphemes, it means *no* or *not.* Consider words such as ***un**faithful,* ***un**reliable,* ***un**interesting.* Does this mean that anytime *un-* appears in a word it is a morpheme? Consider the word *uncle.* In this word, *un-* does not provide meaning but is one part of a two-syllable free morpheme. In the same way, *in-* in the word *indirect* means "not," but in the word *interest, in-* is simply part of a three-syllable free morpheme.

Usually a single sound is not a morpheme, but a sound can be a morpheme. What happens to meaning when we add *s* to the free morpheme *cat* to produce *cats?* The free morpheme *cat* refers to *one cat,* but *cats* refers to *more than one cat.* The *s* in *cats* is a bound morpheme that means *plurality.* The *s* in *cat's box* means *possessive.*

Bound morphemes can be either **derivational** or **inflectional.** Derivational morphemes are added to the front of free morphemes and commonly referred to as *prefixes* or are added to the back of free morphemes and called *suffixes.* Derivational morphemes change the class or category of a word. If, for example, we add the derivational morpheme *-ly* to *slow* to create *slowly,* we have changed an adjective to an adverb. We can change the adjective *sad* to a noun by adding *-ness* to create *sadness.* Inflectional morphemes, which occur only as suffixes, change the meaning of words by marking grammatical adjustments for things such as plurality, possession, and verb tense. When you add *s* to *bat* to make *bats,* or when you add *d* to *dive* to make *dived,* you have used inflectional morphemes.

The child learns to use inflectional morphemes to refine the meanings of words or to make their meanings more exact. When she first begins to produce words, for example, the child might use "cat" to refer to one cat or to several. As she becomes more sophisticated in word usage, she learns that she can add *s* to make *cat* plural. This simple adjustment makes her communication more precise and more meaningful.

Since the child does not begin to use morphemes as grammatical markers until the second of Brown's stages, further discussion about the acquisition of these morphemes is reserved until we reach the second stage. At this point, it is important that you understand what morphemes are, however, because morphemes are counted in determining mean length of utterance, one of the measures used to assess progress in language development (see Figure 4.2).

The term **mean** refers to a statistical average. Assume we have a sample of a child's language containing one hundred utterances. Some utterances consist of single free morphemes. Others consist of four or five morphemes, free and bound. A few utterances contain as many as ten or eleven morphemes. To determine the **mean length of utterance,** count the morphemes in each utterance, add the total, and divide by the number of utterances—in this case, one hundred. Because this is an arithmetic calculation, the MLU is seldom expressed as a whole number. If a child produces a total of 310 morphemes over 100 utterances, his MLU is 3.1.

Stage 1: From Words to Combinations of Words

A child is in the first stage from twelve to twenty-six months, and he has an MLU range of 1.0 to 2.0 morphemes. In practical terms then, the stage opens when the child is producing his first meaningful words, and it closes as he is beginning to put words together. Although an increase of only one morpheme per utterance does not seem to be much progress, this is an exciting and significant stage because the child is moving from prelinguistic to linguistic communication, which represents one giant step in the "Mother May I?" of speech and language development.

Because this is a giant step, with significant changes in language including the transition from one- to two-word combinations at about eighteen months, this stage needs to be divided. We have organized our discussion of stage 1, following Roger Brown's (1973) lead, into early stage 1 and late stage 1.

Early Stage 1 (MLU: 1 to 1.5; Age: Twelve to Twenty-Two Months)

Most of us have been around young children enough to be familiar with what speech sounds like in the beginning. The child's first utterances are single-word productions like "wawa" for "water," "mama" for "mother," and "bye-bye" for "good-bye" or "Let's get out of here!" In these examples, the child's words resemble the adult versions, but this is not always the case. A child one of us observed some years ago referred to cookies and other snacks as "chee-chee." James (1990, p. 40), in her dis-

English Morphemes

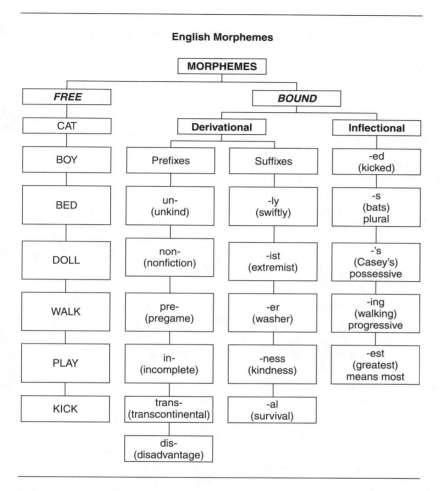

FIGURE 4.2 Morphemes: Types and Examples

cussion of first words, writes about a child who referred to cats as "gee." These productions are common during this first stage of true speech and language development, and caregivers quickly learn what these unique words mean even if other people do not have a clue.

The child's first words are used in reference to the things that matter most in her own world. She does not reflect on current events, and she does not offer criticisms of art and music. She names people, objects, and actions that are of immediate interest. Most of the child's first words consist of one syllable ("up"), two syllables ("doggie"), or one syllable repeated ("wawa"). First words are usually consonant–vowel ("no"), vowel–consonant ("eat"), or consonant–vowel–consonant–vowel ("mama") forms. Consonant–vowel–consonant forms ("hot") may be produced but are rare (Owens,

2005, p. 232). Lewis (1951) studied the first few words of twenty-six children and found that 75 percent of these words were either single-syllable productions or two-syllable productions in which one syllable was simply repeated as in "mama" or "dada." Lewis also found that 75 percent of these first words included consonants produced at the front of the mouth such as *m, b,* and *w.* There is a wider range of vowels than consonants in the early words of children, although some vowels like the *e* in *eat* and the *a* in *mama, dada,* and *wawa* are heard more often than others (Ingram, 1976).

I May Not Mean What You Mean, But I Know What I Mean . . . I Think!

It becomes immediately obvious to anyone who listens to children producing their first words that the meanings attached to these words are often inconsistent with adult meanings. One child we knew, for example, used the word *go-go* in reference to a wide range of motions, but she also used it to refer to cars, trucks, and other objects that moved. A child might use the word "nite-nite" to mean *darkness* as well as *go to sleep* probably because he associates going to sleep with darkness. He might use the word *hot* as a noun, in reference to a flame or the stove, before he uses it as an adjective referring to the temperature of an object.

In our discussion of the child's cognitive development, we identified two processes important to the development of schemata: assimilation and accommodation. We see the child applying these processes in her first words. When the child assimilates horses, cows, pigs, and elephants into her "doggie" schema, the assimilation is reflected in the way she uses the word *doggie.* That is, she uses *doggie* in reference to dogs, horses, pigs, elephants, and probably all other animals with four legs. The application of assimilation to the child's words is called **overextension.** Overextension is very common in the speech of young children. The word *wawa* is often used to refer not only to water but to any liquid. *Mama* may be used to name all women, not just mother. Anything edible might be called a *cookie.*

Sometimes the child will use a word in a sense that is too narrow from an adult perspective. This is called **underextension.** The child might use the word *doggie* only in reference to Fido, the family pet. Other dogs are something else, but they are definitely not "doggie." The word *cookie* might be reserved for chocolate chip cookies only. If there is a raisin or a nut in the dough, it might be edible, it might even be delicious, but it is not a cookie. As children sort out their cognitive categories by assimilating what should be assimilated and by accommodating when new schemata are needed, their words will be more accurately defined and applied in comparison to adult usage.

There is not universal agreement among language experts about how children attach meanings to words, but three basic views seem to exist: the semantic feature hypothesis, the functional core hypothesis, and the prototype hypothesis.

According to the **semantic feature hypothesis** (Clark, 1975), each word is composed of bits of meaning information called *semantic features.* Many words will have some semantic features in common, but each word has its own unique collection of semantic features. The semantic features for a word such as *dog* might include *animal, mammal, furry, four legs, wet nose, tail,* and *barks.* You can easily think of other words that would contain one or more of these semantic features. Some are obvious, but think about *four legs* as a semantic feature for *table* or *barks* as a semantic feature for *seal* or *circus ringmaster*. Consider the possibilities. Words are much more interconnected on the basis of bits of meaning information than they appear on the surface. What must not be missed in this mental exercise, however, is that each word is unique by virtue of its own collection or set of features. Only *dog* includes *all* of the semantic features of *dog,* and it is that set of features that separates *dogness* from *catness, pigness,* and all other words that share some but not all of the semantic features of *dog.*

Clark (1973) suggests that the development of meaning for a particular word is a gradual process. The child begins with one or two semantic features, and this accounts for the way the child uses her first words. If, for example, the only semantic feature she has for *dog* is *four legs,* she will call everything she sees with four legs a *dog.* If the only semantic feature she has for *dog* is *that animal who lives at our house and slobbers all over my face,* she will use the word *dog* in reference to that dog and to no other dog. As the child adds more semantic features, her meanings more closely approximate adult meanings, and she uses words in a more adultlike manner. According to Clark, the semantic features of the child's first words are based on perceptual categories like size, shape, texture, taste, and movement. When the child includes a size feature for dogs, she envisions an animal not as large as a horse or as small as a toad. The size feature is a kind of medium, and this works most of the time because most dogs are roughly the same size, but try to imagine the problems created when the child sees a dog like a Chihuahua that is small enough to put into a coffee mug or a giant Great Dane that is large enough to ride. Suddenly the size feature is not as reliable as it once seemed! Clark contends that even if the child notices size differences that matter to adults, she is not immediately interested in the semantic significance of the differences.

You may recognize that we used the same Chihuahua–Great Dane example in the preceding chapter in the discussion about developing schemata. Developing schemata and acquiring meanings for words by discovering and adjusting semantic features are simply two views of the same process. Cognitive development and the acquisition of language meaning are not so much parallel phenomena as they are integrated phenomena.

Nelson (1974) has rejected the notion that the meanings of first words are based on unchanging perceptual features as suggested by Clark. Nelson has proposed the **functional core hypothesis,** the argument that the meanings of early words are based on the functions or actions of the things these words represent. Whereas Clark suggests that a child categorizes things according to percepts like size and shape, Nelson proposes that the child places things into categories based upon their actions if they are animate objects or on the actions taken upon them if they are inanimate objects. The most appealing aspect of Nelson's hypothesis is that it fits Piaget's explanation of early cognitive development in the sensorimotor phase. That is, the child's first concepts are based on his sensory contacts with objects and on his manipulation of these objects.

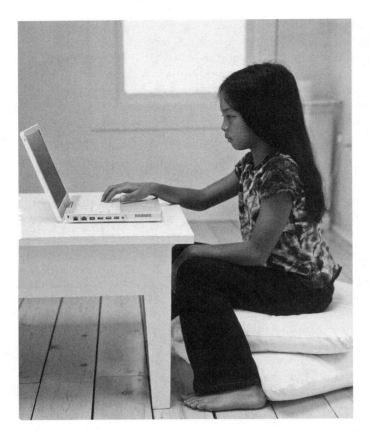

Discovering new things, words, and meanings.

As often happens when there are two substantially different explanations of the same process, someone suggests an option that combines the best features of the opposing views (see Table 4.6). This is essentially what we find in the **prototype hypothesis** developed by Bowerman (1978). Bowerman contends that both the semantic feature hypothesis and the functional core hypothesis are too narrow in their explanations, that the child relies on both perceptual features and functions in developing the meanings of words. She proposes that the child develops a **prototype** to represent a given concept. A prototype can best be understood as a model or standard. The idea is that the child will find a model that best represents a concept. The model for "dog," for example, is much more likely to be a cocker spaniel or a German shepherd than a Chihuahua because these dogs are more doglike in size than the Chihuahua. The child's model for "cat" is likely to be the domestic variety, not a lion or tiger. The prototype for "chair" will be the usual four-legged chair we find in our homes, not the bean bag chair that frequently fills the corner of the family room. The model for "fruit" will be an apple, pear, orange, or peach, not a watermelon, grape, or banana.

Table 4.6 Learning Word Meanings: Three Perspectives

Semantic feature hypothesis (Clark, 1973)	Each word has its own set of semantic features that distinguishes it from other words. Features are perceptual characteristics such as shape and size (e.g., *dog = furry, four legs, tail, barks*).
Functional core hypothesis (Nelson, 1974)	Early word meanings are learned primarily on the basis of the function of objects.
Prototype hypothesis (Bowerman, 1978)	Early word meanings are based on the child's first experience with the object the word represents. This experience forms a model (prototype) against which the child can compare other words and the objects or actions they represent.

The closer an object comes to matching the child's prototype for a given concept, the more likely he will use the name for that concept.

According to this view of meaning acquisition, the child's prototype for a concept will be strongly influenced by the first object or activity he names within the concept. Any new object or activity will be included or not included within the concept depending on how close it comes to fitting the prototype. The child's initial understanding of a concept will be fairly narrow. As his understanding of the concept develops, the meaning expands, and more and more exemplars are included. At some point, therefore, his understanding of "dogness" is sufficiently broad and refined to include all dogs, in all sizes and shapes, but he is also able to exclude wolves and coyotes because while they are similar and share many traits of dogness, they are not domestic pets. Meaning develops, therefore, as the child expands, fine-tunes, and adjusts his prototype for a given concept. For some concepts and the words associated with them, this process continues throughout childhood, adolescence, and into adulthood.

Classifying the Child's First Words

When adults listen to young children producing their first words, they may be tempted to classify these words according to traditional grammatical categories. If the child says "doggie," we think *noun*. If she says "on," we think *preposition*. If she says "go," we think *verb*. If we listen more carefully, however, we will discover that first words do not always fit adult categories. When the child points to the light switch and says "on," she may be using the word like a verb to mean "turn on the light." She might use the word *go* like a noun to name a car, bus, or train. It becomes obvious fairly quickly that since children do not use their first words in the same way that adults do, we should probably not classify or categorize these words according to adult grammatical and semantic standards.

Bloom (1973) suggests, based on analysis of her daughter's first words, that early words are of two basic types: substantive and relational. **Substantive words** refer to classes or categories of objects or events that have perceptual or functional features in common. Words such as *mama, dada, wawa,* and *doggie* are substantive. Substantive words can be divided into two more categories based on action. Those words referring to things that cause action are called *agents,* and words that identify things receiving action are called *objects.*

Relational words reflect the child's understanding of object permanence and causality. Relational words refer to actions or states of being that can affect a variety of categories. For example, the child might use the utterance "Allgone" to mean that her plate is clean or her glass is empty or her Daddy has gone to work. Relational words are most typically used to refer to the appearance or disappearance of objects, the existence or nonexistence of objects, the traits or characteristics of objects, or the location of objects and to note the possession of one object by another (Bloom & Lahey, 1978). Productions such as *more, no, stop,* and *bye-bye* are common relational words in the early vocabularies of children.

Bloom (1973) discovered that when her daughter's speech was confined to single-word productions, she used a limited number of relational words frequently and sustained these words in her vocabulary. She used a much larger number of substantive words, but many of these were not used often and tended to drop out of her vocabulary for weeks or even months. By the time she was about eighteen months old, however, substantive words were no longer dropping out, and since new words were being constantly added, an overall growth in her functional vocabulary took place.

Although Bloom's view of early vocabulary can be considered largely *semantic* in orientation because of her emphasis on the meanings of words, Nelson (1973) interpreted early vocabulary from a *grammatical* point of view. She did not use the traditional adult categories such as noun, verb, adjective, adverb, and so forth, but she did place early words into categories based on grammatical function. Nelson studied the first fifty words of eighteen children and concluded that these words could be placed into five major categories, one of which was divided into two subcategories: (1) nominals (specific and general), (2) action words, (3) modifiers, (4) personal–social words, and (5) functional words. **Nominals** are words used to refer to objects. A **specific nominal** is a word that refers to only one thing, as when a child uses *doggie* in reference to the family pet only. A **general nominal** is used in reference to all objects in a category, as when the child identifies all dogs as "doggie" or all females as "girl." It should be noted that if the child uses *doggie* to refer not only to dogs but to cats, horses, pigs, elephants, and other four-legged animals, the word is still a general nominal. It is just more general than the adult version. Nelson found that these children had more nominals than any other category. In fact, 65 percent of their words were nominals, mostly general nominals. Most of the general nominals referred to objects that moved or could be manipulated in some way, such as *car* or *ball,* or to objects of personal interest to the child such as *doggie* or *light.* These children were far less likely to identify static objects like buildings or pieces of furniture.

The second most popular category, with 13 percent, was **action words.** As the name suggests, these are words used to describe or demand action, such as *go* or *look* or words used to accompany action as when the child says, "Up," as he is being picked up or "Bye-bye" as he waves.

Simple arithmetic indicates that 78 percent, almost eight of every ten words in the early vocabularies of children, are either nominals or action words. What may be surprising is that nominals dominate so much, but this tendency has been noted by a number of researchers, even when environmental differences are taken into account (Schwartz & Leonard, 1984). Perhaps nominals dominate because it is easier for the child to conceptualize things than it is for him to conceptualize how things might be related to one another. In using an action word, he must conceptualize not just an object, but how the object might act or be acted upon.

Nelson found that the other categories accounted for far fewer words. **Modifiers,** words such as *hot, little,* and *mine,* which were used to identify the characteristics or qualities of things or events, accounted for only 9 percent of the total. **Personal–social words,** including *no* and *please,* which express emotions or identify relationships, made up just 8 percent of early vocabularies, and **functional words** such as *for* or *that* accounted for only 4 percent of the words in the vocabularies of Nelson's subjects. Benedict (1979), studying the same grammatical categories, essentially confirmed Nelson's percentages. As the child gets older, the percentage of nouns in her vocabulary continues to increase until she is using about one hundred words (see Table 4.7). At this juncture, the number of verbs relative to the number of nouns begins to increase (Bates et al., 1994; Marchman & Bates, 1991).

Although it is important to stress that the early words of children are predominantly nouns or object words (Gentner, 1982; Schwartz & Leonard, 1984), it is also appropriate to note that not all early vocabularies are the same. Horgan (1981) identifies some children as "noun lovers" and others as "noun leavers." That is, although some children use so many nouns we might assume they love nouns, others use fewer nouns, but even "noun leavers" use more nouns than other categories of words.

Although nouns dominate the early vocabularies of all children, there are small but noteworthy differences among children. As Nelson (1973) noted, although some children seem to use language primarily to describe and categorize things, others seem to give language a major role in their social and personal interactions. These differences can probably be viewed more as preferential or stylistic differences than major variations in language substance, and they may simply reflect early personality differences. That is, children who use language primarily to describe and categorize may be somewhat less social than children who emphasize language usage in their interactions with other people.

Before we move on to the pragmatics of single-word productions, we want to add a few observations about the rate of vocabulary growth in early language development. Many caregivers are overly concerned when their children do not produce their first words by some arbitrarily established developmental deadline. We know that the prototypical, average child experiences rapid vocabulary growth at about the time she hits the 50-word mark, and we know that the rate of growth remains strong from about 18 months to 24 months. The caution, however, and it is a caution that

Table 4.7 Categories of the First Fifty Words: The Results of Two Studies

Grammatical Category	Description	Percentage		Examples
		Benedict (1979)	**Nelson (1973)**	
Nominals—specific	Refer to only one thing	11	14	"Casey" referring to the family's pet dog
Nominals—general	Refer to all members of an object category	50	51	*Doggie, girl, boy, cup*
Action words	Describe or demand an action	19	13	*Go, look, run*
Modifiers	Identify quality or characteristics of things or events	10	9	*Hot, little, mine*
Personal–social	Express emotions or identify relationships	10	8	*No, please*
Functional	Serve a grammatical function	*Note:* Benedict did not include a Functional category.	4	*For, that, this*

Source: Adapted from R. Owens, *Language Development: An Introduction,* 6th ed. (Boston: Allyn & Bacon, 2005), 233.

comes with vigorously waved red flags, is that "normal" children do not all follow the same course. Some normal children acquire their first words earlier than other normal children, and some normal children add words to their vocabularies over the first two years of their lives more quickly than other normal children. There also is a sex difference we can note. Generally speaking, girls acquire their first meaningful words earlier than boys, and, generally speaking, girls acquire their first words more quickly than boys (Bauer, Goldfield, & Reznick, 2002).

The Functions of Single Words: Pragmatics

Earlier in this chapter, in our discussion of infant communication, we introduced pragmatics, the study of the practical aspects of communication. Pragmatics includes the functions, purposes, or intents of communication. According to Halliday (1975), Bates (1979), and others, children show evidence of communicative intent before they begin to use words, but when the child moves from prelinguistic to linguistic communication, pragmatics undergoes a significant evolution. Words allow for more specific intentions than gestures alone, and as we all know from our adult experiences with language, words provide opportunities for many layers of meaning, including layers of pragmatic meaning. As adults, when someone says something to us, we are often more curious about the intentions of the communicator than about the message itself. We are more inclined to ask questions like "What did she mean by that?" or "Why did she say that?" than "What did she say?" Figuring out what someone says is usually fairly easy. Determining motive, purpose, or intention is often much more difficult and, in the final analysis, more important because communication ultimately is about getting things done.

The evolution of pragmatics triggered by the onset of language becomes apparent even in the single-word stage of language development. Whereas Halliday (1975) identified four intents in the nonlinguistic utterances of his son, Nigel, the number of intentions expanded to seven with the introduction of his first words (see Table 4.8). In addition to the earlier functions, which included *satisfying needs and wants, controlling the behavior* of others, *interacting* with others, and *expressing* emotion or interest, Nigel used his early words in his efforts to *explore and categorize* the things in his

Table 4.8 Halliday's Communicative Functions

Function	Explanation	Example
Interacting	Using language to maintain contact with others	Child says, "Mama," while mother is in the room; comparable to Dore's categories of *greeting* and *calling.*
Regulatory	Using language to control the behavior of others	Child says, "Ball," in an attempt to have Mother give him the object; comparable to Dore's category of *requesting an action.*
Personal	Using language to express emotions or interest	Child says, "Whee!" as she plays with toy; comparable to Dore's category of *protesting.*
Heuristic	Using language to explore and categorize	Child sees a new toy and asks "Doggie?"; comparable to Dore's category of *requesting an answer.*
Instrumental	Using language to satisfy needs and wants	Child says, "Milk," in an effort to obtain a drink; comparable to Dore's category of *requesting an action.*
Imagine (pretend)	Using language to accompany her play activity	Child says, "Up," as he puts a doll in a chair.
Informative	Using language to share her knowledge with others	Child points to Daddy's eye and says, "Eye"; comparable to Dore's category of *labeling.*

Source: Adapted from M. A. Halliday, *Learning How to Mean: Explorations in the Development of Language* (New York: Arnold, 1975).

environment, to *imagine* or pretend, and to *inform* by sharing his experiences with others. You will recognize that these are functions of communication that continue throughout one's life, but these are pretty basic functions or intents. As the child matures and his language becomes more sophisticated, his pragmatic functions expand as well.

Halliday's interpretation of early communicative intents takes into account the reactions of listeners. His categories of functions are based on how well the child's communicative attempts work toward accomplishing specified purposes. Dore (1974, 1975), who analyzed the communicative functions of children during the single-word stage of language development, tried to look at these functions from the point of view of the child. That is, what are the child's intentions and reasons for communicating, regardless of whether they work or do not work from the listener's point of view? According to Dore, children in the single-word stage (twelve to eighteen months) produce what he called **primitive speech acts** (PSAs) to communicate their intentions (see Table 4.9). A primitive speech act might be a word, a change in the prosodic pattern, or a gesture. Dore found that children could use these communication skills to *label* objects or events, to *answer* questions, to *request an action or answer,*

Table 4.9 Dore's Primitive Speech Acts (PSAs)

The Act	Communicative Purpose	Child's Behavior
Labeling	Identifies an object	Child points to Mother's eye and says, "Eye."
Answering	Responds to caregiver's inquiry	Caregiver asks, "What's that?" while pointing to a toy dog. Child says, "Doggie."
Requesting an action	Looks at caregiver; produces a word or a prosodic change; waits for a response	Child says, "Ball," in a manner indicating that the caregiver is being instructed to give him the ball.
Requesting an answer	Asks for information from a caregiver	Child says, "Doggie?" and waits for caregiver to respond and confirm identification.
Calling	Attempts to gain the attention of a caregiver	Child says, "Daddy" in an attempt to gain his attention.
Greeting	Acknowledges a caregiver upon entering a room	Child says, "Daddy," as he enters a room.
Protesting	Rejects an object or action	Child says, "No!" when an attempt is made to give him spinach.
Repeating/ Imitating	Produces at least part of what is said by a caregiver	Dad hits his hand with a hammer and says, "Ouch!" Child responds with, "Ouch!"
Practicing	Produces a word or prosodic pattern without anyone being in the room	Child says, "Ball," while playing with a ball.

Source: Adapted from J. Dore, "Holophrases, Speech Acts and Language Universals," *Journal of Child Language 2,* no. 1, (April 1975): 33.

to *address* a person or thing, to *greet* someone, to *protest* or *object*, to *imitate* or *repeat*, and simply to *practice* language.

Bloom and Lahey (1978, pp. 202–203) provide labels that may help clarify what happens to communicative intentions as the child moves from the prelinguistic stage of communication development to the linguistic stage. They suggest that when children are using just a few words in combination with gestures, they are using *primary forms.* When their intentions are more consistently communicated through words, they are using *conventional forms.* In some cases, such as the child's pointing to something she wants, the gesture may be just as effective as making a request in words, but when children begin to use conventional or language-based forms to express their communicative functions, they add many more options to their repertoire of intentions, and they can express their intentions with much greater clarity and specificity.

Presuppositions and Conversational Turn Taking

As the child's communicative intentions become more elaborate, the role of the child in speaker–listener relationships becomes more interesting and complex. During the single-word stage, we see evidence of what are called presuppositions. A **presupposition** is an assumption the speaker makes concerning what the listener knows about the subject of the conversation. In a typical communicative exchange, the child will provide information the listener needs and will not comment on what he believes the listener already knows (Greenfield & Smith, 1976). If the child is preparing to push a toy car, for example, he may make the presupposition that the listener knows that the object in his hand is a car. He might comment on what the speaker does not know, which is that he is about to make the car move, so he says, "Go!" while pushing the car across the floor toward Rex, the previously sleeping, now frantic and scurrying family dog. We should keep in mind, of course, that the adult's ability to interpret what the child says is made a little easier because children at this early stage of language development typically talk about the here and now (Greenfield, 1978). Most adults, given even modest communicative assistance from children, are bright enough to figure out communications that focus on what is happening in the present tense in the present place.

The child in the single-word stage is just beginning to develop presuppositional skills. As we shall see, the child at three and four years is still having difficulty with presuppositions that consider the listener's perspective. Although this aspect of communication begins to emerge early, it continues to develop throughout the preschool and school-age years.

There is evidence of communicative turn taking before the child begins to use words, but as she moves from prelinguistic to linguistic communication, develops specific communicative intentions, and begins to use presuppositions, she begins to develop a turn-taking style more closely resembling adult conversation. By the time the child is eighteen months old, she is demonstrating some of the basic rules of turn taking in her conversations with other people (Bloom, Rocissano, & Hood, 1976). If, for example, the child's conversational partner names an object in the child's possession, the child might make a comment about the object, but she will not repeat the label already identified by her partner. She presupposes this knowledge and uses her turn to describe the object or to explain to her partner what is going to happen next. Her partner might then comment on the action the child has taken, and the child, presupposing knowledge of all that has been said before, uses her turn to contribute additional information or respond directly to her partner's comments. Turn taking, assuming knowledge, and taking into account the partner's perspective are some of the bases of adultlike conversation.

Midstage Review: What Is Happening So Far?

To this point, the child's productions have been mostly single words. Before moving to the combination phase of stage 1, it will be useful to review some of what you have learned so far about the child's earliest language efforts.

The child's first meaningful word appears at about twelve months. By the time he is eighteen months old, he will have about fifty words in his expressive vocabulary, and he will understand many more than that. His first words are mostly nouns, but he does use some action words, and he uses a few modifiers such as *big, bad,* or *hot.* These first words refer to things, events, people, and actions that are of personal interest to the child. They may not be adult forms of comparable words, and they are often used with wider or narrower meanings than adult versions of the same words. The child might call a dog a *gaga,* for example. He might produce an adultlike version such as *doggie,* but he might use *doggie* to refer to all four-legged animals, not just dogs, or he might use the word to refer to just one dog, the family pet.

His first words are used for fairly specific purposes: to name objects or people, to request something, to control the behavior of someone else, or to express emotion. Even though he is typically using only one word at a time, he shows some understanding of conversation. In a limited way, he takes into account what his listener knows about a subject and tends not to repeat redundant information. He engages in a turn-taking style of communication that allows for comment and the contributions of new information on the parts of both conversational partners. By using basic body language and by varying intonation, the child can indicate that he is asking questions, and he can produce a negative communication by shaking his head or using the word *no,* which is likely to show up in his vocabulary very early.

Although it is true that adults must be pretty active interpreters to determine the semantic and pragmatic messages in the child's speech, this is pretty impressive stuff for a communicator whose utterances are mostly single words. Try to imagine what will happen to the child's communicative abilities when he begins to put words together.

The First Combinations: True Syntax or Transitional Productions?

Keep in mind that the child acquiring language has been given no instructions about what she is supposed to do next, and it is often difficult for the observer to figure out what the child is doing as she moves from one stage of language development to the next. In the child's first word combinations, we find a perfect example of this kind of problem. What is going on? What do these combinations tell us about the child's knowledge of syntax, semantics, and pragmatics? Because these first combinations do not follow adult rules of grammar, because they often seem to be words simply strung together, and because they often appear in the midst of unintelligible productions not unlike babbling or vocal play, it is difficult to know what the child is doing and what he knows.

According to some observers, children do go through a transitional stage between single-word productions and multiple-word productions. Bloom (1973) reports, for example, that her daughter included the meaningless production "wida," before and after a wide range of meaningful words. Some children repeat a word but vary prosodic elements such as stress and intonation. Others produce what appear to be merely strings of single-word utterances. Bloom provides the example of the child who, while looking at a picture of another child in a play car, said, "Go, car, ride." Because each word was produced with equal emphasis and ended with a falling pitch, Bloom concludes that these were three single-word utterances, not one multiple-word utterance. She argues that although these productions indicate that the child knows something about relationships among things, people, and actions, they do not suggest an understanding of the syntactic knowledge that results in the production of true sentences.

Not everyone agrees with Bloom's conclusions, however. Branigan (1979) reports that closer examination of what appear to be successive single-word utterances suggests that, although the pauses between words make them sound like distinct and separate productions, there are other prosodic variations that are more sentence-like. In some cases, not all the words end with a falling pitch, and the last word in the series is often produced with longer duration than the preceding words. These variations suggest that the child is putting the words together in some fashion, even if we cannot recognize the rules or the meaningfulness of the combinations.

Two-Word Productions: The Dawning of Syntax in Late Stage 1 (MLU: 1.5 to 2.0; Age: Twenty-Two to Twenty-Six Months)

Whether or not there is a transitional stage between single- and multiple-word productions, we know that the child typically begins to put two words together between the ages of eighteen and twenty-four months. These combinations represent the beginning of language structure, or **syntax.** The child discovers and applies rules for putting words together in a manner that creates meaning greater than the added meanings of the words alone. That's what makes a **sentence.** The meaning of any sentence is the result, not just of the cumulative meanings of the individual words, but of the interactive meanings of words based on their semantic and grammatical relationships with one another, and on how they are ordered in the sentence. The child's two-word utterances do not allow for much complexity in terms of sentence meaning, of course, but they do represent the beginning of syntax and the dramatic extension of meaning made possible by putting words together. Armed with a limited vocabulary and combining only two words at a time, the child is able to make declarative statements ("Daddy go") and to express negation ("No night-night"). Whereas early in stage 1, the child expressed questions by using a rising intonation on single-word productions ("Doggie?" or "Bye-bye?") or single-word productions such as "What?" or "Where?" the child in late stage 1 creates primitive interrogative forms by combining those words with other words in productions such as "What doing?" or "Where go?" These are very simple structures to be sure, but they are the embryos of real syntax.

The significance of two-word utterances can be examined and described on three levels: syntactic, semantic, and pragmatic. We consider each level separately, but keep in mind that this separation is for convenience only. When human beings communicate, whether they are adults or children, they do not fragment their messages into structure, meaning, and purpose. The meanings of words are enriched and clarified by the structuring of words into sentences, and our communicative intentions are facilitated, if we use language well, by choosing the right words with the right meanings and putting them in correct and appropriate relationships with one another in effectively crafted sentences.

The Syntactic Level: Arranging Words Appropriately

There are at least two ways to describe syntax in two-word utterances. Crystal, Fletcher, and Garman (1976) suggest that the child chooses two words from four basic sentence constructions: subject, verb, object, and adverbial. These options allow the child to produce clause-like utterances with subjects and predicates as well as phrase-like constructions that include modifications of a subject or predicate. For example, the child might say, "Car go," a clause-like production in which *car* is the subject and *go* is the predicate. He might then say, "Go fast," a phrase-like construction in which *fast* is an adverbial modification of the verb *go*. He might also produce a phrase such as "Daddy car," in which *Daddy* is used to modify the noun *car*.

Another approach to describing syntax at the two-word level was proposed by Braine (1963). Braine suggested that the child uses a primitive form of grammar called **Pivot-Open Grammar.** According to this view, the child has just two categories of words: open and pivot. **Open words** can be used alone, in combination with other open words, in combination with pivot words, and in either the first or second position of two-word utterances. **Pivot words** cannot be used alone, cannot be combined with other pivot words, but can be used in either the first or second position of utterances. This means then that the child can produce the following kinds of two-word sentences—open + open, pivot + open, or open + pivot—but does not produce pivot + pivot sentences. One cannot assume that a given word will always be an open word or always a pivot word. Two children might use a given word in different ways so that the word is open for one but pivot for the other.

When Braine's grammar was first published, it seemed a promising way to describe and understand the child's early two-word utterances, but by 1970 some of the limitations of this approach were becoming apparent. One of the first language experts to express concern about the Pivot-Open Grammar was Bloom (1970), who criticized the approach because it did not take into account the meanings of the child's two-word productions. She contended that because the Pivot-Open Grammar considers only structure, it does not give children adequate credit for their language knowledge.

Using one child's productions as examples, Bloom contends that in one context, "Mommy sock" was produced when the child picked up one of her mother's socks. On another occasion when the child's mother was putting a sock on the child's foot, the child produced the same two-word utterance, "Mommy sock." Categorizing these productions as combinations of open and pivot words misses much of what is being communicated, according to Bloom. In the first case, "Mommy sock" is used to mean "This sock belongs to Mommy." In the second case, "Mommy sock" certainly seems to mean "Mommy is putting a sock on my foot." The first utterance focuses on possession. The second utterance is primarily concerned with action performed by an agent (mother) on an object (sock). One of Bloom's primary contentions, therefore, is that one cannot determine how a child is using language, what a child knows about language, or what a child means by the language she is using unless one takes **communicative context** into account. Using context to help determine the meanings of a child's utterances is referred to as **rich interpretation** by Brown (1973). This process has helped guide much of the research on the language of children since the early 1970s.

Semantic Level: Determining the Meanings of Early Sentences

Bloom's objections to a strictly syntactic description of the child's early word combinations, and her emphasis on taking communicative context into account, led to a semantic interpretation of early sentences. Bloom and Lahey (1978) assert that early two-word utterances reflect an understanding on the child's part about meaning relations and rules for word order. To take this twofold understanding into account, they suggest that the rules the child uses at this juncture in development be referred to as **semantic-syntactic** rules. One might argue that when the child is producing two-word utterances, there is not much opportunity for creating language structure, just as it would be difficult to structure a wall with only two bricks. On the other hand, we have already discovered that the child is able effectively to communicate complete, and sometimes fairly sophisticated, thoughts with single-word utterances. What kind of messages might the child be able to convey if he puts words together with meaning relationships that, when they interact, communicate far more than the additive values of their meanings?

Language experts have proposed several semantic classification systems they believe will more adequately describe children's two-word combinations. Bloom (1970) was the first expert to identify semantic relations in the early language productions of three American children. A few years later, Brown (1973) examined semantic relations in the early productions of children acquiring a range of languages from English to Samoan. Brown suggests that these early productions reflect what children know about the things and actions in their lives and that the meanings they express are consistent with the level of their intellectual development. The eight amalgamated meanings on page 146 were typical of those produced by the late stage 1 children who were the subjects in Brown's study.

Additional two-term relations have been identified by other researchers (Bloom, 1973; Schlesinger, 1971). For example, the child might use a recurrence + _____ production if she wants something to occur or appear again, as in "More juice!" She

Semantic–Syntactic Relation	Example
demonstrative (*this/that*) + entity	*That ball*
entity + attribute	*Kitty nice*
possessor + possession	*My dolly*
entity + location	*Dolly chair*
action + location	*Put table* (object is being placed on a table)
agent + object	*Baby shoe*
agent + action	*Doggie sit*
action + object	*Drink juice*

might use a nonexistence/disappearance production such as "Allgone juice" to proudly announce that she has finished her drink, that it has disappeared, that it no longer exists. She might use a rejection production such as "No 'tatoes!" when she exercises what she thinks is her right to refuse an order to finish her helping of mashed potatoes. She might use a denial production such as "Not kitty" in response to her mother's incorrect reference to the family dog as a "kitty."

Among the forms children use to express negative semantic relations, nonexistence/disappearance is used by children more frequently than rejection or denial. The use of denial involves some fairly complicated cognitive and perceptual manipulations. That is, the child must compare the object or being described by the caregiver to his own perception and understanding of that object or being in order to make a judgment about the validity of the caregiver's observation or question. If the caregiver points to the family dog, for example, and asks, "Is that a kitty?" the child must compare his understanding about what he sees with his understanding about what a kitty is. If there is a mismatch between what he is being asked and what he knows, he produces the denial "Not kitty!" (Hummer, Wimmer, & Antes, 1993). Researchers have noted that because this kind of production depends on fairly sophisticated perceptual and cognitive processing, it emerges at about twenty to twenty-five months, somewhat later than other productions that are otherwise comparable in terms of meaning and function (Bloom, 1970, 1973; Choi, 1988; Vaidyanathan, 1991).

Research has provided some information about the developmental order of a few semantic relations. According to Wells (1985), for example, when children express **entity + location,** they generally refer to the location of a static or stationary entity or object before they refer to the movement or action of placing an object *in* or *on* something. That is, the child will typically say something such as "Doggie chair," to indicate that a dog is sitting on a chair, before she manages a comment about an activity in progress involving the movement of an object from one place to another. Caregivers must patiently wait for the child to make a statement such as "In box," to indicate that she is in the process of dumping a spoonful of mashed potatoes into her mother's sewing basket. This kind of utterance, in addition to creating a sense of excitement for mother, expresses an entity + location semantic relation in which there is the movement of something (mashed potatoes) from one place (the child's plate) to another (Mom's sewing basket). Wells's (1985) findings suggest that the child will produce location relations by twenty-one months, and the typical child will be using two-word combinations to express attribute (attribute + entity) by the time she is two years old.

Using this kind of analysis, one might reasonably conclude that the child is able to talk about things, where they are, what actions they perform, what actions are performed on them, and who creates these actions. He is also able to identify characteristics or attributes of things, and he can express ownership or possession. We should not lose sight of the fact that the child in early stage 1 can use single-word utterances to express relations such as **existence, nonexistence, disappearance,** and **recurrence,** but the successful communication of these relations during early stage 1 depends heavily on the interpretative powers of adult listeners. When the child begins to use two-word combinations, interpretation remains difficult, but it is somewhat less murky because the child is now employing syntactic rules for ordering words in combination with the stress patterns of his language to help convey his intended meanings. Interpretation is also facilitated by context. That is, if the adult takes into account what was said prior to the utterance being interpreted, and if she considers the nonlinguistic circumstances surrounding the production, she is more likely to interpret the meaning of the child's message correctly.

As the child develops into late stage 1 (twenty-two to twenty-six months), she continues to make steady, if not always dramatic, progress in terms of semantic-syntactic relations. There is evidence that the child will begin to produce three- and even four-word combinations at approximately twenty-four months. Only about half of her productions at this point are two-word utterances (Owens, 2005, p. 255). Productions such as "Baby push truck" (agent + action + object), and "Daddy put box" (agent + action + location, to indicate that Daddy is putting something in the box) are not uncommon utterances for the late stage 1 child.

The Pragmatic Level: An Emphasis on the Functions of Early Sentences

Throughout this chapter, we have cited the work of Dore (1974, 1975) and Halliday (1975) to trace the development of communicative intents during stage 1 of language development. Before the child begins using words, he is able to express four communicative intentions, according to Halliday. When the child uses words, he expands his repertoire of intentions to about seven. When the child begins to put words together, between the ages of eighteen and twenty-four months, we see additional changes in communicative intentions. The child now engages in what can properly be considered dialogue. He understands that in two-way communication, the participants fill and exchange certain roles. One speaks and the other listens, then the listener speaks and the speaker listens. When one speaks, the other sometimes responds to the message expressed by the speaker, sometimes by simply acknowledging the message, sometimes by adding information, sometimes by agreeing or disagreeing. Sometimes the speaker is a questioner and the listener is a responder. There are many roles to be filled in communication, and even with a limited expressive vocabulary and only single-word and two-word utterances, the child is able to fill these roles.

The functions or intentions we identified earlier from Halliday's work are now combined and modified into at least three new functions: pragmatic, mathetic, and informative. The **pragmatic** function of language is undoubtedly the most basic. The child uses language to get things done. She uses language to make requests and demands, to satisfy needs, to interact with and control the behavior of other people.

The **mathetic** function of language is manifested in communications concerned with learning. The child uses language to learn about herself and about her world. She comments, questions, predicts, and remembers. She uses language to express her developing understanding of how people, things, and events are connected. Her language, however limited, is a reflection of her intellectual development.

The **informative** function emerges when the child uses language to give new information to others. Adults often think of the informative function as the most basic function of language and probably the first to emerge, but it is actually one of the last. Why? We cannot use language to inform until we know something others do not or until we think we know something we assume others do not know. In the beginning, everyone knows more than the child! Before stage 1 ends, however, the child is more than happy to use language to tell others what she knows, even if what she "knows" is incorrect, incomplete, or irrelevant. She uses language to inform the dog, brothers and sisters, Mom and Dad, Teddy Bear, and anyone else who cares to profit from her wisdom. This is one of the most delightful functions of early multiple-word utterances. When this child speaks, listen, learn, enjoy, and be prepared to be amazed.

The child at this stage abides by some of the basic rules of conversation. He will address his conversational partner by name to gain his or her attention before speaking. He will listen before he responds, and he understands the turn-taking aspect of conversation. His primary limitation as a conversationalist is a short attention span. He will usually stay on the same topic for only a few turns before he is ready to move on to something else (Bloom, Rocissano, & Hood, 1976). We will see a dramatic change in this aspect of conversation after the child passes his third birthday. It's quite possible that you have already encountered a three-year-old who wanted to talk about a topic long after your knowledge and/or interest was exhausted.

Comprehension and Production: A Critical and Evolving Relationship

Before concluding this description of language development in stage 1, we need to include a brief review of what the child comprehends at this time. Expressive language cannot be separated from receptive language, of course. As children mature, what they understand dramatically impacts what they are able to express and how they express it.

For as long as people have systematically studied language and language development, there have been questions about the relationship between comprehension and production. There is appealing logic in the assumption that comprehension must precede production, and many linguists have held that view through the years. In fact, one notable linguist, Ingram (1974), made the clear assertion that "comprehension ahead of production is a linguistic universal of acquisition" (p. 313). Others are not sure that the relationship is this simple. Bloom (1974), for example, argues that although we do not know the precise character of the relationship between comprehension and production, we know it is a relationship of shared dependence.

Whatever the true nature of this relationship, it seems clear that it changes as language develops, and it is not the same for all components of language. As we noted in the opening section of this chapter, the infant comprehends differences among speech sounds, sequences of speech sounds, and intonational patterns long before he produces sounds and superimposes intonational patterns on sequences of sounds. These discriminations are made within the first half of the first year (Goodsitt et al., 1984; Kessen, Levine, & Wendrich, 1979), while comparable productions do not occur until after the first birthday.

When the child begins to produce his first meaningful words, we see a changing relationship between comprehension and production. The child produces words *before* he has a complete understanding of them. We have already noted, for example, that the child might use the word *doggie* to refer to only the family pet, or he might use *doggie* to refer to any four-legged animal. There is some comprehension associated with this production, of course, but it is not a complete comprehension according to adult standards. Only after the child experiences sufficient intellectual development to understand *doggie* as a category that includes all dogs but only dogs, and only after he acquires additional words in his vocabulary to reflect this understanding will his comprehension of *doggie* be complete. In the meantime, the child's ability to understand is greatly influenced by all the nonlinguistic cues that surround the words spoken to him. Because adults often fail to take this nonlinguistic information into account, they may overestimate what the child really comprehends in the words spoken to him, and they may overestimate, based on the child's language production, the child's real language competence.

According to Benedict (1979), comprehension does precede production to a significant extent for the first fifty words. The eight children in her study comprehended about fifty words before they were able to produce ten words. They comprehended fifty words at thirteen months, but did not produce fifty words until they were nineteen months old. Their receptive vocabularies increased by about twenty-two words per month, but their expressive vocabularies grew by only nine or ten words each month. Based on these findings, it is reasonable to conclude that in early language development, the gap between comprehension and production is substantial.

In the beginning, comprehension is not language based. That is, the child does not understand a word such as *doggie* in reference to a dictionary definition. The child's first understandings are based on nonverbal insights about things, actions, and the relationships among things and actions (Huttenlocher, 1974). Paul (1990) refers to this type of understanding as knowledge based on routines, or scripts of events, in which repetitions of the event itself in combination with adults' repetitive linguistic and nonlinguistic behaviors associated with the event facilitate word comprehension. The child understands important and basic categories of things such as food, people, and pets. She understands basic actions such as eating or sitting and obvious relationships such as putting food into the mouth. The child conceptualizes these things, actions, and relationships apart from language, but as she hears certain sequences of sounds produced in connection with these mental representations, she associates the sequences of sounds, or words, with the things, actions, and relationships. When the connections become established, the words serve to help the child recall the things, actions, and relationships to which the words refer. It is important to notice the sequence in comprehension Huttenlocher is suggesting. The child first understands aspects or characteristics of things and actions in her environment. She then creates mental pictures or concepts of these things and actions, and she gradually associates these mental pictures with spoken words. The words help her to retrieve the mental pictures.

As one might guess, children comprehend names for things and people before they comprehend words that describe actions and relationships. As one might also guess, children understand words for things and people in the here and now before they understand words for things and people that are absent in time or space. The findings of a study of children between the ages of ten and twenty-one months by Miller, Chapman, Branston, and Reichle (1980) suggest a fairly consistent sequence of comprehensions. All of the twelve-month-old subjects understood names for people in sight, and about half understood words for things in their presence. Words describing actions were understood by most of the subjects older than fifteen months. A little more than half of the children between nineteen and twenty-one months understood words referring to people and things not present. Semantic relationships in two- and three-word utterances were understood only by those children over eighteen months. Among the semantic relationships studied, the most often understood was possessor + possession as in "My doggie" or "Mommy shoe."

Just as adults may overestimate the child's understanding of single words, they may overestimate what the child is able to comprehend in the sentences he hears. Chapman (1978) suggests that when the child responds to utterances, he may use comprehension strategies that give the impression of greater understanding than the child actually possesses. For example, when an adult says, "Throw the ball," the child might pick up the ball and throw it. The adult assumes the child understands the words *ball* and *throw* and the relationship between them. If the adult then says, "Hide the ball," or "Kiss the ball," or "Hit the ball," the child is likely to throw the ball again. If the child has selected the ball from among several objects, it might be safe to assume he understands the word *ball*, but he may not understand the rest of the words in any of these sentences. What he does know is that balls are for throwing, so whenever he hears *ball* in an utterance, he throws it. His comprehension strategy, therefore, is to perform the action on an object most commonly associated with that object. Assuming he understands the words *milk, cookie,* and *ball*, he *drinks* milk, *eats* the cookie, and *throws* the ball, no matter what other words happen to surround the words he knows in sentences spoken to him.

Huttenlocher (1974) asserts that when the child *comprehends* language, she uses a word to retrieve the mental image of an object, person, or action. When she *produces* language, she recognizes an object, person, or action, and must retrieve the matching word. Comprehension involves an easier or more direct association between object and word than production, according to Huttenlocher, because the child's understanding of objects, people, and events is more complete than her understanding of the words used to represent them. Adults often have a similar experience with a foreign language. It is easier to comprehend a new language than to speak it because when we listen to the vocabulary of the new language that is not well known, we move to the vocabulary of our native language, which is well understood. When we try to speak the language, we must move from the known to the incompletely known, a much more difficult task. During language development, this difference seems to be reflected in the occurrence of overextensions. The child tends to overextend the meanings of words in production, but not in comprehension. In the example we have used several times, the child overextends the word *doggie* to include not only dogs but cats, horses, cows, and many other four-legged animals. The same child who produces *doggie* to refer to a cow would likely point to the correct animal if, while looking at a cat, dog, and cow, an adult produced each animal's name. In other words, it is easier for the child to retrieve her mental image of an object than to retrieve the word that represents the object.

The Role of the Caregiver in the Acquisition of Early Language

Keep in mind that language does not develop in a vacuum. Children bring to the acquisition process a strong biological drive to develop language, and the emergence of language is closely associated with cognitive development, but they will not acquire language unless they are exposed to language models. There is evidence, too, that simply hearing language is not enough. The child's communicative interactions with his caregivers facilitate vocabulary acquisition (Ahktar, Dunham, & Dunham, 1991) and overall language development. When a caregiver responds to her child's early utterances, she often **expands** them. If the child says, "Mommy work," the caregiver might respond, "Yes, Mommy went to work." The caregiver does not change the order of the words in the child's utterance, and she maintains what she believes is the child's communicative intent, but she expands the utterance into a complete form. According to Hirsch-Pasek, Treiman, and Schneiderman (1984), caregivers expand about 20 percent of their two-year-old children's utterances into more syntactically correct and complete sentences, and children often respond to these expansions by imitating them (Folger & Chapman, 1978).

Although it is not known precisely *what* expansions contribute to language development, Scherer and Olswang (1984) believe they assist the acquisition of language by helping the child better understand the grammatical functions of words and the rules by which words are combined, by keeping the communicative effort focused on subjects the child has selected, and by reinforcing the turn-taking aspect of conversation. Farrar (1990) suggests that the child may derive different benefits from different types of expansion in learning grammatical morphemes. For example, restating the child's utterances with added or revised grammatical morphemes may assist the child in acquiring plurals and possessives, whereas expanding the topic or general intent of the child's utterance may be more helpful in the acquisition of other grammatical morphemes, including tense markers.

Caregiver–child interactions make important contributions to language development.

Apparently caregivers are sensitive to the length and complexity of their own models even before they expand the child's utterances. According to Murray, Johnson, and Peters (1990), caregivers actually produce shorter utterances when they talk to toddlers than when they talk to infants. Furthermore, there seems to be a relationship between these shorter adult utterances during the second half of the child's second year and her receptive language abilities at eighteen months. It appears that when adults sense that the child is old enough to benefit from speech and language models, they pay greater attention to the length and complexity of the models they provide in order to give the child clear and attainable language targets. Then when the child begins to produce her own utterances, adults provide additional assistance through various forms of expansion.

Sometimes a caregiver will do more than expand the child's utterance. In an example similar to the one in a preceding paragraph, the child might say, "Daddy go," and the caregiver responds by saying, "Yes, Daddy went to work." In this case, the caregiver is not only providing a more syntactically accurate model, but she is providing additional semantic information. This kind of response is called **extension.** On other occasions, the caregiver will simply imitate what the child has said. Very often when the adult imitates the child's utterance, the child will imitate the imitation to create a simple form of turn taking. Whether the caregiver expands, extends, or imitates, the child is taking the communicative initiative, but he is being provided models that include enriched syntactic and semantic information. Of no less importance, the child is being encouraged in his language attempts and rewarded for his successful communication connections.

Stage 1: A Brief Look Back and a Glimpse Forward

This stage began with the production of first words and ended with the production of combinations of words. The child produces her first word at about twelve months and begins to combine words at about eighteen months. Her expressive vocabulary grows from one word at the beginning of the stage to 200 to 300 words by the end of the stage. Her first words are mostly nouns used to name people or objects. By the end of the stage, she is producing two-word and even some three- and four-word utterances to make statements, ask questions, express negatives, and make demands. She is using language to get things done, manipulate the behaviors of other people, and exchange information in a rudimentary form of conversation, complete with turn-taking and presuppositional skills, although these skills are just beginning to emerge and are quite primitive by adult standards (see Table 4.10).

During the remaining stages, the child will learn to produce a greater variety of sentences and to make them more elaborate. She will learn how to put simple sentences together to produce compound sentences and how to put sentences into one another to make complex sentences. She will also become a more sophisticated conversationalist, and, of course, her vocabulary will grow, and her understanding of the meanings of words and word combinations will increase. As exciting and full as stage 1 has been, the child's language development has truly just begun!

Review Questions

1. Before they have language, how do children communicate? What are the limitations of these prelinguistic communications?

2. Identify and discuss the infant's perceptual abilities. How do these early perceptual abilities apparently prepare the child for speech production?

3. Describe the prelinguistic interactions of infants and adults. What arguments might be developed to support the importance of infant–adult interactions in communication development?

4. Trace communication production during the infancy months from cries to words. How does each progression appear to build on behaviors produced earlier to make oral communication more sophisticated and adultlike?

5. What is the value of a *stage* view of language development? What are the potential dangers of adhering too rigidly to this view in studying the development of any set of behaviors in human beings?

6. Define and provide examples for each of the following: morpheme, free morpheme, bound morpheme, derivational bound morpheme, and inflectional bound morpheme.

7. What is *mean length of utterance,* and what is its value in tracing early language development?

8. Briefly describe the following views concerning how children attach meanings to words: semantic feature hypothesis, functional core hypothesis, and prototype hypothesis.

9. Assuming it is not appropriate to classify the child's first words into

Table 4.10 Stage 1 Highlights

Typical Age Range: 12–26 Months
MLU: 1.0–2.0 Morphemes

First Words
- Do not always sound like adult words
- Used in reference to things of greatest importance to the child: people, objects, actions of immediate interest
- Most are single-syllable words or single-syllables repeated.
- May infrequently exhibit overextended or underextended meanings.

Pragmatics
- Uses nonverbal and verbal communication to satisfy needs and wants, control the behavior of others, interact with others, express emotion or interest, explore and categorize, imagine, and inform
- Demonstrates primitive presuppositional and turn-taking skills

Multiword Productions
- The combining of two words typically begins at eighteen to twenty-four months.
- Three-word and some four-word combinations appear when about half of the child's utterances are two-word productions.
- These productions can be interpreted at three levels: syntactic, semantic, and pragmatic.

Sentence Types
- In early stage 1, the child uses a rising intonation on single words to pose *yes/no questions* and may use approximated forms of *what* or *where* to ask questions.
- In late stage 1, the child combines two and three words, but still using a rising intonation to pose *yes/no* questions, as in "*That +* ___?" *Wh* interrogative words are still limited to *what* and *where*.
- In early stage 1, words such as *no, gone,* and *allgone* appear. One of these words may be used in combination with another word (negative + ___).
- In late stage 1, the words *no* and *not* are used interchangeably at the beginning of word combinations (e.g., "No bye-bye!")
- In early stage 1, declarative statements are limited to two constructions: agent + action and action + object.
- In late stage 1, the child forms declarative statements by combining subject + verb + object.
- In late stage 1, the prepositions *in* and *on* are embedded in a sentence.
- In late stage 1, the child uses *and* to form conjoined sentences.

Comprehension
- Comprehension probably precedes production for the first fifty words.
- Understanding names for things and people precedes understanding of words describing actions and relationships
- Understanding of early words appears to be facilitated by knowledge of event routines or scripts

Role of Caregiver
- Provides models for language development and opportunities for communicative interactions
- Assists by expanding and extending the child's utterances

traditional grammatical categories, how can they be classified?

10. What functions are filled by the child's first words?

11. What does the stage 1 child seem to understand about conversational techniques?

12. What are the developmental changes in communication functions associated with the perlocutionary, illocutionary, and locutionary stages?

13. What are the primary semantic-syntactic rules the child expresses in stage 1?

14. How do children construct the following sentence types as they progress through stage 1: declaratives, interrogatives, negatives, and conjoined?

15. What is the importance of joint referencing in the development of child language?

16. What language knowledge might be reflected in the child's first word combinations?

17. Discuss the evolving relationship between comprehension and production during early language development.

18. Describe Dore's categorization scheme for children's early utterances.

19. What is the role of the child's caregiver during stage 1 of language development?

References and Suggested Readings

Acredolo, L., & Goodwyn, S. (1998). *Baby signs.* Chicago: Contemporary Books.

Ahktar, N. (2002). Relevance and early word learning. *Journal of Child Language, 29,* 677–686.

Ahktar, N., Dunham, F., & Dunham, P. (1991). Directive interactions and early vocabulary development: The role of joint attentional focus. *Journal of Child Language, 18,* 41–49.

Aslin, R., Pisoni, D., & Jusczyk, P. (1983). Auditory development and speech perception in infancy. In M. Haith & J. Campos (Eds.), *Handbook of child psychology: Vol. 2. Infancy and developmental psychobiology.* New York: Wiley.

Austin, J. (1962). *How to do things with words.* London: Oxford University Press.

Barrett, M., Harris, M., & Chasin, J. (1991). Early lexical development and maternal speech: A comparison of children's initial and subsequent uses of words. *Journal of Child Language, 18,* 21–40.

Bates, E. (1979). *The emergence of symbols: Cognition and communication in infancy.* New York: Academic Press.

Bates, E., Bretherton, L., Shore, C., & McNew, S. (1983). Names, gestures and objects: The role of context in the emergence of symbols. In K. Nelson (Ed.), *Children's language* (Vol. 4). Hillsdale, NJ: Erlbaum.

Bates, E., Camaioni, L., & Volterra, V. (1975). The acquisition of performatives prior to speech. *Merrill-Palmer Quarterly, 21,* 205–216.

Bates, E., Marchman, V., Thal, D., Fenson, L., Dale, P., Reznick, J., Reilly, J., & Hartung, J. (1994). Developmental and stylistic variation in the composition of early vocabulary. *Journal of Child Language, 21,* 85–123.

Bauer, D., Goldfield, R., & Reznick, J. (2002). Alternative approaches to analyzing individual difference in the rates of early vocabulary development. *Applied Psycholinguistics, 22,* 313–335.

Baumwell, L., Tamis-LeMonda, C., & Bornstein, M. (1997). Maternal verbal sensitivity and child language comprehension. *Infant Behavior and Development, 20,* 247–258.

Benedict, H. (1979). Early lexical development: comprehension and production. *Journal of Child Language, 6,* 183–200.

Bernstein, D. (1989). Language development: The preschool years. In D. Bernstein & E. Tiegerman (Eds.), *Language and communication disorders in children* (2nd ed.). Upper Saddle River, NJ: Merrill/Prentice Hall.

Blake, J., & deBoysson-Bardies, B. (1992). Patterns of babbling: A cross-linguistic study. *Journal of Child Language, 19,* 51–74.

Bloom, L. (1970). *Language development: Form and function of emerging grammars.* Cambridge, MA: MIT Press.

Bloom, L. (1973). *One word at a time: The use of single-word utterances before syntax.* The Hague: Mouton.

Bloom, L. (1974). Talking, understanding, and thinking. In R. Schiefelbusch & L. Lloyd (Eds.), *Language perspectives: Acquisition, retardation and intervention.* Baltimore: University Park Press.

Bloom, L., & Lahey, M. (1978). *Language development and language disorders.* New York: Wiley.

Bloom, L., Rocissano, L., & Hood, L. (1976). Adult–child discourse: Developmental interaction between information processing and linguistic interaction. *Cognitive Psychology, 8,* 521–552.

Bowerman, M. (1978). The acquisition of word meaning: An investigation into some current conflicts. In N. Waterson & C. Snow (Eds.), *The development of communication.* New York: Wiley.

Braine, M. (1963). The ontogeny of English phrase structure: The first phrase. *Language, 39,* 1–13.

Branigan, G. (1979). Some reasons why successive single word utterances are not. *Journal of Child Language, 6,* 411–421.

Brazelton, T., & Cramer, B. (1990). *The earliest relationship: Parents, infants, and the drama of early attachment.* Reading, MA: Addison-Wesley.

Brent, M., & Siskin, J. (2001). The role of exposure to isolated words in early vocabulary development. *Cognition, 81,* B33–B44.

Bretherton, I. (1988). How to do things with one word: The ontogenesis of intentional message-making in infancy. In M. Smith & J. Locke (Eds.), *The emergent lexicon: The child's development of a linguistic vocabulary.* San Diego, CA: Academic Press.

Bridger, W. (1961). Sensory habituation and discrimination in the human neonate. *American Journal of Psychiatry, 117,* 991–996.

Brown, R. (1973). *A first language: The early stages.* Cambridge, MA: Harvard University Press.

Bruner, J. (1975). The ontogenesis of speech acts. *Journal of Child Language, 2,* 1–19.

Bruner, J. (1981). The social context of language acquisition. *Language and Communication, 1,* 155–178.

Bushnell, I., Sai, F., & Mullin, J. (1989). Neonatal recognition of the mother's face. *British Journal of Developmental Psychology, 7,* 3–15.

Butterworth, G., & Morissette, P. (1996). Onset of pointing and the acquisition of language in infancy. *Journal of Reproductive and Infant Psychology, 14*, 219–231.

Campbell, A., & Namy, L. (2003). The role of social referential context and verbal and nonverbal symbol learning. *Child Development, 74*, 549–563.

Carpenter, K. (1991). Later rather than sooner: Extralinguistic categories in the acquisition of Thai classifiers. *Journal of Child Language, 18*, 93–113.

Carter, A. (1975). The transformation of sensorimotor morphemes into words: A case study of the development of "more" and "mine." *Journal of Child Language, 2*, 233–250.

Caselli, M. (1990). Communicative gestures and first words. In V. Bolterra & C. Erting (Eds.), *From gesture to sign in hearing and deaf children* (pp. 56–67). New York: Springer.

Chapman, R. (1978). Comprehension strategies in children. In J. Kavanaugh & W. Strange (Eds.), *Speech and language in the laboratory, school, and clinic*. Cambridge, MA: MIT Press.

Childres, J., & Tomasello, M. (2002). Two-year-olds learn novel nouns, verbs, and conventional actions from massed or distributed exposures. *Developmental Psychology, 38*, 967–978.

Choi, S. (1988). The semantic development of negation: A cross-linguistic longitudinal study. *Journal of Child Language, 15*, 517–531.

Clark, E. (1973). What's in a word? On the child's acquisition of semantics in his first language. In T. Moore (Ed.), *Cognitive development and the acquisition of language*. New York: Academic Press.

Clark, E. (1975). Knowledge, context and strategy in the acquisition of meaning. In D. Dato (Ed.), *Developmental psycholinguistics: Theory and application*. Washington, D.C.: Georgetown University Press.

Clarke-Stewart, K. (1973). Interactions between mothers and their young children: Characteristics and consequences. *Monographs of the Society for Research in Child Development, 38* (Serial No. 153).

Crystal, D., Fletcher, P., & Garman, M. (1976). *The grammatical analysis of language disability: A procedure for assessment and remediation*. London: Arnold.

Davis, B., & MacNeilage, P. (1990). Acquisition of correct vowel production: A quantitative case study. *Journal of Speech and Hearing Research, 33*, 16–27.

deVilliers, J., & deVilliers, P. (1978). *Language acquisition*. Cambridge, MA: Harvard University Press.

D'Odorico, L. (1984). Nonsegmental features in prelinguistic communications: An analysis of some types of infant cry and noncry vocalizations. *Journal of Child Language, 11*, 17–27.

D'Odorico, L., Cassibba, R., & Salerni, N. (1997). Temporal relationships between gaze and vocal behavior in prelinguistic and linguistic communication. *Journal of Psycholinguistic Research, 26*, 539–556.

Dore, J. (1974). A pragmatic description of early language development. *Journal of Psycholinguistic Research, 3*, 343–350.

Dore, J. (1975). Holophrases, speech acts and language universals. *Journal of Child Language, 2*, 21–40.

Ebeling, K., & Gelman, S. (1994). Children's use of context in interpreting "big" and "little." *Child Development, 65,* 1178–1192.

Eimas, P., Siqueland, E., Jusczyk, P., & Vigorito, J. (1971). Speech perception in infants, *Science, 171,* 303–306.

Eisenberg, R. (1976). *Auditory competence in early life: The roots of communicative behavior.* Baltimore: University Park Press.

Farrar, M. (1990). Discourse and the acquisition of grammatical morphemes. *Journal of Child Language, 17,* 607–624.

Fernald, A. (1985). Four-month-old infants prefer to listen to motherese. *Infant Behavior and Development, 8,* 181–195.

Fernald, A. (1994). Human maternal vocalizations to infants as biologically relevant signals: An evolutionary perspective. In P. Bloom (Ed.), *Language acquisition: Core readings.* Cambridge, MA: MIT Press.

Fernald, A., & Morikawa, H. (1993). Common themes and cultural differences in Japanese and American mothers' speech to infants. *Child Development, 64,* 637–656.

Ferguson, C. (1978). Learning to pronounce: The earliest stages of phonological development in the child. In F. Minifie & L. Lloyd (Eds.), *Communicative and cognitive abilities—Early behavioral assessment.* Baltimore: University Park Press.

Folger, J., & Chapman, R. (1978). A pragmatic analysis of spontaneous imitations. *Journal of Child Language, 5,* 25–38.

Gelman, S., Coley, J., Rosengran, K., Hartman, E., & Pappas, A. (1998). Beyond labeling: The role of maternal input in the acquisition of richly structured categories. *Monographs of the Society for Research in Child Development, 63*(253).

Gelman, S., Croft, W., Fu, P., Clausner, T., & Gottfried, G. (1998). Why is a pomegranate an *apple?* The role of shape, taxonomic relatedness, and prior lexical knowledge in children's overextensions of *apple* and *dog. Journal of Child Language, 25,* 267–291.

Gentner, D. (1982). Why nouns are learned before verbs: Linguistic relativity versus natural partitioning. In S. Kuczaj (Ed.), *Language development: Vol 2. Language, thought, and culture.* Hillsdale, NJ: Erlbaum.

Ginsberg, G., & Kilbourne, B. (1988). Emergence of vocal alternation in mother–infant interchanges. *Journal of Child Language, 15,* 221–235.

Goldfield, B. (2000). Nouns before verbs in comprehension vs. production: The view from pragmatics. *Journal of Child Language, 27,* 501–520.

Goldfield, B., & Reznick, J. (1990). Early lexical acquisitions: Rate, content, and the vocabulary spurt. *Journal of Child Language, 17,* 171–183.

Goldstein, M., King, A., & West, M. (2003). Social interaction shapes babbling: Testing parallels between birdsong and speech. *Proceedings of the National Academy of Sciences, 100,* 8030–8035.

Goodsitt, J., Morse, P., VerHoeve, J., & Cowan, N. (1984). Infant speech recognition in multisyllabic contexts. *Child Development, 55,* 903–910.

Gopnik, A., & Choi, S. (1990). Language and cognition. *First Language, 10,* 199–216.

Gopnik, A., & Meltzoff, A. (1984). Semantic and cognitive development in 15- to 21-month-old children. *Journal of Child Development, 11,* 495–513.

Gopnik, A., & Meltzoff, A. (1986). Relations between semantic and cognitive development in the one-word stage: The specificity hypothesis. *Child Development, 57,* 1040–1053.

Gopnik, A., & Meltzoff, A. (1987). The development of categorization in the second year and its relation to other cognitive and linguistic developments. *Child Development, 58,* 1523–1531.

Greenfield, P. (1978). Informativeness, presupposition, and semantic choice in single-word utterances. In N. Waterson & C. Snow (Eds.), *The development of communication.* New York: Wiley.

Greenfield, P., & Smith, J. (1976). *The structure of communication in early language development.* New York: Academic Press.

Grieser, D. L., & Kuhl, P. (1988). Maternal speech to infants in a tonal language: Support for universal prosodic features in motherese. *Developmental Psychology, 24,* 14–20.

Halliday, M. (1975). *Learning how to mean: Explorations in the development of language.* New York: Arnold.

Hammer, C., & Weiss, A. (1999). Guiding language development: How African American mothers and their infants structure play interactions. *Journal of Speech, Language, and Hearing Research, 42,* 1219–1233.

Harding, C. (1983a). Acting with intention: A framework for examining the development of intention. In L. Feagans, C. Garvey, & R. Golinkoff (Eds.), *The origins and growth of communication.* Norwood, NJ: Ablex.

Harding, C. (1983b). Setting the stage for language acquisition: Communication development in the first year. In R. Golinkoff (Ed.), *The transition from prelinguistic to linguistic communication.* Hillsdale, NJ: Erlbaum.

Hickey, T. (1993). Identifying formulas in first language acquisition. *Journal of Child Language, 20,* 27–41.

Hilke, D. (1988). Infant vocalizations and changes in experience. *Journal of Child Language, 15,* 1–15.

Hirsh-Pasek, K., Treiman, R., & Schneiderman, M. (1984). Brown and Hanlon revisited: Mother's sensitivity to ungrammatical forms. *Journal of Child Language, 11,* 81–88.

Hoff, E., & Naigles, L. (2002). How children use input to acquire a lexicon. *Child Development, 73,* 418–433.

Horgan, D. (1981). Rate of language acquisition and noun emphasis. *Journal of Psycholinguistic Research, 10,* 629–640.

Hummer, P., Wimmer, H., & Antes, G. (1993). On the origins of denial. *Journal of Child Language, 20,* 607–618.

Huttenlocher, J. (1974) The origins of language comprehension. In R. Soslo (Ed.), *Theories in cognitive psychology: The Loyola symposium.* New York: Wiley.

Ingram, D. (1974). The relationship between comprehension and production. In R. Schiefelbusch & L. Lloyd (Eds.), *Language perspectives— Acquisition, retardation, and intervention.* Baltimore: University Park Press.

Ingram, D. (1976). *Phonological disability in children.* London: Arnold.

James, S. (1990). *Normal language acquisition.* Austin, TX: PRO-ED.

Jusczyk, P. W. (1997). *The discovery of spoken language.* Cambridge, MA: MIT Press.

Kaplan, P., Bachorowski, J., Smoski, M., & Hudenko, W. (2002). Infants of depressed mothers, although competent learners, fail to learn in response to their own mothers' infant-directed speech. *Psychological Science, 13,* 268–271.

Karrass, J., Braungart-Rieker, J., Mullins, J., & Lefever, J. (2002). Processes in language acquisition: The roles of gender, attention, and maternal encouragement of attention over time. *Journal of Child Language, 29,* 519–543.

Kaye, K. (1977). Towards the origin of dialogue. In H. Schaffer (Ed.), *Studies in mother–child interaction.* London: Academic Press.

Kaye, K. (1979). Thickening thin data: The maternal role in developing communication and language. In M. Bullowa (Ed.), *Before speech.* New York: Cambridge University Press.

Kaye, K. (1980). Why we don't talk "baby talk" to babies. *Journal of Child Language, 7,* 489–507.

Kessen, W., Levine, J., & Wendrich, K. (1979). The imitation of pitch in infants. *Infant Behavior and Development, 2,* 93–100.

Legerstee, M., & Barillas, Y. (2003). Sharing attention and pointing to objects at 12 months: Is the intentional stance implied? *Cognitive Development, 18,* 91–110.

Lewis, M. (1951). *Infant speech: A study of the beginnings of language.* New York: Humanities Press.

Lynch, M., Oller, K., & Steffens, M. (1989). Development of speech-like vocalizations in a child with congenital absence of cochleas: The case of total deafness. *Applied Psycholinguistics, 10,* 315–333.

Marchman, V., & Bates, E. (1991). *Vocabulary size and composition as predictors of morphological development* (Technical Report No. 9103). University of California, San Diego: Center for Research in Language.

Marchman, V., & Bates, E. (1994). Continuity in lexical and morphological development: A test of the critical mass hypothesis. *Journal of Child Language, 21,* 339–366.

Marcos, H. (1987). Communicative function of pitch range and pitch direction in infants. *Journal of Child Language, 14,* 255–268.

Masataka, N. (1992). Pitch characteristics of Japanese maternal speech to infants. *Journal of Child Language, 19,* 213, 213–223.

Masataka, N. (1993). Effects of contingent and noncontingent maternal stimulation on the vocal behavior of three- to four-month-old Japanese infants. *Journal of Child Language, 20,* 303–312.

McCathren, R., Warren, S., & Yoder, P. (1996). Prelinguistic predictors of later language development. In K. Cole, P. Dale, & D. Thal (Eds.), *Assessment of communication and language.* Baltimore: Brookes.

Meadows, D., Elias, G., & Bain, J. (2000). Mother's ability to identify infants' communicative acts. *Journal of Child Language, 27,* 393–406.

McDonough, L. (2002). Basic-level nouns: First learned but misunderstood. *Journal of Child Language, 29,* 357–377.

Mervis, C., & Mervis, C. (1988). Role of adult input in young children's category evolution: An observational study. *Journal of Child Language, 15,* 257–272.

Messinger, D., & Fogel, A. (1998). Give and take: The development of conventional infant gestures. *Merrill-Palmer Quarterly, 44,* 566–590.

Miller, J., & Chapman, R. (1981). The relation between age and mean length of utterance in morphemes. *Journal of Speech and Hearing Research, 24,* 154–161.

Miller, J., Chapman, R., Branston, M., & Reichle, J. (1980). Language comprehension in sensorimotor stages V and VI. *Journal of Speech and Hearing Research, 23,* 284–311.

Mitchell, P., & Kent, R. (1990). Phonetic variation in multisyllabic babbling. *Journal of Child Language, 17,* 247–265.

Moon, C., Bever, T., & Fifer, W. (1992). Canonical and non-canonical syllable discrimination by two-day-old infants. *Journal of Child Language, 19,* 1–17.

Murray, A., Johnson, J., & Peters, J. (1990). Fine tuning of utterance length to preverbal infants: Effects on later language development. *Journal of Child Language, 17,* 511–525.

Nakazima, S. (1975). Phonemicization and symbolization in language development. In E. Lenneberg & E. Lenneberg (Eds.), *Foundations of language: Vol. 1. A multidisciplinary approach.* New York: Academic Press.

Nazzi, T., Bertoncini, J., & Mehler, J. (1998). Language discrimination by newborns: Toward an understanding of the role of rhythm. *Journal of Experimental Psychology: Human Perception and Performance, 24,* 756–766.

Nelson, K. (1973). Structure and strategy in learning to talk. *Monographs of the Society for Research in Child Development, 38.*

Nelson, K. (1974). Concept, word and sentence: Interrelations in acquisition and development. *Psychological Review, 31,* 267–285.

Oller, D. (1980). The emergence of the sounds of speech in infancy. In G. Yeni-Komshian, J. Kavanagh, & C. Ferguson (Eds.), *Child phonology: Vol. 1. Production.* New York: Academic Press.

Oller, D., & Eilers, R. (1988). The role of audition in infant babbling. *Child Development, 59,* 441–449.

Oller, D., Eilers, R., Bull, D., & Carney, A. (1985). Prespeech vocalizations of a deaf infant: A comparison with normal metaphonological development. *Journal of Speech and Hearing Research, 28,* 47–62.

Owens, R. (1991). *Language disorders: A functional approach to assessment and intervention.* Upper Saddle River, NJ: Merrill/Prentice Hall.

Owens, R. (1996). *Language development: An introduction* (4th ed.). Boston: Allyn & Bacon.

Owens, R. (2001). *Language development: An introduction* (5th ed.). Boston: Allyn & Bacon.

Owens, R. (2005). *Language development: An introduction* (6th ed.). Boston: Allyn & Bacon.

Paul, R. (1990). Comprehension strategies: Interactions between world knowledge and the development of sentence comprehension. *Topics in Language Disorders, 10*(3), 63–75.

Penman, R., Cross, T., Milgrom-Friedman, J., & Meares, R. (1983). Mothers' speech to prelingual infants: A pragmatic analysis. *Journal of Child Language, 10,* 17–34.

Petitto, L. (1984). *From gesture to symbol: The relationship between form and the meaning in the acquisition of personal pronouns in American Sign Language.* Unpublished doctoral dissertation, Harvard University, Cambridge, MA.

Petitto, L. (1985a). *"Language" in the prelinguistic child* (Technical Report No. 4). Montreal: McGill University, Department of Psychology.

Petitto, L. (1985b, October). *On the use of prelinguistic gestures in hearing and deaf children.* Paper presented at the 10th Annual Boston University Conference on Language Development, Boston.

Petitto, L. (1986). *From gesture to symbol: The relationship between form and the meaning in the acquisition of personal pronouns in American Sign Language.* Bloomington: Indiana University Linguistics Club Press.

Petitto, L. (1987). On the autonomy of language and gesture: Evidence from the acquisition of personal pronouns in American Sign Language. *Cognition, 27*(1), 1–52.

Petitto, L. (1988). "Language" in the prelinguistic child. In F. Kessel (Ed.), *Development of language and language researchers: Essays in honor of Roger Brown* (pp. 187–221). Hillsdale, NJ: Erlbaum.

Petitto, L., & Marentette, P. (1990, October). *The timing of linguistic milestones in sign language acquisition: Are first signs acquired earlier than first words?* Paper presented at the 15th Annual Boston University Conference on Language Development, Boston.

Pettito, L., & Marentette, P. (1991, April). The timing of linguistic milestones in sign and spoken language acquisition. In L. Petitto (Chair), *Are the linguistic milestones in signed and spoken language acquisition similar or different?* Symposium conducted at the Biennial Meeting of the Society for Research in Child Development, Seattle, WA.

Petrovich-Bartell, N., Cowan, N., & Morse, P. (1982). Mothers' perceptions of infant distress vocalizations. *Journal of Speech and Hearing Research, 25,* 371–376.

Phillips, J. (1973). Syntax and vocabulary of mothers' speech to young children: Age and sex comparisons. *Child Development, 44,* 182–185.

Prutting, C. (1979). Process: The action of moving forward progressively from one point to another on the way to completion. *Journal of Speech and Hearing Disorders, 44,* 3–30.

Reed, V. (Ed.). (1986). *An introduction to children with language disorders.* New York: Macmillan.

Rees, N. (1972). The role of babbling in the child's acquisition of language. *British Journal of Disorders in Communication, 4,* 17–23.

Robb, M., & Saxman, J. (1990). Syllable durations of preword and early word vocalizations. *Journal of Speech and Hearing Research, 33,* 585–593.

Rollins, P. (2003). Caregivers' contingent comments to 9-month-old infants: Relationship with later language. *Applied Psycholinguistics, 24,* 221–234.

Rondal, J., & Cession, A. (1990). Input evidence regarding the semantic bootstrapping hypothesis. *Journal of Child Language, 17,* 711–717.

Ryan, J. (1974). Early language development: Towards a communicational analysis. In P. Richards (Ed.), *The integration of a child into a social world.* London: Cambridge University Press.

Sachs, J. (1989). Communication development in infancy. In J. Berko-Gleason (Ed.), *The development of language.* Upper Saddle River, NJ: Merrill/Prentice Hall.

Samuelson, L., & Smith, L. (1998). Memory and attention make smart word learning: An alternative account of Akhtar, Carpenter, and Tomasello. *Child Development, 69,* 94–104.

Scherer, N., & Olswang, L. (1984). Role of mothers' expansions in stimulating children's language production. *Journal of Speech and Hearing Research, 27,* 387–396.

Schlesinger, I. (1971). Production of utterances and language acquisition. In D. Slobin (Ed.), *The ontogenesis of grammar.* New York: Academic Press.

Schlesinger, I. (1977). The role of cognitive development and linguistic input in language acquisition. *Journal of Child Language, 4,* 153–169.

Schwartz, R., & Leonard, L. (1984). Words, objects, and actions in early lexical acquisition. *Journal of Speech and Hearing Research, 27,* 119–127.

Searle, J. (1965). What is a speech act? In M. Black (Ed.), *Philosophy in America.* New York: Allen & Unwin, Cornell University Press.

Searle, J. (1969). *Speech acts.* Cambridge: Cambridge University Press.

Siegel, G., Cooper, M., Morgan, J., & Renneise-Sarshad, R. (1990). Imitation of intonation by infants. *Journal of Speech and Hearing Research, 33,* 9–15.

Singh, L., Morgan, J., & Best, C. (2002). Infants' listening perferences: Baby talk or happy talk? *Infancy, 3,* 365–394.

Smith, B., Brown-Sweeney, S., & Stoel-Gammon, C. (1989). A quantitative analysis of reduplicated and variegated babbling. *First Language, 9,* 175–189.

Snow, C. (1977). The development of conversation between mothers and babies. *Journal of Child Language, 4,* 1–22.

Snow, C., Perlmann, R., Berko-Gleason, J., & Hooshyar, N. (1990). Developmental perspectives on politeness: Sources of children's knowledge. *Journal of Pragmatics, 14,* 289–305.

Stark, R. (1978). Features of infant sounds: The emergence of cooing. *Journal of Child Language, 5,* 1–12.

Stark, R. (1979). Prespeech segmental feature development. In P. Fletcher & M. Garman (Eds.), *Language acquisition.* New York: Cambridge University Press.

Stark, R. (1980). Stages of speech development in the first year of life. In G. Yeni-Komshian, J. Kavanagh, & C. Ferguson (Eds.), *Child phonology: Vol. 1. Production.* New York: Academic Press.

Stark, R. (1981). Infant vocalizations: A comprehensive view. *Infant Mental Health Journal, 2,* 118–128.

Stark, R. (1986). Prespeech segmental feature development. In P. Fletcher & M. Garman (Eds.), *Language acquisition: Studies in first language acquisition.* New York: Cambridge University Press.

Stark, R. (1989). Temporal patterning of cry and non-cry sounds in the first eight months of life. *First Language, 9,* 107–136.

Stark, R., Bernstein, L., Demorest, M. (1993). Vocal communication in the first 18 months of life, *Journal of Speech and Hearing Research, 36* (3), 548–558.

Stoel-Gammon, C. (1988). Prelinguistic vocalizations of hearing-impaired and normally hearing subjects: A comparison of consonantal inventories. *Journal of Speech and Hearing Disorders, 53,* 302–315.

Stoel-Gammon, C., & Otomo, K. (1986). Babbling development of hearing-impaired and normally hearing subjects. *Journal of Speech and Hearing Disorders, 51,* 33–41.

Sullivan, J., & Horowitz, F. (1983). The effects of intonation on infant attention: The role of the rising intonation contour. *Journal of Child Language, 10,* 521–534.

Tomasello, M. (1999). Social cognition before the revolution. In P. Rochat (Ed.), *Early social cognition: Understanding others in the first months of life* (pp. 301–314). Mahwah, NJ: Erlbaum.

Tomasello, M., Conti-Ramsden, G., & Ewert, B. (1990). Young children's conversations with their mothers and fathers: Differences in breakdown and repair. *Journal of Child Language, 17,* 115–130.

Trotter, R. (1983, August). Baby face. *Psychology Today, 17*(8), 14–20.

Vaidyanathan, R. (1988). Development of forms and functions of interrogatives in children: A language study of Tamil. *Journal of Child Language, 15,* 533–549.

Vaidyanathan, R. (1991). Development of forms and functions of negation in the early stages of language acquisition: A study of Tamil. *Journal of Child Language, 18,* 51–60.

von Raffler-Engle, W. (1973). The development from sound to phoneme in child language. In C. Ferguson & D. Slobin (Eds.), *Studies of child language development.* New York: Holt, Rinehart & Winston.

Wells, G. (1985). *Language development in the preschool years.* New York: Cambridge University Press.

Wolff, P. (1969). The natural history of crying and other vocalizations in early infancy. In B. Foss (Ed.), *Determinants of infant behavior IV.* London: Methuen.

5

The Saga Continues: Language
Development through the Preschool Years

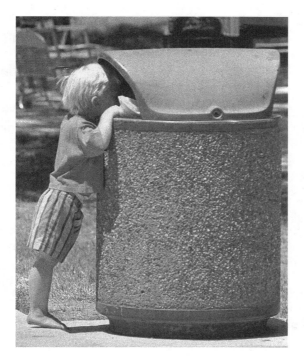

CHAPTER OBJECTIVES

Welcome to the wild and wonderful preschool years, a time of inexhaustible energy, limitless curiosity, and explosive communication development. In this chapter, we examine the phenomenal changes in the child's communication abilities as he runs, jumps, and shrieks through four more stages of language development. At the close of the preceding chapter, the child was just beginning to combine words. By the close of this chapter, she will be an enthusiastic and reasonably competent conversationalist. She will also begin to show evidence of a communication skill we have not seen to this point. She will begin to tell stories, a skill commonly referred to as *narration*. Her narrative skills mature during the school years, but they begin to emerge during the preschool years. Specifically, this chapter is designed to facilitate understanding of the following topics:

Stage 2 (Twenty-Seven to Thirty Months)

- Emergence of grammatical morphemes, pronouns, and auxiliary verbs

- Using phrases and clauses to create more adult-like sentences

- Early versions of negation, the interrogative form, and imperatives

- Cognitive development reflected in vocabulary and semantic advances

- Struggles with conversational skills such as turn-taking and repair

Stage 3 (Thirty-One to Thirty-Four Months)

- More consistent use of grammatical morphemes, pronouns, and auxiliary verbs

- Elaboration of noun phrases in both subjective and objective positions of sentences

- More adult-like versions of negation and the interrogative form

- Slow progress on the conversational front

Stage 4 (Thirty-Five to Forty Months)

- Elaboration of sentences by embedding

- Improvements in turn-taking, topic maintenance, and presuppositional

skills, and learning the art of indirect requests

Stage 5 (Forty-One to Forty-Six Months)

- Mastery of a majority of grammatical morphemes

- Noun and verb phrases do not increase significantly in length but are more complete and correct, according to adult standards

- Multiple embeddings and clausal conjoining

- Struggling with rules of conversational etiquette

- The beginnings of narrative discourse

- Understanding language

- Language comprehension and production supported by cognitive development

- Understanding active and passive sentences

- Learning English word order: Does comprehension precede production?

- Understanding words that identify spatial, temporal, quantity, and dimensional relationships

---

The "twos" may be terrible for the parent trying to keep track of her increasingly active child, but the twos and threes and the remainder of the preschool years are wonderful and exciting from a language development point of view. As children exit stage 1, they are already talking, but over the next few years they will experience unbelievable gains in language ability. In this chapter, we trace those changes through four more stages of language development. You will notice that virtually all of these changes are elaborations of abilities that emerged in stage 1.

Stage 2: Elaborating Structure and Refining Meaning

The child is typically in this stage from twenty-seven months to about thirty months, and his MLU is 2.0 to 2.5 morphemes. Brown (1973) has suggested that the greatest change occurring during stage 2 is what he calls the **"modulations of meaning"** in simple sentences, which is accomplished by the use of grammatical morphemes. To modulate means to modify or regulate, and both of these synonyms are helpful in understanding what occurs when grammatical morphemes are added to base words. By adding *-ed* to a verb such as *show,* we can modify the tense from present to past. We use grammatical morphemes to regulate or govern forms of words so that we create the precise meaning we want to express. The timing of *to show* may be just as important to the message as the meaning of the verb itself. In some circumstances, it might be important to distinguish between having one husband or two husbands. In other cases, prepositions such as *on* or *in* become critically important to meaning. Did he put my daughter *on* the car or *in* the car? See what we mean?

Most of the terms used to describe grammatical morphemes will be familiar, but some supplementary explanations and terminology may be useful. The term **inflection** is sometimes used to refer to a change in a word created by the addition of a grammatical morpheme. We can inflect nouns, for example, to make them plural or possessive. We can inflect verbs to make them past tense or to make them present progressive. The term **present progressive** is used to describe an action of limited duration that is taking place right now. Think about how you use words such as *running, writing, eating.* These are present progressive forms of common verbs. We make some verbs past tense by adding *-ed.* This is known as **regular** past tense. *Looked* is a regular past tense form. Other verbs such as *run, sit* and *go* are made past tense, not by inflection but by word changes. These words require **irregular** past tense changes resulting in *ran, sat,* and *went.* The verb *to be* presents some special problems of its own. This verb can be a **main** verb or **copula** as in "He is my dog," or "I was a bad boy." The verb *to be* can also be used as a helping or **auxiliary** verb as in sentences such as "He is running," or "I was eating." Note that when the verb *to be* is used as an auxiliary, the grammatical morpheme *-ing* is always attached to the main verb that follows the auxiliary. The child must sort out which verb forms can be **contracted** or reduced and which forms cannot be contracted. In our examples, it is proper to contract *He is* in either the copula or auxiliary form to *He's,* but it is not acceptable to contract *I was.* There is much to learn in the acquisition of grammatical morphemes, and unfortunately the rules sometimes do not make much sense. That children sometimes produce forms that do not match adult forms is not surprising. That they master most of the basic grammatical morphemes by the time they are four years old is a miracle!

Although some grammatical morphemes begin to emerge in the latter part of stage 1, their primary development begins in stage 2. Several studies have focused on fourteen grammatical morphemes. Brown (1973) and James and Khan (1982) examined the development of these morphemes in longitudinal studies, and de Villiers and de Villiers (1973) looked at them in a cross-sectional study. Although there are some differences among the three studies, especially with regard to the acquisition of irregular past tense, regular past tense, and the contractible copula, the results suggest the following order of acquisition for the fourteen targeted morphemes:

Grammatical Morpheme	Example	Age Range of Mastery
Present progressive	She runn*ing*.	19–28
In (preposition)	Milk *in* cup.	27–30
On (preposition)	Doggie *on* bed.	27–30
Regular plural	Girls playing.	27–33
Irregular past tense	Mommy *went* work.	25–46
Possessive	Billy*'s* ball.	26–40
Uncontractible copula	Billy *was* bad.	27–39
Articles *(the, a)*	Daddy eating *the* cookie.	28–46
Regular past tense	Mommy look*ed*.	26–48
Regular third person singular	She *eats*.	26–46
Irregular third person singular	Daddy *has* cookie.	28–50
Uncontractible auxiliary	I *was* eating.	29–48
Contractible copula	Billy*'s* bad.	29–49
Contractible auxiliary	He*'s* running.	30–50

Adapted from R. Brown (1973); J. Miller (1981)

In all three studies, the criterion for mastery was 90 percent correct usage in *obligatory contexts*. That is, when an utterance *requires* the use of a given grammatical morpheme, and the child uses the appropriate morpheme, she has met the grammatical requirement or obligation for that context. An obligatory context can be linguistic or nonlinguistic. If, for example, the child is watching his mother jump rope, and the mother says, "What is Mommy doing?" a correct response from the child would include the present progressive form of "jump." If the child says, "Mommy jumping" or "Mommy jumping rope," or even if the child says "hopping" or "bouncing" or "running," he has produced the correct grammatical morpheme for that context. The mother's language set up a linguistic obligatory context. The obligatory context might be nonlinguistic, however. Assuming the child has just eaten a cookie and is prepared to comment on this masterful feat of mastication and deglutition, she *should* use the past tense and say something like, "Ate cookie?" If she uses *ate*, she has met the obligation for irregular past tense in an opportunity set up not by the utterance of someone else but by her own nonverbal, but decidedly oral, actions.

Although researchers have identified age ranges for the mastery of each of these morphemes, it may be more helpful to emphasize what we know about acquisition in general than to focus attention on specific ages. It is important to note, for example, that all of these morphemes begin to emerge during the latter months of stage 1 and throughout stage 2. We see mastery of the earliest grammatical morpheme, present progressive, in some children as young as nineteen months. Emergence of the latest of these selected grammatical morphemes, including irregular third person forms of verbs and the correct sorting of contractible and uncontractible copula and auxiliary verb forms, does not occur until about twenty-eight to thirty months. It is also important to stress that although all of these morphemes appear in stage 2, they are not mastered by some children until stage 5 and beyond. It might be appropriate to remind the reader that some grammatical morphemes are never correctly used by some adults. How often, for example, do adults use the words *data* and *media* as though they are singular noun forms when they are actually plural forms of the words *datum* and *medium?*

One of the interesting, though not surprising, things that happens as children begin to master some of these grammatical morphemes is that they **overextend** or **overgeneralize** their use. When the child begins to make nouns plural by adding *s* to *cat* to make *cats* or the sound *"z"* to *dog* to make *dogs,* he logically concludes that this rule for plural should work on all nouns. His plural form of *man* is *mans* and his plural form of *child* is *childs.* At some point in his language development, he is likely to overextend past tense to produce forms such as *goed, runned, throwed,* and *eated.* Imagine his confusion when he has to learn that the plural of *deer* is *deer* and the plural of *moose* is *moose* or when he learns that the past tense of *burst* is *burst.* Because these productions are unusual and because they catch our attention, we may conclude that they are commonplace in the speech of children at this age.

Chapman, Streim, Crais, Salmon, Strand, and Negri (1992, p. 7), in reviewing Cazden's (1968) original data, found that only about 5 percent of the utterances in the speech samples of her subjects contained overextensions. While it is true, therefore, that a child might occasionally produce an utterance such as, *"Him eated it,"* productions that include overextensions are rare. Keep in mind that while the child is making her own productions, she is listening to the productions of others, and we assume she makes comparisons. In the process of comparing her productions with the productions of those models in her environment who have greater language competence than she does, she will eventually determine how to apply conventional rules. She will figure out, for example, that in some cases the past tense of verbs is indicated by the addition of a grammatical morpheme, as in *tip—tipped.* She will understand that in other cases, past tense is indicated by changing the whole word, as in *run—ran,* and that there are some cases in which the word does not change at all, as in *hurt—hurt.*

Why does the child use overextensions at all? Although it is tempting to view the occurrence of overextensions as evidence that the child is searching for rule-governed patterns, this conclusion is still being debated (Chapman et al., 1992). No matter what all this means at this particular stage of development, it is fair to reach at least one conclusion. Regular rules make language functional. The exceptions make language interesting and prevent us from becoming overconfident.

Pronouns: Words Used to Represent Nouns

We adults use pronouns so easily we probably do not consider how difficult these words are for children acquiring language. The traditional definition of pronoun in English grammar textbooks reads something like this: "A **pronoun** is a word used in place of a noun." Actually, there is much more involved than this, and it is the "much more" that should help you understand why children begin to use pronouns in stage 1 or 2 but may not master the use of some pronouns until stage 5 and beyond. In fact, it is not uncommon for adults to struggle with some pronoun forms, and some of us never get them right!

Consider all the language information conveyed by pronouns. Pronouns convey information about gender or the lack of gender. The child must use pronouns such as *she* and *her* to refer to females and *he* and *him* to refer to males, and he must use *it* when the gender is not known or not important. Pronouns convey information about the number of referents, so the child must know the difference between *I* and *we* and between *he* or *she* and *they*, and then there is that ever popular distinction between *you* singular and *you* plural we all love. The child must learn that pronouns differ depending on whether they are used as subjects in sentences or as objects. The pronouns *I, she, he,* and *they,* for example, are **subjective** pronouns, and their **objective** counterparts are *me, her, him,* and *them.* The child must be able to put the right pronoun in the right part of the sentence. This is not an easy task, and it takes the child some time before he gets it right. According to Wells (1985), most subjective and objective pronouns are not mastered until about thirty-six months, which places the child in stage 4.

In addition to knowing where subjective and objective pronouns belong in the structures of sentences, the child must learn that the number represented by the pronoun determines the verb form to be used. She must say "He is" and "She is" but "They are" and "I am." She must learn the possessive forms of pronouns such as *hers, his, mine, their,* and *your* and when and when not to use reflexive pronouns such as *yourself, himself,* and *herself.* The task becomes even more daunting when one considers that the child must understand that when a pronoun is included in a sentence, the meaning of that sentence will be obscured, or lost entirely, if the listener does not know the informational content of the preceding statement or statements. For example, in order for a listener to properly decode the meaning of the pronoun *it,* as in the sentence "John bought it," he must have heard the previous sentence "John loved that sweater." This type of reference, in which a pronoun is used to refer to something in a preceding utterance, is called an **anaphoric** reference. In the example used here, try to imagine what the listener might conclude without the anaphoric reference. Based on his understanding of common slang expressions, the listener, hearing only that, "John bought it," might conclude that John died, and that would not be a good thing, especially for poor John. This is complicated business! Is it any wonder children get confused and say things like "Me wanna go outside," "Her is eating mine cookie," and "Him wants my ball for hisself"?

Fortunately, there is some order to the potential pronoun chaos. As with all dimensions of language, the child acquires pronouns in a progressive and fairly predictable manner, and we will follow this progress as we move through the remaining stages. In general, you will notice that children acquire subjective pronouns such as *she* and *he* before acquiring objective pronouns such as *her* and *him.* They will then acquire pronouns indicating possession such as *his, hers, their,* and *our,* and, finally, they will use reflexive pronouns such as *myself, yourself* and *themselves.*

Within the context of stage 2, we can say this much. Before the child even enters stage 2, he has probably been using a few pronouns including *I, it,* and *this* and *that*. During stage 2 he will add *my, mine, me,* and *you*. Be aware that the child might not use these pronouns correctly in all situations. He might say, "My ball," one time and "Mine ball" at another time. He might use *me* correctly as an objective pronoun when he says, "Kiss me, Mommy," but he might also use *me* as a subjective pronoun when he says, "Me kiss Mommy." It takes time to get all this, that, and the other sorted out.

Auxiliary Verbs

As mentioned earlier, an auxiliary verb is a helping verb. There are **primary** auxiliary verbs such as *have* and *do,* and there are secondary auxiliary verbs such as *can, shall, may,* and *will,* which are also called **modals.** During stage 2, the child begins to use the verbs *have* and *do* as main verbs and as auxiliary verbs. She also produces what are considered "semiauxiliary" verb forms such as *hafta, gonna,* and *wanna* as in "I hafta go potty," and "I wanna go bye-bye."

As we will continue to emphasize with many language forms, children begin to use auxiliary verbs within a wide range of ages (Wells, 1985). So variable are the ages of acquisition that Wells identified the ages at which only 50 percent of the children studied were producing selected forms. The earliest forms to be used by half of these subjects were *do* and *have,* at about twenty-seven months. *Can, be,* and *will* were being produced at about thirty months, and the last two forms to be used by these children were *shall* at thirty-nine months and *could* at forty-two months, ages that extend beyond stage 2.

Developing the Parts of Sentences: Phrases and Clauses

Many of us have probably pondered that strange and unanswerable question: "Is our universe just one cell in the fingernail of some greater creature?" It is interesting to consider the parts that make up wholes, and the more we learn about anything, the more we appreciate the smaller parts and the greater wholes. In the production of language, we are confronted with the parts and wholes issue. We have considered morphology, which is the study of the meaning units of language. We have established that a **morpheme** is the smallest unit of language that has meaning. Words are made up of one or more morphemes, but morphemes are made up of smaller parts called **phonemes** or speech sounds, and as we shall see in a later chapter, phonemes are made up of even smaller bits called **distinctive features.**

At this point, we want to move from the small parts of language to the larger parts. At the end of stage 1, the child was combining words in ways that suggested sentences. In stage 2, he will produce combinations of words that are more recognizable as sentences. To do this, the child must develop an understanding of the basic parts or components of sentences. We call these components *phrases* and *clauses*.

A **phrase** is a combination of words that are related to one another, and the combination serves a grammatical purpose, but a phrase does not contain a subject and a predicate. There are two kinds of phrases: noun phrases and verb phrases. As the name suggests, a **noun phrase** contains a noun and words that describe or modify the noun. There are four kinds of modifiers in noun phrases: determiners, adjectivals, initiators, and postmodifiers (see Table 5.1). A **determiner** is the first unit in a noun phrase and is an article *(a, the)*, possessive pronoun *(my, his, her)*, demonstrative pronoun *(this, that, these, those)*, or a qualifier *(some, most, any)*. An **adjectival** modifies a noun and can be an adjective *(pretty, tall)*, an ordinal *(second, last)*, or a quantifier *(one, couple, few)*. An **initiator** comes before a determiner and places a limit on the noun *(only, all, both, just)*. A **postmodifier,** as its name suggests, is a modifier that comes after the noun. A postmodifier might be a prepositional phrase as in "The fish *in the little tank* is Fred," or it might be a clause as in "The man *who called last night* is my uncle." Although the child is producing noun phrases in stage 2, he tends to use only determiners and adjectivals as modifiers in these phrases. Not until the end of stage 4 will he consistently use initiators and postmodifiers (Bernstein, 1989, p. 112).

To the surprise of no one, a **verb phrase** contains a verb, and it might contain some other supporting or qualifying words (see Table 5.2). In the sentence "The boy is running," the verb phrase is *is running.* The main verb is *run*, which is in the present progressive form and is supported by *is.* A verb phrase might also contain a **modal,** which is a word indicating the "attitude" of the verb. Common modals are *can, will, must, shall,* and *may.* Notice the difference in the attitudes of the verb phrases in these sentences when we just change the modal: (1) "John will go to the party," and (2) "John may go to the party." The only verb phrase elaboration to be mastered in stage 2 is the present progressive form, but the child does produce primitive infinitive verb forms such as "wanna" and "gonna" (Miller, 1981), and by the end of stage 2, the child is typically creating the negative versions of these forms when she produces those sentences we all love to hear: "I can't" or "I won't." The child does not consistently use modals until stage 4, and she makes further elaborations in her verb phrases in stage 5 (Bernstein, 1989, p. 112). Once again, we see that what begins at an early age is often not finished for many months or several years.

Table 5.1 Possible Constituents of a Noun Phrase

Initiator	Determiner	Ordinal	Quantifier	Adjective	Noun	Postmodifiers
Includes words such as *only, nearly, almost, all*	Includes words such as *the, a, this, that, my, his*	Includes words such as *first, last, final*	Includes words such as *one, two, fifteen*	Includes words such as *big, blue, little*	Includes words such as *boy, girl, dog*	Includes prepositional phrases such as *in the middle, on the chair*
Example: Only	the	last	six	little	dogs	on the chair

Note: Additional adjectives could be incorporated into the noun phrase to make it even longer.

Table 5.2 Possible Constituents of a Verb Phrase

Other than tense, number, and a verb, the remaining elements of a verb phrase are optional in a simple, grammatically acceptable sentence. Optional elements have been placed in parentheses.

Tense and Number	(Modals)	(Perfect Aspect)	(Progressive)	Main Verb	(Noun Phrase)
All sentences are either present or past in *form*.	*Can, may, must, shall, will, could, might, should, would*	*have + en*	Auxiliary verb *to be + -ing:* as in "is running." *Is, are, was, were,* or *am + -ing*	*Run, kick, play*	The noun phrase can be a prepositional phrase, noun phrase, noun complement, or adverbial phrase.

Note: In the example sentence below, the verb is in the past tense and all of the optional constituents identified above are used. The production of this sentence is based on Chomsky's transformational generative grammar. To generate the example sentence, a rule called the "affix" or "hopping" rule enables the speaker to move constituents that can be moved. According to the rule, the speaker can move or "affix" these members to the stationary member on the right.

In the example sentence, the movable members are tense, the participle ending -en that accompanies perfect aspect, and the progressive ending -ing that is progressive aspect.

The boy   may   have + *en*   be +   *-ing*   + run   + in the field.

(NP)   (past tense) (modal) (perfect)   (progressive)   (verb)   (prepositional phrase)

After the affix rule is applied, we end up with the sentence *"The boy might have been running in the field."*

A **clause** is a collection of related words with both a subject and a predicate. Some clauses, called **independent clauses,** can stand alone as simple sentences. When two independent clauses are joined by conjunctions like *and* or *but,* they become one **compound sentence.** A **subordinate clause** has a subject and predicate, but it cannot stand alone as a sentence. When a teacher marks a collection of words on an essay as "incomplete," she is often referring to a subordinate clause. In the sentence "John wondered if his life would have meaning when his Harley stopped running," the subordinate clause is *when his Harley stopped running.* The subordinate clause must be attached to an independent clause to create a complete sentence. The successful merging of an independent clause and a subordinate clause results in a **complex sentence.** Obviously, the stage 2 child is a long way from producing complex sentences. What he does understand by the end of stage 2 is that a sentence must contain a noun phrase and a verb phrase. This knowledge allows the thirty-month-old child to produce and understand simple declarative sentences such as "Mommy going work," "Johnny throw ball," and "Doggie eat gerbil!"

Putting the Pieces of Sentences Together

As the child learns to produce and elaborate phrases and clauses, she produces sentences that are more and more complete, syntactically and semantically. Although the most dramatic changes in sentences will not occur until stage 3 and beyond, the child in stage 2 is producing sentences that contain three, four, and more words. Keep in mind that the upper end of the MLU range in this stage is 2.5. The child is still producing single-word utterances, but she is producing fewer of these short utterances and more multiple-word utterances. Her sentences become longer because she is expanding her noun phrases and verb phrases. Her noun phrases include personal pronouns such as *my* and *mine*, demonstrative pronouns such as *this* and *that*, and the articles *a* and *the*. Her verb phrases include the present progressive form marked by *-ing* as well as semiauxiliary verb forms such as *gonna* and *wanna*.

Producing Sentences to Say "No!"

By late stage 1, the child begins to express negation, even in sentences as short as two or three words. In an early study of the development of negation, Klima and Bellugi-Klima (1971) identified three periods. In the first period, their subjects expressed negation by putting *no* at the beginning of a statement as in "No kick that!" In the second period, the negative element was placed in front of the verb as in "I no like that!" In the final period, the auxiliary was added and the child transformed the sentence into its proper negative form as in "Daddy is not going to work."

The three periods of negation noted by Klima and Bellugi-Klima (1971) emerge in a time frame that roughly corresponds to the stages described by Brown (1973). That is, the first of these forms of syntactic negation is typically produced by the child in late stage 1 and early stage 2 when the MLU range is from approximately 1.5 to about 2.25. The second period of negation is produced by the child in late stage 2 and early stage 3 when the MLU range is from 2.25 to 2.75. It is in stage 3 that the child is likely to position the negative element between the subject and predicate, an accomplishment Brown considers to be one of the major highlights of stage 3. The development of additional auxiliaries along with the negative form begins to appear in Klima and Bellugi-Klima's final period, which includes Brown's late stage 3 and early stage 4 in which the MLU ranges from 2.75 to 3.5. Would it be correct to assume that the child has mastered syntactic negation by the time he reaches stage 4? Not hardly! The child is probably going to be beyond his preschool years before he starts using questions that contain negative forms, such as in the sentence "Why don't you like spinach?" (Owens, 2005, p. 319).

According to Bloom (1970), the child in stage 2 understands the concept of negation well enough to express three variations of the negative theme. He can express the *nonexistence* of something as when he says, "Cookie allgone." He can *reject* as when he says, "No nite-nite," to indicate that he does not want to go to bed, and he can express *denial* as when he says, "No doggie," to indicate that the object being identified by his conversational partner as a "dog" is not a dog. This child does not differentiate between *no* and *not,* and sometimes one must consider the situational context to determine what the *no* or *not* really means. For example, the child's mother might say to the child, "Let Mommy put you in your chair," and the child responds, "No Daddy." This could mean that the child is rejecting assistance from his father, but depending on the child's body language and the prosodic variations of his speech, it could mean "I want Daddy to put me into my chair."

By late stage 2, the child is using *no, not, can't,* and *don't* in an undifferentiated manner, but he is beginning to put the negative form between the subject and predicate. You should note that even though the child is using *can't* and *don't* in stage 2, he does not use their positive forms, *can* and *do,* until later (Brown, Cazden, & Bellugi, 1969). It is not appropriate, therefore, to conclude that the stage 2 child understands that *don't* is a contracted form of *do not.* He simply uses *don't* and *can't* as forms of negation, and he might use *can't* when it should be *don't* and vice versa.

Asking Questions: The First Interrogative Forms

Before we consider what the stage 2 child is able to do in creating question forms of sentences, we should consider the functions of questions. Speakers can ask essentially two kinds of questions. They can ask questions that elicit *yes* or *no* answers, and they can ask questions beginning with *who, whose, whom, what, where, which, when, why,* or *how.* Questions that begin with *wh*-words or *how* require answers that provide information. If you ask "What time is it?" your friend will consult his cell phone and provide you invaluable information about the time of day. Knowing the difference between *yes/no* questions and *wh*-questions should help you understand why the following exchange can be funny: A man asks, "Can you tell me where Grand Central Station is?" The second man answers, *"Yes."* The first man intended a *wh*-question because he needed information, but the second man perceived a *yes/no* question. Well, guess you had to be there.

A *yes/no* question is usually created by moving an auxiliary verb in front of the subject and closing the sentence with a rising intonation. The sentence "He was going to the store" is transformed into a *yes/no* question by moving the *was* in front of the *he* to create "Was he going to the store?" If the statement to be transformed does not have an auxiliary verb, the speaker must add the appropriate form of *do,* so that "You have my steak," becomes "Do you have my steak?" or "John plans to come home" becomes "Does John plan to come home?" A *wh*-question is formed by inverting the subject and auxiliary and adding the appropriate *wh*- word or *how* to the beginning of the sentence. "He is sitting" can be transformed into "Where is he sitting?" "How is he sitting" or "Why is he sitting?"

The stage 2 child is obviously not ready for the sometimes convoluted questions adults ask, such as, "Where is he sitting, with whom, and why?" She is asking questions, however, and some of these questions call for more than *yes* or *no.* Klima and Bellugi-Klima (1971) have identified three periods in the development of interrogative forms. The first of these periods occurs in the latter part of stage 1 and early stage 2 of language development, when we would expect to see MLU values of 1.75 to 2.25.

New experiences, new discoveries, and neverending questions.

In period 1, between the ages of twenty-five and twenty-eight months, the child is still asking *yes/no* questions by adding rising intonations to simple declarative sentences, the same method she used at the single-word stage of development. By adding a rising intonation to the end of "Go bye-bye," she transforms a statement or demand into a question meaning "Are we going bye-bye?" or "Can we go bye-bye?" In this first phase, she is also asking a few simple *wh*-questions, such as "What this?" or "Where Mommy?" "What" and "where" questions are most common, probably because they focus on two of the most prominent semantic categories the child uses at this age, naming and locating. In turn, these may be popular semantic categories because they relate to the child's immediate environment and because they are frequently used by the child's caregiver to stimulate speech.

The second period of interrogative development occurs during the latter months associated with late stage 2 and early stage 3. When the child is approximately twenty-six to thirty-two months, and MLU values range from 2.25 to 2.75, he continues to use a rising intonation as the primary means by which he expresses *yes/no* questions. In addition to increased use of *what* and *where* questions, he now adds the infamous *why* question, which will become one of his favorite language forms over the next year or so. The child's questions at this point are more elaborate and typically have subjects and predicates, although he still omits auxiliaries. He poses questions such as "Where Daddy go?" "What Mommy doing?" and "Why he eat that?" Throughout the first two phases, the child experiences some confusion with *wh*-questions. Until he is about two years old, he interprets most *wh-* questions as *where* questions. After two years, he still responds to some *why* questions as though they are *what* questions. The child, for example, throws his food on the floor. The adult asks, "Why did you do that?" The child responds, "I throwed cookie." In this second phase, the child is still forming *yes/no* questions by using rising intonations at the end of statements, but we will see appropriate inverted questions before he reaches his third birthday.

Imperative Sentences: Requests and Demands

Since the child has been making requests and demands even before she started to use language, you may wonder when the imperative form of sentences emerges. The child is about thirty-one months old before she begins to form true imperative sentences (McCormick, 1990, p. 89). The imperative form has an implied subject and uses an uninflected verb. If you say, "Turn off the light," it is understood that the subject of the sentence is the person to whom the command is given. The child in stage 1 and 2 certainly uses the imperative function in her communication system. Her body language and prosodic variations are sufficient to make her request, demand, or command obvious to the listener. When the child in the single-word stage says, "Mommy!" with her arms stretched out and urgency in her voice, the imperative message is clear. When the stage 2 child says, "Go bye-bye" while tugging on his mother's skirt and motioning toward the door, the imperative message is also clear.

Semantic Development in Stage 2

When the child begins to put words together, his vocabulary grows rapidly. Carey (1978) estimates that between the ages of eighteen months and six years, the child adds an average of nine new words every day and by the age of six may have a comprehension vocabulary that reaches approximately 14,000 words. That becomes impressive when you consider how slowly vocabulary grows when the child creeps into adulthood. If you added just one word per day over the next year, you would add 365 words to your vocabulary. I doubt you have had that kind of vocabulary bonanza in more than a few years. The child at twenty-four months has about 200 to 300 words in his expressive vocabulary. The child in the latter months of stage 2 will probably have a productive vocabulary of about 400 words.

There are undoubtedly many factors that account for how the child apparently acquires so much information about words so quickly, and it will be many years before we identify all of them. Part of the explanation may be inherent in a process called **fast mapping** (Carey & Bartlett, 1978). The foundation for fast mapping is laid when the child first encounters a new word. Even if he does not understand the word completely, he is able to quickly gather information about the word from the context in which it is introduced. There might be information in the surrounding language, for example, that provides the child some insights about what the word means. There may be clues in the discourse in which the word was used. The child stores this information, no matter how fragmented and incomplete it may be in the beginning, in long-term memory. When he encounters the same word in the future in a different context, he gathers additional information that makes his understanding of the word more complete. Keep in mind that the child is repeatedly exposed to communicative routines and that his caregivers are constantly providing him reviewed and new information, factors Crais (1992) believes contribute to word learning. Many of the principles of learning that apply to word mastery are the same as those that apply to learning of any kind. That means, for example, that if a child is exposed to a new word many times over several days, he will learn the components and nuances of its meaning more quickly and completely than if he experiences the same number of exposures in just one day (Childers & Tomasello, 2002). If we put all of these factors together, we understand that what appears to be a rapid acquisition of word knowledge may be somewhat illusory. That is, the child apparently understands and uses a wide range of words quickly, but he may actually understand only bits and pieces of these words. He understands enough of the bits and pieces to decode them and to use them, but we should not assume that just because words are included in the child's receptive and productive vocabularies at a young age that he understands them in the same way that adults understand them. What may be so rapidly acquired, therefore, are pieces of information about many words, and that is very different from complete understandings of many words.

The increase in word knowledge that occurs during stage 2 impacts virtually all language components. As was true in stage 1, the stage 2 child talks about people, objects, actions, and events, and multiple-word utterances reflect her understanding of relational meanings. In stage 2, however, she is using longer and more elaborate sentences resulting in meanings that are more elaborate and increasingly refined.

One development of note in this stage is that the child's cognitive grasp of emotionality is reflected in his language. Some children as young as eighteen months begin to talk about emotions (Bretherton, Fritz, Zahn-Waxler, & Ridgeway, 1986), and by twenty-four months most children are including references to emotion in their language. The stage 2 child identifies emotions, those he is feeling as well as those being experienced by others, and he talks about emotions experienced in the past. As he approaches the end of this stage, he understands that emotions are causative factors in human behavior. If he sees someone crying, for example, he might say, "She sad," reasoning that sadness causes crying. The time is rapidly approaching when the child will begin to use emotional language to manipulate the behavior of others. Is it difficult to imagine the late preschool child saying to his caregiver, "I love you," in the hope that this show of affection will translate into an ice cream cone?

The child's general understanding of causality is reflected by the appropriate use of the words *because* and *so* as early as thirty months (McCabe & Peterson, 1985). It will be another year before the child is able to provide the language detail consistent with a complete understanding of how a causal factor produces a given circumstance. During stage 2, for example, the child might say, "Milk allgone cause me," whereas in the next stage she might say, "I spilled milk Daddy shirt." Beyond the obvious language differences, we see a more precise understanding of the cause and the effect.

Because it is difficult to isolate the development of understanding within each stage, there is a general discussion of comprehension as it relates to cognitive devel-

For the stage 2 child, communication is still heavily nonverbal.

opment and language production at the close of this chapter. This section has provided a preview of the relationships we will examine. That is, as children's understanding of things, people, and events increases, they acquire the vocabulary to name and describe these things, people, and events. As they develop the intellectual capacity to understand concepts, object permanence, causality, and means–ends, they acquire the language by which they can express these understandings. As we established earlier and as we have emphasized throughout this book, it is difficult to separate language and cognitive development. After we complete our examination of stages 2 through 5, we consider this critically important, interactive relationship once again, this time within the context of children's language abilities as they have developed through the preschool years.

Pragmatics: Small Steps toward Conversational Competence

We do not see dramatic changes in pragmatics in stage 2, although in the stages that follow there are significant developments. In stage 2, the child continues to use language to request objects from other people, to request that certain actions be taken, to obtain information by asking questions, and to respond to the questions or comments of others. One interesting development during this stage centers on the word *please*. The child between the ages of twenty-four and thirty-six months uses *please* in her requests with some discretion. She is more likely to include *please* if she perceives the listener to be older, more dominant, and less familiar, or if the listener has something she really wants (Ervin-Tripp & Gordon, 1986).

Perhaps the most significant change in the child as a conversationalist in this stage is that he simply talks more. There are fewer nonverbal responses. His verbal responses are more frequent, and because of the other changes in his language we have already noted, his responses are more elaborate (Mueller, Bleier, Krakow, Hegedus, & Cournoyer, 1977). The stage 2 child is also more adept at gaining his listener's attention, and he is able to provide more complete and meaningful responses to his conversational partner's comments and questions (Wellman & Lempers, 1977). In this case, more is better!

In addition to increased verbal output, the child is showing greater skill in introducing new topics into the conversation, although she is still not able to sustain a topic for more than a turn or two. One of the problems the adult listener sometimes faces in conversations with a very young child is trying to figure out exactly what the topic is. Foster (1986) suggests that the child between twenty-four and thirty-six months is beginning to create understandable topics. Since the stage 2 child is still changing topics after only one or two turns, it is still a constant struggle for the adult partner to stay tuned to what the child is trying to say. This, however, is part of the magic of conversations between adults and toddlers. Some adult-to-adult conversations seem to never end. Adult-to-toddler conversations may be confusing and exasperating, but these exchanges have so many beginnings and quasi-endings they are never boring!

The child in this stage still has much to learn about turn taking and the common courtesies of conversation. Although she is able to participate in conversations with one or two partners, the child does not always allow the speaker to complete his turn before she tries to speak. Ervin-Tripp (1979) has noted that most of these interruptions occur at syntactic junctures or when the speaker's prosody seems to signal conversational right-of-way. Whereas adults allow about one second between turns, the stage 2 child allows longer pauses. By the time she reaches her third birthday, however, she learns that these longer pauses can be interpreted to mean that no response will follow, so she shortens her response time to maintain her turn.

One of the skills all conversationalists must learn is **conversational repair.** If you say something to a listener that you believe the listener has not understood, you will revise or repair your message to increase the chances of successful communication. Gallagher (1977) studied conversational repairs in children between the ages of twenty and thirty months, a span that includes stages 1 and 2. During conversations with these children, an adult listener indicated a lack of understanding by saying "What?" following a child's utterance. More than 75 percent of the requests for clarifications were followed by revised utterances from the children. Shatz and O'Reilly (1990) found that even though their subjects in this age range tried to repair, only about 38 percent of their repair attempts were successful. It is important to note that although children throughout this age range regularly try to repair when their listeners do not understand, their approach changes as their language abilities become more sophisticated. According to Gallagher, the younger child is most likely to repair by changing a speech sound. If the child says, "More cookie," and the adult does not understand, the child might say, "More tookie!" The child at twenty-five or twenty-six months tends to revise by deleting a word from his original statement. If his original utterance "That little doggie" is not understood, he might say, "That doggie" or "Little doggie." By the end of stage 2 or the beginning of stage 3, the child is more likely to repair by changing words. He might revise "She drink milk" to "She drink it" or "Mommy drink milk." It is important to note that a revision or repair is not necessarily more accurate or more correct. In the case of *tookie* for *cookie*, for example, the revision is clearly incorrect.

The idea of conversational repair, however, for the child or even the adult is to try something different in order to make a communicative connection, and different is not always better. Listen carefully to the attempted repairs of adults, and you will hear some fascinating attempts to clarify. Sometimes the harder we try to make something clear, the more confusing or embarrassing our communications become. Consider the following conversational exchange in an episode of the original Bob Newhart television series. Bob, a psychologist, is just leaving his apartment. He has been asked to lead a workshop for people whose marriages are in trouble because of sexual problems. The omnipresent next-door neighbor, Howard, is entering the apartment just as Bob is leaving. Howard addresses Bob's wife: "Where's he going, Emily?" Emily answers, "Bob's going to a sex workshop." Howard responds with a series of statements separated by startled, disbelieving looks from Emily. He says, "I'm sorry to hear that Emily. I didn't know you were having those kinds of problems. Can I help . . . ? I mean, can I be of any service . . . ? I mean, can I function in any way as a friend . . . ? I didn't mean any of those things . . . If you want me, I'll be in bed. . . ." These are conversational repairs based not on lack of clarity in the words themselves but on a lack of clarity in the communicative intentions of the speaker or, more accurately, what the speaker perceives as possible lack of clarity from the viewpoint of his listener.

It is interesting that even though young children consistently respond to requests for clarification from their listeners, they make few requests for repairs when they listen to adult speakers (Gallagher, 1981). Perhaps these children are so accustomed to understanding only portions of the utterances of adults that they do not feel a need to request clarification, or perhaps, as Gallagher suggests, they are reluctant to imply that adult speakers have not produced clear and effective messages. (See Table 5.3 for a summary of stage 2 characteristics.)

Stage 3: Producing Longer, More Adultlike Sentences

The child is typically in stage 3 between the ages of thirty-one and thirty-four months and has an MLU of 2.5 to 3.0. By the time she reaches the end of this stage, the child knows that every sentence must have a verb or predicate, and within a few more months she understands that every sentence must also have a subject. Armed with this basic syntactic knowledge, the child can create complete simple declarative sentences, and she is acquiring knowledge of the rules for changing declarative

Table 5.3 Stage 2 Highlights

Typical Age Range: Twenty-Seven to Thirty Months
MLU: 2.0–2.5 Morphemes

Grammatical Morphemes
- Brown's (1973) fourteen specified grammatical morphemes emerge during the latter months of stage 1 and throughout stage 2.
- As these morphemes develop, the child overextends their use (e.g. child → child**s**; *go* → *go**ed**.*).

Pronouns
- Enters stage 2 using *I, it, this*, and *that*
- Adds *my, me, mine*, and *you*

Verbs
- Uses *have* and *do* as main verbs and as auxiliary verbs
- Produces semiauxiliary forms: *hafta, gonna, wanna*

Noun Phrases
- Uses only determiners and adjectivals as modifiers
- Elaborates in the object position of sentences

Verb Phrases
- Uses present progressive forms of common verbs

Sentences
- Understands that a sentence contains a noun phrase and a verb phrase
- Produces negation by putting *no* or *not* at the beginning of a sentence
- Produces a *yes/no* question by adding a rising intonation to the end of a sentence
- Asks *what, where*, and *why* questions
- Produces the imperative function but not the imperative form

Pragmatics
- Continues to use language to request, to obtain information, and to respond
- Fewer nonverbal responses than in stage 1
- Sustains topic for one or two turns
- Attempts conversational repairs when the listener does not understand

sentences into negative and question forms. We saw the beginning of these forms in stage 2, but they were primitive versions. In stage 3, the child produces more advanced, adultlike negative, interrogative, and even imperative sentences.

Morphological Development Continues

Many of the morphological elements that emerged in stage 2 continue to develop in stage 3, including the fourteen grammatical morphemes we highlighted. In addition, the stage 3 child is more consistent in the use of personal pronouns such as *your, yours, she, he,* and *we* (Owens, 2005, p. 285), the demonstrative pronouns *this, that, these,* and *those,* as well as the articles *a* and *the* (Brown & Bellugi, 1964). Among the modifiers the child uses are a few quantifiers, including *two, some,* and *a lot.* The child is also using common adjectives such as *big, little, good,* and *bad.*

Although the stage 2 child was producing some auxiliary verbs, the stage 3 child is using these verbs, including *can, will,* and *do* more consistently. She is also using the verb *to be* as an auxiliary and as a copula, although in both cases, it may not correctly indicate person or number. She might say, "They is running," "She am my Mommy," or "We is here."

Phrases and Clauses: Construction Continues

The stage 2 child elaborated noun phrases when they were in the object position. The stage 3 child elaborates noun phrases in both the subjective and objective positions of sentences (Brown & Bellugi, 1964). He elaborates by adding the words we identified earlier. He adds demonstrative pronouns *(this, that, these, those),* possessive personal pronouns *(my, your),* quantifiers *(some, a lot),* articles *(a, the),* and adjectives *(big, little, pretty).* He now produces noun phrases such as "My doggie," "Good cookies," and "Little boys."

The child is producing verb phrases that include auxiliary verbs such as *can, do,* and *will* and is also including the auxiliary form of the verb *to be.* As we noted earlier, however, the verb *to be* in both the auxiliary and copula forms may not correctly indicate person and number, and it may not be properly marked for tense. The child might say, "I *is*," for "I *am*" or he might say, "She *is*," when he really means "She *was*." He will also overextend the regular past tense when he is using irregular verbs so that he will say, "She runned away," or "I falled down" (Miller, 1981).

More Changes in Sentence Forms

The child was creating primitive forms of negative and question sentences in stage 2. In this stage, she produces forms that are more adultlike in that she is including auxiliary verbs and the copula, and she is inverting words when they should be inverted.

In stage 2, the child usually creates the negative form by adding *no* or *not* to the beginning of a simple declarative sentence. The negative version of "Go nite-nite" is "No go nite-nite." In stage 3, the child places the negative element between the subject and predicate to produce an adultlike version. Instead of "No Daddy go bye-bye," for example, she says, "Daddy no go bye-bye." The child is also adding auxiliary verbs to negative forms as in "Doggie *don't* bite." As indicated by this example, the child is producing contracted negative forms such as *can't, don't,* and *won't.* Since she is also producing the affirmative forms of these verbs, we can assume that these contractions are based on the application of a rule and are not simply imitations of whole constructions. It is noteworthy that Brown (1973) considered the changes in the negative form to be one of the most important advances to occur in stage 3.

The stage 2 child was creating questions by adding rising intonations to the ends of sentences. In stage 3, he is including the auxiliary verbs we hear in adult speech, and he is inverting words according to adult production rules. Instead of "She go bye-bye?" with rising inflection, or even "She can go bye-bye?" (which includes the uninverted auxiliary verb), the stage 3 child says, "Can she go bye-bye?" The yes/no question is common in this stage, in sentences that include auxiliary verbs and in sentences that include copula verbs. Instead of the earlier question "I am good boy?" the child will ask, "Am I good boy?" with the subject and copula properly inverted.

The most frequent *wh*-words used in stage 3 are *what* and *where*, but the child will also use *why, who,* and *how* (Tyack & Ingram, 1977). According to some researchers, the *wh*-questions during this stage are not inverted, but more recent evidence suggests that *most* of the child's *wh*-questions in stage 3 are inverted (Klee, 1985). The child might say, "Where the cookie is?" but she is more likely to produce the properly inverted form, "Where is the cookie?" She will also include some, though not all, of the required auxiliary verbs. She might say, "*Can* I go bye-bye?" but she might also say, "Why Bobby kick me?" instead of "Why *did* Bobby kick me?"

In this stage we see the adult version of the imperative form. The child seems to enjoy this form and appreciates its power. In its proper form, the verb is not inflected and the subject is implied. The child says things such as "Pick me up," "Give me a cookie," and "Turn on the light." As mentioned earlier, the child has been producing the imperative function from the beginning of his communicative life, long before the emergence of language, but in stage 3, for the first time, he is using the syntactically correct form of imperative sentences.

Pragmatic Development: Slow Progress in the Art of Conversation

During stage 3, the child's dialogues are still relatively brief. She continues to devote only about two turns per conversational topic, and she has difficulty conversing about things that are absent or events in the past. When the child does talk about things or events not in the present, her comments often catch the adult listener off guard because the comments do not seem to be connected to the immediate conversational context (Keenan & Schieffelin, 1976). The difficulty in talking about things and events that are not in the present is that the speaker and the listener must rely solely on language. With a limited vocabulary and limited language skills, the child can talk about things in the present because she can rely on nonverbal communications to fill her language gaps.

The child also has difficulty maintaining a conversational topic. Whereas adults maintain conversation by adding or seeking new information in each turn or by using one comment to prompt a new but related response, the child in stage 3 is not very adept at these skills. His primary strategy for maintaining conversation is to repeat. He will repeat part or all of the utterance just produced by his conversational partner. This strategy of exactly matching the topic of one's partner is called **topic collaborating** (Keenan & Schieffelin, 1976).

The child in this stage will also maintain a conversational topic by responding to questions asked by the partner. Adults quickly learn that this is an effective way to keep a young child talking, so the conversational exchange consists of questions from the adult and answers from the child. The limiting factor in this kind of dialogue might be the adult's ability to keep asking questions about a relatively uninvolved topic. How many questions can you ask a child about a chocolate chip cookie? "What is that?" "Is it good?" "What are the brown things?" "Did it break?" "What do you suppose is the fat content of a single cookie, and how will that affect your eating habits for the rest of this day?" "If cookies are bad for you and spinach is good for you, why are wax beans yellow?"

The child in stage 3 continues to repair her conversational statements by changing words. As we noted in the previous stage, these changes do not always result in more correct statements, but the changes do indicate that the child knows her message was not clear, and she is trying to fix it. As her vocabulary grows and understanding of how words are related increases, her repairs will be more effective. If you say, "He is morose," and you receive a quizzical look from your listener, you may repair the comment to "He's sad." The child's ability to make this kind of repair is obviously related to her language knowledge and skills so that conversational repair skills develop in a parallel manner with overall language development. In stages 2 and 3, the child repairs by using a different word, even if it is not a more appropriate word.

Although adults take into account what the child knows in adult–child conversations, the child's presuppositional skills remain relatively undeveloped. As long as the topic is immediately present, the adult will know the child's conversational focus, but the child often uses pronouns when their referents are not identifiable, and he provides little assistance to his listener except for supplying some details about the topic which might enhance understanding (Owens, 2005, p. 266). (See Table 5.4 for a summary of stage 3 highlights.)

Stage 4: Elaboration by Embedding

The child is typically in stage 4 between the ages of thirty-five and forty months and has an MLU of 3.0 to 3.75. As the MLU increase from stage 3 to stage 4 indicates, the child continues to elaborate by adding words to his utterances, but in this stage we see elaboration take a new and exciting turn. In the previous stages, the child made phrases and clauses longer by adding modifiers or auxiliary verbs. In stage 4, he places a phrase within a clause, and he combines two or more clauses into one clause. This combining process, called **embedding,** results in complex sentences, and it is one of the most important syntactic developments in this stage (Brown, 1973). An embedded phrase or clause becomes a grammatical element within a larger sentence. A phrase, for example, might function as a noun, an adjective, or an adverb.

Phrases: Embedding for Specific Grammatical Functions

There are essentially four kinds of phrases: (1) prepositional phrases, (2) participial phrases, (3) infinitive phrases, and (4) gerunds. You should not assume that when the child exits stage 4, she is producing all of these phrases as embedded forms. Phrasal and clausal embedding are complex processes that develop over a long period of time. The child begins to develop prepositional phrases by using words such as *in* and *on* as early as stage 2, but she does not produce true infinitive forms until stage 5 and beyond (Bloom, Tackeff, & Lahey, 1984; Miller, 1981).

Table 5.4 Stage 3 Highlights

Typical Age Range: Thirty-One to Thirty-Four Months
MLU: 2.5 to 3.0 Morphemes

Grammatical Morphemes
- Continue to develop

Pronouns
- More consistent in use of *you, your, yours, she, he, we, this, that, these,* and *those*

Verbs
- Uses the modal verbs *can, will,* and *do* more consistently
- Uses the verb *to be* as both copula and auxiliary, although makes mistakes in terms of person and number

Noun Phrases
- Uses a few quantifiers: *two, some, a lot*
- Elaborates in the subject and object positions of sentences

Verb Phrases
- Elaborates by using modals and the auxiliary forms of *to be*
- Overextends the regular past tense form to irregular verbs (e.g. "He runn*ed* away")

Sentences
- Produces negation by putting *no* or *not* between the subject predicate to create an adultlike form, also uses contracted negative forms: *can't, don't*
- Questions include auxiliary verbs, and the elements are properly inverted (e.g., "She go bye-bye." → "Can she go bye-bye?")
- In addition to *what, where,* and *why,* produces questions with *who* and *how,* often properly inverted
- Produces the imperative form of sentences

Pragmatics
- Most exchanges are still limited to one or two turns per topic.
- Primary strategy for maintaining a topic is repeating part or all of the utterance produced by her partner.
- Continues to attempt conversational repairs, usually by using a different word even if it is not a more appropriate word.

As the name suggests, a **prepositional phrase** contains a preposition such as *in, on, under, over,* or *onto,* together with an object of the preposition and accompanying modifiers or articles. In the phrase *under the old car, under* is the preposition and *car* is the object. The child will add prepositional phrases to the ends of his sentences early in stage 4.

Verb forms, usually ending in *-ing, -ed, -en,* or *-t,* that function as adjectives are called **participles** in the following examples: *babbling* brook, *pickled* egg, *shaven* head, and *past* Wednesday. A **participial phrase** contains a participle and functions as an adjective. In the sentence "The woman calling my name is Aunt Bertha," the participial phrase, *calling my name,* functions as an adjective describing *woman.*

Most of us are familiar with the term **infinitive** because we learned we are not supposed to split infinitives when we speak and write. An infinitive is a verb form introduced by the word *to* or the phrase *in order to*. In the sentence "I called to confirm my reservation," the infinitive is *to confirm*. In the sentence "I called to, after trying to remember the date, confirm my reservation," the infinitive is split. An improved version of the same sentence would be "After trying to remember the date, I called to confirm my reservation." Infinitive phrases can function as nouns, adjectives, or adverbs. In the sentence "Daddy wanted to go to the store," the infinitive phrase *(to go to the store)* functions as a noun and is the object of the verb *wanted*. In the sentence "Because of my job, I have little energy to devote to my hobbies," the infinitive phrase *(to devote to my hobbies)* modifies *energy* and functions as an adjective. In the sentence "My father exercises to increase his physical fitness," the infinitive phrase *(to increase his physical fitness)* functions as an adverb in modifying the verb *exercises*.

The child is using forms such as *gotta* and *wanna* as early as thirty months, and these productions certainly sound like infinitive forms as in "I wanna (want to) go bye-bye." Many language experts refer to these productions as **semiauxiliaries** and do not consider them to be true infinitives (James, 1990, p. 83). Simple infinitives in which the subjects are the same as the subjects of the main sentence emerge in stage 4, and more difficult infinitives in which the subjects are different from the subjects of the main sentence emerge in stage 5 (Paul, 1981). In stage 4, for example, the child might say, "Mommy want to eat cookie." The subject of the sentence and the infinitive ("to eat") is "Mommy." In stage 5, the child might say, "I want the kitty to go outside." In this case, the subject of the sentence is *I*, but the subject of the infinitive *(to go)* is *kitty*.

When a verb ending in *ing* functions as a noun, as either a subject or an object, it is called a **gerund.** In the sentence "Sleeping is the most vigorous exercise of my day," *sleeping* is a gerund and the subject of the sentence. In the sentence "Mary dislikes walking," *walking* is a gerund and the object of the verb *dislikes*. When a verb phrase operates as a noun, it is called a **gerund phrase.** In the sentence "Compulsive eating is a serious health problem," *compulsive eating* is a gerund phrase and is the subject of the sentence. According to Paul (1981), gerund phrases tend to emerge later than infinitives. When her subjects had MLU's above 4.5, more than 90 percent were producing simple infinitive forms, but only about 50 percent were producing sentences that included gerunds. Keep in mind that an MLU of 4.5 places the child within stage 5.

Clauses within Clauses: Complex Sentences

As we noted earlier in this chapter, a complex sentence is created when the speaker embeds one clause into another. A compound sentence is created when the speaker joins or conjoins two independent clauses. Even though the order might seem to violate common sense, the child engages in serious clausal embedding before she becomes proficient in clausal conjoining. There is evidence of some clausal conjoining in stage 4, but Brown (1973) identifies clausal conjoining primarily with stage 5.

According to Brown (1973), there are three types of embedded clauses: (1) object complement clause, (2) *wh*-question clause, and (3) relative clause. In a sentence with an object complement clause, there is an independent clause containing a verb such as *think, hope, know, guess, mean,* or *need,* followed by a noun phrase that functions as an object. In the sentence "I think you know what I mean," the subordinate clause (*you know what I mean*) functions as the object of the verb *think*. The object complement clause emerges during stage 4.

The embedded *wh-* clause also emerges during stage 4, and these clauses also function as objects. Consider the following examples:

"I know what you did."

"He showed me where to get one."

"You probably know when he'll come back."

Since the child is learning to use these words in question sentences, it is not surprising that he sometimes produces sentences that seem to mix the inverted structure of the interrogative form and the embedded *wh-* clause. He might say, for example, "Show me where can I get one," instead of the more proper construction, "Show me where I can get one."

A relative clause is introduced by *who, whom, whoever, whomever, whose, which,* or *that* and modifies the preceding noun. A problem for many speakers, including adults, is determining which relative pronoun should be used in a given sentence. Identifying and discussing the rules for selecting the proper pronoun is beyond the scope of this book, but a few examples may help you understand some of what the child must learn about pronoun usage:

"He is the man who helped me last week."

"He's the boy whose finger was broken when he was hit in the nose."

"The ball that broke the window was thrown from a passing car."

Although we are introducing the concept of relative clauses as part of our explanation of clausal embedding, be aware that the child does not begin to use relative clauses until stage 5 and beyond.

As one might guess, the first conjunction used to link two or more independent clauses is *and.* By the time the child is twenty-five to twenty-seven months old, she is using *and* correctly to join words (Bloom, Lahey, Hood, Lifter, & Fiess, 1980). Even though she begins to conjoin clauses in stage 4, the child does not consistently conjoin clauses with *and* and other conjunctions until late in stage 5 (Miller, 1981). It is interesting, though not surprising, that even after the child has acquired many conjunctions and is beyond her fifth birthday, she continues to favor *and* (Bennett-Kaster, 1986).

What's Happening on the Morphemic Front?

Although no dramatic developments in morphology are unique to stage 4, keep in mind that overall growth in vocabulary is rapid throughout the five stages of language development we are describing. The fourteen grammatical morphemes we identified as emerging in stage 2 are continuing to develop. The stage 4 child is consistently using the pronouns *they, us, her, hers, his,* and *them* (Owens, 2005, p. 285). He is also using modifiers such as *some, something, other, more, one, two,* and *another* (Miller, 1981). The child's sentences are likely to include some past tense forms of common modals such as *could, should,* and *would* (Chapman, 1978), and he is putting *be* and the *-ing* form of verbs together to create sentences such as "He is running" (Chapman, Paul, & Wanska, 1981). As the child acquires more words, he incorporates them into his sentences to make them longer and more elaborate.

Elaboration of Noun Phrases and Verb Phrases

The stage 4 child understands that a sentence must have a noun or a pronoun as a subject (Ingram, 1971). Recall that the child was elaborating noun phrases as subjects and objects in the previous stage; she continues to elaborate in much the same way in stage 4. That is, she usually adds only one modifier in front of the noun. She will produce sentences such as *"The* boy took *my* ball" or *"That* doggie ate *his* bone." In looking ahead to the inclusion of several modifiers in front of a noun, think about what the child must learn. If we use three modifiers to describe the noun *house,* we do not arrange the modifiers in random order. There are rules for sequencing modifiers. Take a moment to think about this intriguing little puzzle: You want to say, *"There are* _____ , _____ , _____ *houses on this street,"* and you are going to insert the modifiers *white, three,* and *big.* What is the proper order? The answer, of course, is *"Three big white. . . ."* If you put them in any other order, the phrase does not make sense. At some point in the child's language development, she learns the rules for ordering modifiers. In this example, number modifiers precede size modifiers, which precede color modifiers. Learning these rules takes time, time that extends well beyond stage 5.

The stage 4 child is expanding his verb phrases by including the auxiliary *do* in negative and question forms and by including modals such as *would, could, should, might,* and *must* (Chapman, 1978). Although the child has been using modals since stage 2, he is now using them more consistently and appropriately. Remember that a modal reflects the speaker's attitude about what is happening in the sentence (Broderick, 1975, p. 81). In this stage, the child demonstrates by use of modals that he understands the difference between using *might* to indicate that something is *possible* and using *must* to indicate that the something is *required* or *obligatory.* You will notice, however, that the meanings of some modals are troublesome for children, and even adults, for a long time. For example, *can* means *ability* and *may* signals *permission,* but many speakers ask a question such as *"Can* I throw the ball?" when what they really mean is *"May* I throw the ball?" This particular confusion occurs so commonly that *can* is now considered to be an acceptable modal to express permission in informal social contexts (Broderick, p. 82). Sorting out what modals mean and how they should be used begins in earnest in stage 4, but like so many aspects of language development, the learning and sorting will continue for many years.

The child was overextending the regular past tense in stage 3, and she continues this overextension in stage 4. Since she is now using present and past tense modals, however, we see some interesting constructions in which past tense is marked twice. The child might say, for example, "She couldn't catched the ball." Compare this construction with the correct version, "She couldn't catch the ball." Since the modal is marked for past tense, the main verb is not inflected. These are tricky rules! The main verb must be inflected to mark past tense *except* when the modal is marked for past tense, in which case the main verb remains in the present tense. That's not a fair rule! The child must also learn, of course, that some verbs are marked for past tense in the *regular* manner, some verbs undergo complete changes such as *go—went* or *see—saw*, and some verbs do not change at all, *hit—hit*. These examples are provided to help you understand why the child overextends and why it takes so long to understand all the rules and at least most of the exceptions.

Progress on Negative and Interrogative Forms

Prior to stage 4, the child indicates negation by using the words *no* and *not* and by using the contractions, *can't, don't*, and *won't*. By the end of stage 2 or the beginning of stage 3, the child is properly placing the negative element between the subject and predicate. Although he is using words such as *can't* and *won't* as early as stage 2, these are probably not true contractions until stage 3, when he begins to use the positive forms of the modals involved in these contractions. By the end of stage 4, the child has added the following negative contractions: *didn't, doesn't, isn't*, and *aren't* (Miller, 1981). Once again the progress is slow but true. From the caregiver's point of view, the progress may actually seem slower than it really is. When the child produces a form such as *can't* as early as twenty-seven to thirty months, the caregiver may assume the child understands the modal *can*, the negative element *not*, and the rule for producing the contraction. In fact, the child at this point is producing the word *can't* as a whole unit, without understanding its parts and the rule that makes the parts a new whole. He uses *can't* when he should use *won't* and vice versa. In fact, he often does not differentiate among any of the terms he uses to indicate negation. Over the next ten to twelve months, he is learning a great deal that is not apparent to the caregiver. He learns what a modal is and which modal works in which context. He learns that modals can be contracted with negative elements to produce *can't, won't*, and so forth. He learns to place the negative form between the subject and predicate. Over the course of stages 2, 3, and 4, therefore, he learns a great deal about creating negative forms, but the caregiver still hears only *can't* and *won't*, and may have no idea that the *can't* of stage 2 is very different from the *can't* of stage 4.

We see similar progress with interrogative forms. In stage 2, the child signals a question by using a rising intonation at the end of a declarative statement. In stage 3, she is including some auxiliary verbs, and she is learning to invert words properly to move from the declarative form of a sentence to the interrogative form of the same sentence. By the time the child reaches the end of stage 4, she is producing adultlike questions in their inverted forms and with the appropriate auxiliary verbs. Prior to this stage, most of her *wh-*questions were introduced by *what* or *where*. By the end of stage 4, she is consistently creating questions initiated by *why, who*, and *how*, which were used sparingly in the preceding stage, and she is using *when*. The order in which *wh-*questions emerge may be explained according to how the words are used in sentences (Wootten, Merkin, Hood, & Bloom, 1979).

Questions introduced by *what, where,* and *who* are among the earliest to emerge, perhaps because these words are **interrogative pronouns.** If the child says, "What is that?" the *what* is a pronoun representing a specific thing. *Who* represents a specific person, and *where* represents a specific location. Throughout his language and cognitive development, the child has managed to deal more effectively with things, people, and events in his immediate environment than with abstract concepts or with things, people, and events that are remote in time and space. Consider the problems created by words such as *why, how,* and *when,* which are acquired later than *what, where,* and *who.* There are no easy and specific referents for these words. Even as adults, we may have trouble responding to some *why* and *how* questions. If someone asks, "Is the sky blue?" we can provide a simple and direct answer, but the question "Why is the sky blue?" is much more difficult. Economists make a living trying to answer *why* and *how* questions such as "Why does the value of the dollar affect the balance of trade?" or "How do the Dow-Jones averages measure the strength of the American economy?" What substitutes for the *why* and *how* in these questions can fill books. *When* questions are fairly easy for adults because we have a sense of the present in the relative context of past and future, but the child at two, three, or four years is still grappling with the concept of time in its past and future dimensions.

Pragmatic Development: Becoming a Better Conversationalist

Early in stage 4, at about three years, the child learns a simple but important lesson about time in the art of conversation. She recognizes that there is a difference between a pause of less than one second and a pause greater than one second. Think about this for a moment. In your conversations with other adults, when there is a pause of several seconds, what does that mean? It could mean, of course, that the other person is thinking about his response, but if there is no nonverbal evidence of pondering, you are likely to conclude that no response is forthcoming. The stage 4 child has learned this lesson, that a pause greater than one second means that the conversational partner is probably not going to respond (Craig & Gallagher, 1983). Short pauses, those less than one second in duration, mean that exchanges on this topic will continue. As adults, we are so sensitive to this time factor that long pauses in conversations, especially with people we do not know well, are very uncomfortable. In fact, as we become skilled conversationalists, we learn to overlap our responses so that there are no pauses.

By the end of stage 4 or the beginning of stage 5, at about forty-two months, the child is able to maintain a topic for more than two turns (Bloom, Rocissano, & Hood, 1976). Not surprisingly, based on everything we know about children, the child is more likely to maintain a topic for several turns if the conversation centers on something in her immediate environment and if the topic interests her. Most adults respond in a similar way. When someone tries to engage me in a conversation about opera, there is usually only one exchange because my response is *"Don't like it,"* but if someone wants to talk to me about baseball, football, or basketball, there is the potential for many turns. Part of the art of conversation, therefore, is finding a topic that interests your partner, and a good conversationalist is not necessarily someone who has a great deal to say, but someone who knows how to get others to talk about what interests them. The lesson to be emphasized at this point, with the stage 4 child, is that the adult, by choosing topics that interest or fail to interest the child, usually determines how long child–adult conversations will last.

Before the child's third birthday, his presuppositional skills have been limited. Unless the topic of conversation is immediate, the adult often has difficulty following shifts in the conversation because the child does not provide the information the listener needs to keep abreast of the changes. During stage 4, following his third birthday, the child begins to make some meaningful and helpful presuppositions in his conversations. The stage 4 child understands what the listener needs to know about the topic, and he can determine how much information he needs to provide (Shatz, Wellman, & Silber, 1983; Wellman & Estes, 1987).

The child adjusts the amount of information she provides depending on whether the listener can directly observe the topic of conversation and depending on what the child assumes the listener knows or understands about the topic. That is, if the listener is looking at the object of the conversation or the child believes the listener already knows what he needs to know about the object, the child knows that little additional information is needed. If, however, the child is talking about something that is not present or she believes the listener lacks the information he needs to make sense of the communication, the child provides more information. As the child moves past her third birthday, she becomes increasingly proficient in making these presuppositional decisions. Several specific skills emerge at about this time, including the use of *anaphoric references, deixis,* and *grammatical ellipsis.*

Anaphoric reference should sound familiar, because we discussed this term earlier in this chapter under the heading *Pronouns: Words Used to Represent Nouns.* In that section, we pointed out that an anaphoric reference is used to refer to something in a preceding utterance. Where does presupposition fit into anaphoric reference? Consider a simple example. If the child says, "I played baseball with my new mitt," and then says, "It is just like the one Sammy Sosa uses," we know several things: (1) We know that the *it* in the second sentence refers to the *mitt* in the preceding sentence. (2) We know that the child assumes the listener will know that the *it* in the second sentence references the *mitt* in the first sentence, and (3) We know that Sammy Sosa is making some extra money in an endorsement deal. The child, at three and four years, makes more anaphoric references, not only because he understands this form of pronoun, but because he is developing the presuppositional skill that allows him to use fewer words in utterances that follow the introductory utterance if he has properly established the information necessary for the listener to follow his train of thought and if he properly assumes the listener will make the necessary connections that tie words together and make some linguistic redundancies unnecessary.

A common thread woven through maturing suppositional skills is the ability to process information from the perspective of another person. We see this thread very clearly in **deixis.** Contrary to what you might expect, this word was not invented for the purpose of describing an emerging presuppositional skill. The word *deixis* comes from the Greek word *deiknunai,* which means *to show.* In the context of presuppositional skills, the child uses *deixis* when she demonstrates an understanding that certain words are interpreted differently depending upon who speaks them. It is easiest to understand *deixis* if we identify what are called *deictic word pairs.* Examples include *here/there, this/that,* and *I/you.* Imagine conversational partners seated across from one another at an ice cream parlor. One person says, "I bet *this* ice cream tastes better than *that* ice cream." Depending upon which speaker makes this statement, *this* and *that* refer to different bowls of ice cream. Let's throw in another deictic word pair to make the point even clearer. Assume that the two speakers are *you* and *I,* and you are eating vanilla ice cream, and I am eating chocolate ice cream. If you are speaking, *this* is vanilla ice cream and *that* is chocolate ice cream, but if I am speaking, *this* is chocolate ice cream and *that* is vanilla. As is obvious to anyone who has watched a child progress though language development, she does not master the complexities of deixis in one neat step. In fact, she appears to move through three phases in learning that deictic word pairs have opposing meanings (Clark & Sengul, 1978). In the first phase, the child uses the members of a deictic pair as though they are synonyms. For example, she will use *this* and *that* as though they mean the same thing whether she is pointing to something in her grasp or something someone sitting ten feet away is holding. Please note that she understands the basic meaning of *deixis,* which is *to show* or *point to.* What she is not getting is the speaker's perspective that dictates which word is appropriate in a given context. In the second phase, the child will use one of the two words more often that the other, so that she uses it correctly in some cases but incorrectly in others. In the third phase, she learns when to use each word, depending upon who the speaker is and depending upon the context in which the word is used. Not surprisingly, the child masters deictic pairs that are more absolute in nature, such as *I/you* and *my/your,* before she masters those that are spatial or more relative, such as *here/there* and *this/that.* The child does well with the absolute deictic pronoun pairs by the time she is thirty months old (Owens, 2005, p. 271), but she may not master the spatial or relative pairs until she is in her early elementary school years. Consider the potential uncertainty in a pair such as *here/there.* How proximal must something be in order to be considered *here* and not *there*? Even for an adult this can be problematic. If someone asks "How long have you lived *here*?" how do you know what *here* means— this house, this neighborhood, this city, this state, this country, this planet? Even words such as *this* and *that* can be confusing if the listener sees an array of objects to which the *this* or *that* could refer. It takes time for the child to sort out the general parameters that should be applied when using these terms and the parameters she can assume the listener applies in interpreting messages the child sends.

When presuppositional skills are mature, the speaker has some degree of awareness about what the listener knows about the subject of their conversation. There are times for all of us when we assume too much knowledge or too little, but as mature speakers, we can adjust our presuppositions depending upon the kind of response we get. When a teacher assumes a level of understanding, for example, in explaining a new concept to students, and the reactions of his students range from puzzled looks and gasps to panic-induced fainting, he adjusts his explanation by assuming a lower level of understanding. The child must develop the basic skill—that is, learning to assume understanding, and eventually he must learn the art of adjusting his assumptions of understanding.

A language behavior that directly reflects this developing understanding is **grammatical ellipsis.** When a speaker uses grammatical ellipsis, she deletes information when she assumes the listener already possesses it. She might use this device if she believes the information has been established in prior communicative exchanges, or if she believes the information is obvious because of the nonverbal context in which the communication is taking place. Consider the following scenario: A couple is taking a trip. They stop to eat lunch at a fast food restaurant. Within minutes after leaving the restaurant, the wife says "Where's my purse?" The husband says "Probably in the restaurant." He does not need to provide additional language detail because the context provides all the supporting information the wife needs to make sense of his response. Grammatical ellipsis is not as simple, however, as this example might make it seem. As this skill matures, the speaker develops a clearer and more complete understanding about what can be omitted in a communicative exchange and how the number and nature of omissions might need to be amended depending upon who the listener is (Bloom and Lahey, 1978). Very young children often produce abbreviated sentences. Are they using grammatical ellipsis? Most likely, these shortened utterances reflect developing but incomplete syntactic skills, not emerging presuppositional skills. The evidence suggests that grammatical ellipsis emerges slowly after the child is three years old and is gradually mastered during the school years (Bloom, Miller, & Hood, 1975; Owens, 2005, p. 264).

At the same time that the child is mastering these elements of presupposition, she is also adjusting her speech according to the age of her listener. She uses very basic syntax and vocabulary when talking to a younger child and uses more sophisticated language when talking to adults or to children her own age. The child adjusts the amount of information she provides depending on whether the listener can directly observe the topic of conversation. That is, if the listener is looking at the object of the conversation, the child knows that little additional information is needed, but if the child is talking about something not present, she provides more information.

Keep in mind that presuppositional skills depend not only on the speaker's sensitivity to what the listener may need to know but on the speaker's cognitive and linguistic abilities to convey information the listener needs. Although the stage 4 child's presuppositional skills have improved, she is still limited in these skills by what she knows and what she is able to express. If the child has a firm cognitive grasp of the topic and if she has the vocabulary and language ability to talk about the topic, she is likely to provide the information necessary. If the topic is beyond her understanding and language abilities, she will have trouble providing the information the listener needs. Even adults run into this problem. If you were talking to someone about the operation of the engine in your Toyota, say, you might be very sensitive to your listener's informational needs, but beyond identifying what you think are spark plugs, the air filter, and the oil dip stick, you would probably use the word *thing* quite often, and your listener would never have adequate information. Presuppositional skills, you see, depend on knowledge, insight, understanding, vocabulary, syntax, and all the other elements of communication. As a conversationalist, the stage 4 child is perfectly willing to help, and she wants to help, but she will help only to the extent that she can help. Otherwise, she can only say, "Help!"

As mentioned earlier, *pragmatics* is concerned with using language to get things done. Adult speakers are often very direct in making requests or demands. If you say, for example, "Close the door," there is no question about what is meant and the language is unequivocal. This is a *direct* request. You might say, "Can you close the door?" On the surface, this seems to be a question about the ability of the listener to close the door, but it is really an *indirect* request to close the door. You assume the listener has the ability, but you choose this manner to make your request because it is more polite and does not have the edge of a direct order. You can give the request an even softer edge if you say, "There seems to be a little breeze in here," or you can give it a harder, sarcastic edge if you say, "Were you raised in a barn?!" These examples are even less direct, but the request is still being made. The child's ability to use language to make requests and demands, and to change the manner in which the requests are made, must evolve. This evolution is not rapid.

Prior to the emergence of language, the child indicates needs and makes requests by gesturing, crying, and producing speech-like noises. By the time he is two years old, he is able to accompany these nonverbal communications with some words, but his efforts to gain attention and have his requests met often fail (Ervin-Tripp, O'Connor, & Rosenberg, 1987). He will use words such as *mine, want,* and *more* (Newcombe & Zaslow, 1981), and when he begins to combine words, he will make requests such as "I want cookie," "I need blankie," or "Give me ball" (Ervin-Tripp, 1977). At this point, virtually all requests are direct.

The stage 4 child has developed an understanding of the meanings of most common modals; she is now using these modals to make *indirect* requests. She might say, for example, "Could you give me a cookie?" or "Can you pick me up?" Just as she has learned the power of *please* with adults (Ervin-Tripp & Gordon, 1986), so has she learned that these indirect and more polite requests are often more effective, or at least more warmly received, than their direct equivalents. This is a small but important example of how pragmatic skills advance as a direct result of greater language ability. The child cannot make an indirect request until she has the language required for such a request, and we witness only the first step in indirect requests in this stage. As the child matures and as her language becomes more sophisticated, she will be able to make requests so subtly and indirectly that she will make her listener believe the satisfaction of the request is the listener's idea, not the child's. We all know a few people, children and adults, whose talents in this area of pragmatics are amazingly effective! (See Table 5.5 for highlights of stage 4.)

Stage 5: Polishing the Act

As we have suggested throughout this chapter and the preceding chapter, these five stages do not finish the acquisition of speech and language. The child still has much to learn when he completes stage 5, but he has certainly learned all that can be considered basic in speech and language by the end of this stage. The child is typically in this stage between the ages of forty-one and forty-six months and has an MLU range of 3.75 to 4.5. During stage 5, the child reaches closure on some language behaviors, elaborates

Table 5.5 Stage 4 Highlights

Typical Age Range: Thirty-Five to Forty Months
MLU: 3.0 to 3.75 Morphemes

Grammatical Morphemes
• Still developing, slowly but surely

Pronouns
• More consistent in use of *they, us, his, her, hers*, and *them*

Verbs
• Uses past tense of common modals: *could, should, would*

Noun Phrases
• Continues to elaborate by adding only one element in front of the noun

Verb Phrase
• Elaborates by including *do* in negative and question forms and by including modals such as *could, would, might*, and *must*
• Continues to overextend the regular past tense form to irregular verbs

Sentences
• Adds the following contractions in his productions of negative sentences: *didn't, doesn't, isn't*, and *aren't*
• More consistent in use of *why, who*, and *how* questions, also asks *when* questions

Pragmatics
• Learns that short pauses mean that exchanges will continue; long pauses, that responses are not forthcoming
• By the end of stage 4, is able to sustain conversation for more than two turns
• Developing primitive presuppositional skills (i.e., understanding what the listener needs to know and providing appropriate information)
• Beginning to make indirect requests (e.g., "Can you pick me up?")

---

on others, and is still struggling with other aspects of language. The process of acquiring and learning about speech and language will continue throughout childhood and adolescence, and even into adulthood. It is certainly a reasonable hope that five years from the day you read these words you will know more about language than you do now, that you will use language more skillfully in writing and speaking, and that you will be more sophisticated in the art of conversation. The stage 5 child has come a long way in his quest for communicative competence, but beyond his fourth birthday, he still has miles and miles to go.

Morphemic Development: The Acquisition Continues

If we consider the aggregate findings of Brown (1973) and Miller (1981), we can conclude that nine of the fourteen specified grammatical morphemes are mastered by the close of stage 5. The remaining five are mastered by fifty months, just four months beyond the upper age limit we have used to mark stage 5. More specifically, the stage 5 child masters or is close to mastering the irregular past form of common verbs, the contractible copula, the uncontractible auxiliary, and the regular and irregular markers for third person singular.

The regular past tense of verbs is created by adding *-ed*. Verbs that are made past tense by some other change are considered irregular. Although English has relatively few irregular past tense verbs, they are used frequently and pose an immediate problem for the child learning English. In stages 3 and 4, the child manages this problem by overextending the regular past tense form to these irregular verbs. He says, *catched* instead of *caught* and *throwed* instead of *threw*. Early in language development, the child might give the appearance of understanding some irregular past tense forms. He might say, for example, "Daddy went work," but a few months later he might say, "Daddy wented work." This might seem like a regression to the caregiver, but it is actually a step forward in the child's understanding of past tense. He continues to have a problem, however, knowing the difference between regular and irregular past tense forms, so he uses the regular form on all verbs. By the end of stage 5, he understands the difference, at least for commonly used irregular past tense forms such as *sat, went, broke, ate, ran,* and *fell*. He may continue to have problems with verbs such as *hit* and *put* that do not change when they move from present to past tense. He might also try to find regularity where there is none. For example, he might reason that if the past tense of *sing* is *sang* and the past tense of *ring* is *rang,* then the past tense of *bring* must be *brang*. He would, of course, be wrong, but eventually he will get most of the exceptions and irregularities figured out.

To this point we have used the terms *contractible* and *uncontractible* in reference to the copula and auxiliary forms of the verb *to be* with little explanation. Although these terms seem to be self-explanatory, the issue of contractibility may be more complex than you imagine. The speaker must learn that sometimes it is permissible to contract and sometimes it is not, and the rules for contractibility are not always clear. We can say, "He is tall," or we can contract this copula form to "He's tall." This is a **contractible** copula form. If the same copula form is in an answer to a question, adult usage suggests that a contraction is not acceptable. If you ask, "Is he tall?" the response is "He is," or "Yes, he is tall," but the answer, *"He's,"* does not sound right because it violates a rule of contractibility based on usage. In this case, the copula is **uncontractible.** Consider contractibility in a question such as "Do you know how tall he is?" It would not be acceptable to say, "Do you know how tall he's?" although you could say, "He's tall, isn't he?" You can say, "He's tall," or "He isn't tall," but you cannot say, *"He'sn't tall,"* because it is not acceptable to contract a form that is already contracted. It is also not permissible to contract the copula when it is in the past tense. You can say, "He's tall," but in the past tense, you must say, "He was tall." Children must learn when it is permissible to contract and when it is not. It is not surprising that they are still struggling with contractible and uncontractible forms of the copula and auxiliary versions of *to be* as they enter stage 5.

Although the child is producing some uncontractible copula forms as early as stage 2 or 3, she does not master the uncontractible copula until stage 5. The child masters the contractible copula even later, toward the end of stage 5 or beyond (Miller, 1981). According to Brown (1973), a copula is contractible even if it is not actually contracted in a given production. You might say, *"He's tall,"* or *"He is tall."* In both cases, you have used a contractible copula. The child must not only learn when the copula is contractible and when it is not, but also must learn the forms of the copula that reflect **person** ("I *am*," "She *is*"), **number** ("I *am*," "We *are*"), and **tense** ("I *am*," "I *was*") and the various combinations of these. If there are several people, not including you, and you are referring to the past, you will say, "They were." If there are several people, including you, and you are referring to the future, you will say, "We will." It takes the child considerable time to learn all the copula's variations, how they combine with nouns and pronouns, and to determine when it is acceptable to contract and when it is not.

The child must also learn when it is permissible to contract the auxiliary forms of *to be*. As with the copula, the child uses the uncontractible form of the auxiliary before the contractible form. The auxiliary form is uncontractible when it is past tense. The sentence "He was running away," cannot be contracted to "He's running away," because *He's* is interpreted in the present tense. If someone asks, "Who is running away?" the contraction *He's* would not be an acceptable answer, whereas *He is* would be acceptable. In response to the question "Is he running away?" you might respond "He isn't running away" or "He's not running away," but you cannot combine the contractions into *He'sn't*. The child masters the uncontractible auxiliary during stage 5. The contractible auxiliary is mastered beyond stage 5, and as with the copula, the child masters the *is* and *are* forms before mastering the *am* form. That is, she will say, "He's running," or "They're running," before she says, "I'm running."

In English, the person(s) performing the action of the verb is indicated by the person and the number of the noun or pronoun. Using the verb *eat*, we can create sentences such as "I eat," "We eat," "You eat," and "They eat." The verb stays the same regardless of the person or number of the subject, but notice what happens when we have a third person singular subject. We now produce sentences such as "He eats," "She eats," and "John eats." The only marker we use to indicate **third-person singular** on the present tense forms of regular verbs is the addition of *s*: "He sings," "She jumps," "Mary writes," "John stands." A few verbs require irregular adjustments to reflect third-person singular. We say "I do," "You do," and "They do" but add *-es* to say "He does." We say "I have," "You have," and "They have" but say "He has." The regular and irregular forms of third-person singular markers on verbs emerge in stage 2, but they are not mastered until stage 5 and beyond (Trantham & Pederson, 1976).

The stage 5 child is producing the personal pronouns *its, our, ours, him, their, theirs, myself*, and *yourself* in sentences such as these:

"The dog has something in *its* ear."

"It's *our* house."

"Do you have a doggie like *ours*?"

"I like *him*."

"*Their* Mommy is nice."

"We have a tree like *theirs*."

"I can do it *myself*."

"You can watch TV by *yourself*."

During the late preschool years and into the early elementary years, the child learns how to change the meanings of words by adding suffixes. Certain adjectives can be changed to **comparative** or **superlative** forms by adding *-er* and *-est*, respectively. The comparative form of *big* is *bigger,* and the superlative form is *biggest.* The stage 5 child understands the superlative forms of common adjectives, but she does not understand the comparative form until she is about five years old, well beyond the end of stage 5 (Carrow, 1973).

It should also be emphasized that the child *understands* these forms before she *uses* them. Even after she understands the comparative and superlative concepts, she may struggle for many years with some adjectives because she does not know or remember whether comparative is marked with *-er* or with *more* and superlative is marked with *-est* or *most.* Does this sound like a familiar problem? The general rule is that if the descriptive adjective is one syllable, use *-er* and *-est.* Two-syllable adjectives often require *more* and *most,* and adjectives of three or more syllables usually require *more* and *most.* The comparative and superlative forms of single-syllable adjectives such as *tall* and *cold* are *taller—tallest* and *colder—coldest,* but consider the following:

beautiful—more beautiful—most beautiful

ridiculous—more ridiculous—most ridiculous

Using *-er* and *-est* on these words would be awkward. Some children, and even adults, get so carried away with the comparative and superlative concepts that they say things like "It was the most ugliest dog I have ever seen," or "She is more shorter than I am." When my youngest daughter was five years old, she loved the word *ridiculous* and used it often, but she had trouble with the comparative and superlative forms. She produced delightfully entertaining sentences such as, "It was the most ridiculousest thing I ever saw," and that's not easy to say!

The stage 5 child is just beginning this struggle. It will be years before he uses the comparative and superlative forms of some adjectives correctly, and he may continue into adulthood with doubts about some. He must learn, for example, that it is not proper to produce comparative and superlative forms of *absolute adjectives.* There are no degrees of *dead* or *perfect,* so it is improper to say "He was the most perfect man I ever met." Likewise, it makes no sense to say "Max the goldfish is deader than Xanadu the mouse," and there is no such thing as *more pregnant.* Let's see now, is it *more lucky* or *luckier?*

During the same preschool period, the child learns to produce the noun versions of certain verbs by adding *-er.* A person who runs, for example, is a *runner,* and a person who plays is a *player.* These are called **agentive** forms. When the child is two or three years old, he usually creates this form by adding *man* to the verb to produce words such as *runman,* or *runningman.* He understands and uses the regular agentive form when he is about five years old.

Noun and Verb Phrases: Still Adjusting the Pieces of the Puzzle

Not much happens in stage 5 relative to the elaboration of noun and verb phrases—nothing at least that is unique to this stage. The child's sentences are a little longer, on average, as indicated by the increase in MLU from stage 4 to stage 5. Nevertheless, the construction of the child's noun phrases is much the same as in stage 4. That is, she continues to use only one element in front of the noun. This element might be a demonstrative pronoun ("*That* cat . . ."), a possessive pronoun ("*My* Mommy . . ."), an article ("*The* doggie . . ."), or an adjective ("I saw a *big* car"). The child continues to have difficulty matching the number of the subject and the verb in this stage and well beyond this stage (Miller, 1981). She will produce sentences such as "The doggies is eating my sandwich," and "Joey and Billy is playing baseball."

It may seem a simple task to establish subject–verb agreement in terms of number, but even many adults struggle with this requirement in certain situations. When the subject of a sentence is conjoined, one might assume the verb should be plural, and in most cases the verb should be plural, but not always. It is correct to say "The pitcher and catcher are important members of the team," but in the sentence "The director and star of the movie is Rock Hunk," the verb is singular because *director* and *star* refer to one person. When *or* or *nor* conjoin singular words, the verb should be singular, as in "Neither George nor Ralph needs the job." When *or* or *nor* conjoin plural words, the verb must be plural, as in "Forks or spoons are stored in this drawer." When a gerund phrase containing a plural noun is the subject of a sentence, the verb is singular, as in the sentence "Collecting baseball cards is my favorite hobby." Some nouns are plural in form but singular in meaning, and they require a singular verb—"Politics is a dirty business." In some cases, a sum of money or a unit of time requires a singular verb. We would say "Three dollars were found on the sidewalk," but we would also say, "Forty thousand dollars is too much to spend for that car," or "Four months is plenty of time to paint the house." Indefinite pronouns such as *all* or *few* can require singular or plural verbs depending on how they are used. We would say "A few of these are spoiled," but we would also say "A few is all he could eat at one time." These are just a few examples of the problems that face the speaker on the single issue of subject–verb agreement. The stage 5 child is still struggling with the most basic of these problems. As she moves through her school years and into adulthood, she will have many opportunities to wrestle with the more difficult challenges of subject–verb agreement.

The changes we see in verb phrases in stage 5 occur as a result of the child's acquisition of the grammatical morphemes we identified earlier. As the child progressively masters irregular past tense forms, the contractible copula, the uncontractible auxiliary, and the markers for regular and irregular third person singular, his verb phrases become more adultlike. His verb phrases are not necessarily longer, but they are more correct according to adult language standards.

Sentence Construction: Negatives, Questions, Embedding, and Conjoining

By the close of stage 5, the child is using negative past tense forms of the verb *to be,* as in the sentence "He wasn't a good boy." Although they do not appear often, he also produces the negative past tense of common modals, including *wouldn't, couldn't,* and *shouldn't* (Miller, 1981), resulting in sentences such as the following:

"Mommy couldn't open the can."

"She wouldn't eat her soup."

"Bobbie shouldn't do that."

Progress in the creation of negative sentences in stage 5 centers on the use of past tense and appropriate modals, and we see the same adjustments as the child continues to develop the interrogative form of sentences. The child is producing correctly inverted question forms in stage 4, but is somewhat inconsistent in making the required inversions. In this stage, he is much more consistent in moving from a declarative statement such as "He is playing baseball," to the interrogative version, "Is he playing baseball?

We also see the appearance of the **tag question** in stage 5, an interrogative form not frequently used in American English (Klee, 1985). The easiest and most common form of tag question is acquired in stage 5. In this version, the speaker adds a tag like *huh* or *OK* to the end of a sentence, as in "I'm going to leave now, OK?" or "You're going to buy me some ice cream, huh?" Beyond stage 5, the child learns a somewhat more difficult form of tag question, not including a negative element, as represented in the sentence "You're going to buy me some ice cream, are you?" Within the next few years, he is producing the adult form of tag questions, complete with a negative element, as in the sentence "You're going to buy me some ice cream, aren't you?" The progression from *huh* to *are you* to *aren't you* sounds subtle, but each step reflects a more sophisticated use of language (Reich, 1986).

During stage 5, the child begins to embed relative clauses in the object position of sentences. According to Menyuk (1977), she will not embed relative clauses into subjects until she is beyond the age of five years. As indicated earlier in this chapter, a relative clause is introduced by a relative pronoun such as *who, which, what,* or *that.* In the sentence "The man who came to dinner with Sally is my brother," the clause *who came to dinner* is embedded into the subject to describe or modify *man.* The child's earliest relative clauses are used to describe **empty nouns.** These are nonspecific nouns such as *thing* or *one.* Using these nouns, the stage 5 child produces sentences containing object-embedded relative clauses such as "She's the one *that I kissed,*" or "That's the thing *that I broke.*" By the end of this stage, the child will produce a few sentences in which the relative pronoun is omitted and understood, but still only in the object position. Without the relative pronouns, our example sentences would be produced as follows: "She's the one I kissed," and "That's the thing I broke." Perhaps because the relative pronoun helps preserve the meaning of the sentence, preschool children are less likely to delete it than adults (Menyuk, 1977).

The first relative pronoun the child is likely to use in all circumstances is *that.* Whereas the adult would say, "She's the one *who* came to the party," the child in stage 5 will probably say, "She's the one *that* came to the party." Even when the child adds other relative pronouns to his repertoire, he often uses them incorrectly. He might continue to use *that* for *who* for some time, and he might use *what* for *who* or even for *that,* resulting in sentences such as the following:

"George is the one *what* broke the window."

"The glass is the thing *what* spilled."

By the close of stage 5, the child is producing multiple embeddings (Miller, 1981). She might produce a sentence that embeds an infinitive into a subordinate clause that serves as the object of the sentence: "I think I want to eat all the cake." The clause "I want to eat all the cake" is the object of the verb *think*. The infinitive *to eat* is embedded in this clause, so we have a sentence that contains an embedded subordinate clause that, in turn, contains an embedded infinitive. This is only the beginning of the possibilities. As the child moves into the school years, she will produce sentences with even more elaborate embeddings, and she will learn to embed and conjoin at the same time. That sounds illegal, doesn't it?

Although the child uses the conjunction *and* as early as the end of stage 1 and adds other conjunctions such as *but, so, if,* and *or* in stage 3, he does not conjoin clauses until stage 4, and he does not really get serious about clausal conjoining until stage 5 (Brown, 1973). The child's favorite conjunction is *and,* and he continues to favor it in combining clauses well beyond stage 5 (Bennett-Kaster, 1986).

According to Bloom, Lahey, Hood, Lifter, and Fiess (1980), the semantic relations conveyed in conjoined sentences emerge in an identifiable sequence. In the beginning, the child uses *and* to express all of these semantic relations. The first conjunctive relation to emerge is **additive,** a relation we are most likely to associate with *and.* In an additive sentence, the child combines two clauses that are independent of one another. She might say, "I went to Billy's house, and I'm a big girl." In this sentence, the combined meaning is the same as the added meanings of the separate clauses. The child then uses *and* to express **temporal** relations. In the sentence, "I went to Billy's house, and I played with his toys," the child is talking about one event that follows another in time. The child then expresses the **causal** relation. One clause expresses an action or state of being, and the other clause provides a reason or describes the effect. The child might say, "I ate all the cake, and my tummy is full." The combined meaning in this sentence is clearly greater than the sum of the meanings of the separate clauses. The child then expresses the **adversative** relation in her conjoined sentences. In this case, the two parts of the sentence represent a contrast. The child says, "This doggie big, and this one little." The children in this study also used *and* to connect a clause that described or elaborated on the subject of the preceding clause. The child might say, "I got a baseball bat, and you play baseball with it." The authors called this semantic relation **object specification.** They conclude that the child is using *and* to link subjects and objects appropriately in a listing sense by the end of stage 1 or the beginning of stage 2.

As already noted, some children conjoin clauses with *and* as early as stage 4, but we usually do not see clausal conjoining until the end of stage 5 (Miller, 1981). Although the dominant conjunction continues to be *and* for some time, the child is using *if* to conjoin clauses by the close of stage 5. Other conjunctions, including *because, but, so,* and *when* do not emerge until after stage 5 when the child's MLU is about 5.0 (Owens, 2005, p. 325).

Pragmatic Development:
The Conversational Fine-Tuning Continues

We generally think of the child's becoming a social creature between the ages of three and four. This maturity seems to be reflected in the stage 5 child's conversation, which is becoming increasingly social. When she speaks to others, her utterances are appropriately structured, understandable, and designed to meet her listeners' conversational needs (Mueller, 1972).

In stage 4, we observed that the child develops a sensitivity to the time factor in conversational exchanges. That is, when there is a time delay of less than one second, he concludes that exchanges will continue, but if the delay is longer than one second, he concludes that no response is forthcoming (Craig & Gallagher, 1983). In stage 5, the child's turn taking continues to be affected by his interpretations of short and long pauses. As is true of the adult in conversation, the child uses the pause as a cue for initiating his turn (Garvey & Berninger, 1981). Perhaps of even greater significance, he takes into consideration what is likely to be included in the next turn. That is, he shows an awareness of what is being discussed in the present turn, and he anticipates how this topic will be completed in succeeding turns (McTear, 1985). He is sensitive to problems his partner may have in finishing her turn, and when he senses his partner is having difficulty, he will attempt to help by completing what he perceives to be his partner's thought. In addition, he is developing a sensitivity to the problems created by simultaneous talking. When he senses that information will be lost when he and his partner are talking at the same time, he is willing to give up his turn to preserve the conversational topic. By the time the child is ready for school, he has developed considerable turn-taking skills, but conversational inadequacies remain.

Some preschool children are able to handle conversations involving two partners but struggle with three-party conversations (Ervin-Tripp, 1979). Interruptions remain a problem for young communicators for some time. Remember that interruptions are sometimes necessary to capture one's turn in a conversation. The child must learn how and when to interrupt according to the "rules" of conversational etiquette. Sachs (1982) found that the preschool child typically does not use polite verbal or nonverbal strategies for gaining the attention of her listener. That is, she does not say, "Excuse me," or does not gently tap her listener's shoulder or lean forward or gesture in a manner that suggests she wants to say something. She simply yells at her listener. Only 36 percent of the utterances produced by Sachs's subjects, who ranged from forty to sixty-six months, were at a conversational loudness level. Not surprisingly, only the oldest subjects in this study were sensitive to their proximity to their listeners. The older children did not try to initiate conversation until they were within an appropriate range. Even then, they yelled. The younger children just yelled. If you have spent much time around children in this age range, you are probably saying, "Yep, that just about captures it!"

Over the course of the preschool years, the child improves his ability to initiate and sustain a conversation. As we have mentioned, the child does not maintain a topic for more than two turns until he is about forty-two months, which marks the beginning of stage 5 (Bloom et al., 1976). By the time the child is five years old and well beyond stage 5, he maintains a topic for an average of five turns compared to the eleven turns on average by adult speakers (Brinton & Fujiki, 1984). Even when the preschool child is maintaining a topic through three or four turns, he is not contributing much new information. He maintains the conversation primarily through repeating part of what his partner has already said or by asking questions about his

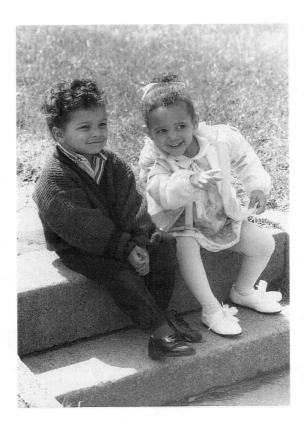

Learning the art of conversation.

partner's comments. Even when the child is in the early elementary school years, he seldom adds significant information to a conversation (Brinton & Fujiki, 1984). In this sense, he remains a conversational follower.

We see no radical changes in conversational repairs during stage 5, although as the child's overall language skills improve, she is better able to respond to requests for clarification. As early as stage 1 or 2, the child has shown an awareness of the need for conversational repairs. Throughout the five stages of language development, she tries, within the limits of her intellectual and linguistic abilities, to provide the information her conversational partner finds lacking or confused. Even as stage 5 closes, however, she sometimes has difficulty identifying the part of the message that needs to be repaired (Brinton & Fujiki, 1989, p. 92), and she still responds readily to requests for repairs more than she makes requests for repairs from her conversational partners.

We noted that the child's presuppositional skills in stage 4 depend on his knowledge of the topic and his language skills. Nothing has changed in this regard as he moves into stage 5. Naturally, his presuppositional skills improve as he moves toward his fourth birthday, but the limitations are the same. Several studies requiring young children to describe stimuli to listeners have demonstrated these limitations. When preschool and even kindergarten children have tried to describe blocks of varying sizes, colors, and geometric shapes to listeners so that the listeners could choose the correct blocks, they did not perform well. They were not able to provide the information the listeners needed. In their study, Krauss and Glucksberg (1977) had two four-year-old children sitting at a table and separated by a screen so they could not see one another. Each child had an identical set of blocks of unfamiliar geometric shapes. The speaker's task was to describe one of the blocks so that the listener could successfully select it. The following exchange occurred:

CHILD 1: It's a bird.
CHILD 2: Is this it?
CHILD 1: No.

One could conclude, of course, that the speaker in this situation simply had inadequate presuppositional skills, but there is another and perhaps more reasonable interpretation. This task was beyond the cognitive abilities of these children. They did not know these shapes, and the speaker was unable to retrieve an image from his mental bank that was a close enough match to the block he was trying to describe to help his partner who was also unfamiliar with these shapes. Two adults, unfamiliar with the Chinese alphabet, might have similar problems if one were trying to describe a Chinese character to the other. The adults would have the advantage of larger vocabularies, more sophisticated language abilities, and greater experience with a wider range of stimuli that might be similar in important respects to the Chinese character, but it would still be a difficult task. The point is, the stage 5 child might appear to have inadequate presuppositional skills when the real problem is a lack of knowledge. When he is talking about things he knows and understands, he is much more adept at providing the information his listener needs.

The stage 5 child continues to increase her use of indirect requests, although indirect requests are still far less frequent than direct requests. Between forty-two and fifty-two months, less than 10 percent of children's requests are indirect, but we see a dramatic increase in use of the indirect form beyond stage 5 at about fifty-four months (James & Seebach, 1982; Wilkinson, Calculator, & Dollaghan, 1982). The child will make requests such as "Don't forget to get my cookie," or "Why don't you get me some candy?" These are clearly requests, but they are more subtle and more polite than "Give me a cookie," or "Get me some candy." When the child increases her use of indirect requests, she will also include rationalizations for her requests. She might say, for example, "I ate all my peas. . . . Don't forget to get my cookie," a polite and indirect way of saying that she has been a good girl, has fulfilled the obligations of her dinner-eating contract, and now wants a reward.

As early as four years, the child's requests are shaped by his sensitivity to the roles and viewpoints of his listeners and the need to be polite (Gordon & Ervin-Tripp, 1984), and he responds appropriately to indirect requests made to him (Carrell, 1981). He has been using *please* since he was twenty-four to thirty-six months old, but in the beginning, he uses it mostly with people who are older or more dominant (Ervin-Tripp &

Gordon, 1986). By the time he is four years old, *please* has become the magic word that can be used with almost anyone to get almost anything, and over the next few years, he will learn to use the magic word even more effectively.

Pragmatic Development: The Beginnings of Narrative Discourse

In addition to learning the technical skills and artistic nuances of conversation, the child is soon confronted with a new discourse challenge: She must learn how to tell a story, a common narrative form. As is true of a conversation, a narrative consists of a series of sentences, not juxtaposed randomly but appearing in an orderly and interconnected sequence. The sequence of sentences allows the speaker to convey information about events or experiences in a systematic manner, each sentence building on the preceding sentence. Unlike a conversation in which the communicative responsibility is shared by all participants who take turns as speakers and listeners, the narrative form is essentially a monologue in which the responsibility for conveying the message belongs almost exclusively to the speaker. Just as there are rules governing conversation, so are there rules, or principles, for structuring a narrative so that it is a cohesive and effective communication entity.

We will address narrative skills in their more fully developed form in Chapter 6. In this section, we will consider the basic constructs of narratives that develop during the preschool years. These narrative fundamentals will form the foundation for the more complete and complex narrative skills that develop during the school years.

If you listen carefully to a child who is two to three and a half years old, you will hear what are called **protonarratives.** A protonarrative is a primitive story about something that has happened to the child. As we have already noted, the child at this age has been repeatedly exposed to familiar routines or scripts in the common events of her life. While the child at this age cannot accurately and completely describe what happened during an event, she will often produce a series of utterances that, taken together, have a storylike quality. Visualize a very common routine, mealtime. The child is eating one of her least favorite foods, and she and her caregiver go through their usual tortuous exchange of words and actions related to her consumption of this food. That evening, Aunt Mary comes over for a visit, and she asks her about dinner. The child says to Aunt Mary, "It made me sick. I throwed it away. It was lumpy. I don't like oatmeal!" We suspect that the caregiver's version of this event would be quite different and certainly more detailed than the child's version, but the child does convey a message that bears some resemblance to a story, even if it is a little short on detail and even if her description is not exactly on target. Miller and Sperry (1988) note that between the ages of twenty-four and thirty months, children use protonarratives with increasing frequency, and they improve their ability to put events into simple sequences.

When the child develops his first narratives, he uses two basic strategies to provide their organizational structure. One strategy, called **chaining,** involves ordering events that share one or more features in common. Each event in the chain logically follows the preceding event. The second strategy, called **centering,** involves building a story around a central theme. Each item or action in the narrative is connected to the central theme by an attribute that is related to the theme, however marginal that relationship might seem to an adult observer.

According to Sutton-Smith (1986), the child will begin to produce his own stories sometime between the ages of twenty-four and thirty-six months, and, if he is a typical child, most of his earliest narratives will be built around central themes. The central themes of these early stories tend to focus on unusual or upsetting events that have had a significant impact on the child's life (Ames, 1966). An adult, listening to this kind of story, may want to understand exactly what happened to the child, when it happened, and why it happened. The adult listener is likely to be disappointed. In his earliest stories, the child does not take into consideration the listener's need for background information. In fact, even at forty-two months, he does not provide much information about the participants in his narratives (Peterson, 1990). Even if the adult listener is struggling to make sense of it all, the child remains excited about telling his story, and it does not seem to matter much if the listener has a complete grasp of what happened or not. As we mentioned, the child's earliest narratives tend to be centered, or central theme, stories, but by the time he is three years old, he may be using the chaining strategy as often as he uses the centering strategy (Owens, 2005, p. 274).

The child's narrative skills noticeably improve during the preschool years. When she is two years old, the child organizes a narrative by generating a series of brief, unrelated statements connected only by a common originating stimulus. The process the child uses to get from one utterance to the next is something like the free association used by psychotherapists. The critical difference, of course, is that the child is prompting herself and the therapist is prompting a client, but the prompting principle is the same. The therapist instructs the client to say the first thing that comes to her mind, resulting in an exchange such as the following:

THERAPIST: Dog.
    CLIENT: Animal.
THERAPIST: Animal.
    CLIENT: Linebacker.
THERAPIST: Linebacker.
    CLIENT: Overpaid.
THERAPIST: Overpaid.
    CLIENT: Therapist.
THERAPIST: Our time's up. That'll be $100.
    CLIENT: Dog!

Despite the silliness of the example, the reader should be able to sense that these responses are connected, but not in a categorical or cause–effect sense. They are connected, very loosely, in that one response prompts another. A set of unrelated statements connected by a common originating stimulus produced by the two-year-old child is called a **heap.** When he creates a heap, the child uses a basic sentence structure and simply adds or chains one bit of information onto another, prompted by his own observations. In the following example of a heap, you will not find a meaningful organization, even though you should be able to figure out the association that prompts each succeeding utterance. Notice, too, that you could rearrange these utterances into any order without affecting the overall meaning of the heap. Why is the overall meaning of the heap not affected by a reorganization of the utterances? And the answer is . . . there is no overall meaning. This narrative is like an abstract Swedish movie from the 1960s. It's going nowhere.

> Mommy sit here. Baby go "Waa!" Kitty go "meow." Doggie play ball.

At the next level of narrative development, the child's stories have a little more cohesion and a bit more focus. That is, the child's statements reflect a characteristic that several things have in common, or they reflect several events that were juxtaposed by time. Even though she may talk about several things that took place within the same general time frame, the child's statements are not organized in a temporal manner in the sense that the first statement refers to the first thing that happened, the second statement refers to the second thing that happened, and so forth. Neither is there the suggestion of a cause–effect organization. The child's statements are simply chained, or added together, which means that they can still be reorganized into any pattern of presentation without affecting the integrity of the story. An example of this kind of narrative follows:

> Daddy threw a straw. Suzie ate ice cream. I had a Pepsi.

Sometime between the ages of three and five years, the child is producing narratives that have at least a rudimentary temporal organization (Owens, 2005, p. 275), but the glue that holds this kind of narrative together is still the central theme. The child's story statements convey what happened and in what order, but the emphasis is clearly on the essence of the event itself. That this is still a primitive form of narrative is made clear by the absence of a plot and by the absence of cause–effect references. An example of this kind of narrative follows:

> Mommy took me to the zoo. There was a lion. He made a noise. There was a monkey. And I got some popcorn. And we drived home.

The child's narratives will not typically include causality organization until he is five years old (Owens, 2005, p. 276). When he adds this dimension to his stories, his narratives will change dramatically. We will consider these changes and the continued maturation of the child's narrative skills in Chapter 6. (See Table 5.6 for highlights of stage 5 and Tables 5.7 and 5.8 for summaries of negation and question forms, respectively, in Brown's five stages.)

Understanding Language: Cognition, Comprehension, and Production

As has been noted at a number of junctures in this book, it is not possible to separate intellectual growth from language development, and it is not possible to separate the

Table 5.6 Stage 5 Highlights

Typical Age Range: Forty-One to Forty-Six Months
MLU: 3.75–4.5 Morphemes

Grammatical Morphemes
- Nine of the fourteen specified morphemes are mastered by the close of stage 5.
- The remaining five morphemes (irregular past tense, contractible copula, uncontractible auxiliary, regular third person, and irregular third person) are mastered by fifty months.

Pronouns
- More consistent in use of *its, our, ours, him, their, theirs, myself, yourself*

Adjectives
- Understands the superlative forms of common adjectives but does not understand comparative forms until she is about five years old

Noun Phrases
- Continues to elaborate by adding only one element in front of the noun

Verb Phrases
- Continues to have difficulty matching the number of the subject and the verb
- Verb phrases become more adultlike as the child masters verb-related grammatical morphemes.

Sentences
- Using negative past tense forms of *to be* (e.g., *weren't, wasn't*)
- Occasionally uses negative past tense modals (e.g., *wouldn't, couldn't*)
- More consistent in creating questions by properly inverting words (e.g., "He is playing baseball." → "Is he playing baseball?")
- Produces primitive tag questions (e.g., "I'm going now, OK?")
- Embeds relative clauses into the object position of sentences (e.g., "That's the plate *that I broke.*")
- Conjoins clauses, usually with *and*

Pragmatics
- Conversational skills improve as a direct result of more sophisticated language.
- Increases use of indirect requests, although direct requests are still far more common.

---

comprehension of language from the production of language. These processes are inextricably connected, and they have interactive relationships. The child thinks before she has language, but language eventually facilitates and shapes thought. As common sense suggests, comprehension generally precedes production, but production can also assist understanding. That is, sometimes we learn lessons about how language works by producing the language behaviors that illustrate the lessons. As we observe children acquiring language, it appears that some lessons are learned in a dramatic flash of illumination while others are learned more slowly, in an evolution of understanding that is steady but progresses in small steps.

We should also keep in mind that language often reflects what one understands about the things, people, and events in reality, and language production often reflects

Table 5.7 The Development of Negation in Brown's Five Stages

Brown's Stages	Development of Negation	Examples
Early stage 1 12–22 months	Uses single words such as "No!" "Gone!" "Allgone!" to express rejection, denial, nonexistence, and disappearance	"Allgone!" to indicate that he ate all of his spinach
Late stage 1 22–26 months	Uses either *no* or *not* as the first element in constructing a simple sentence	"Not cookie!" "No milk."
Early stage 2 27–28 months	No changes	
Late stage 2 28–30 months	Uses *no, not, don't, can't*, and may place the negative element between the subject and predicate	"Daddy can't go."
Early stage 3 31–32 months	More likely to use *no, not, don't*, and *can't* between subject and predicate	"I can't play." "Baby not cry."
Late stage 3 33–34 months	Uses the contraction *won't*	"Mommy won't play."
Early stage 4 35–37 months	Begins using negation with auxiliary verbs	"He will not run away." "Daddy is not playing."
Late stage 4 38–40 months	Begins using *isn't, doesn't, aren't*, and *didn't*	"That isn't my bike." "The boy didn't run."
Stage 5 41–46 months and beyond	Begins using *wouldn't, couldn't, wasn't*, and *shouldn't*	"The boy wouldn't help me." "The doggie wasn't there."

what one is able to comprehend in language. Even college students are inclined to say, "I know what I mean, but I just can't express it," when the truth is probably closer to "I wish I knew what I mean, but since I don't know, I'll use words that clearly express my confusion and benign ignorance." Although there are exceptions, it is generally true that clear thinking results in clear speaking or writing, and muddled communications reflect muddled or incomplete thinking. If adults struggle with the interactions among cognition, comprehension, and production, imagine how the relationships among these processes affect the child between the ages of two years and four years, the approximate age span between stages 2 and 5. The child must know the words that represent the things, people, places, and events in his environment, of course, but he must also know how to change nouns to reflect plurality and possession; how to replace nouns with pronouns; how to mark verbs to indicate present, past, and future; how and when it is appropriate to contract; how to embed phrases and clauses to elaborate or indicate relationships; and so on and so on. There is much to understand about the world, much to understand about language, and much to

Table 5.8 The Development of Question Forms in Brown's Five Stages

Brown's Stages	Yes/No Questions	Examples	*Wh*-Questions	Examples
Early stage 1 MLU = 1–1:5 Age = 12–22 months	Uses a single word with a rising intonation	"Doggie?"	Uses *What* and *Where* with a rising intonation. *What* and *Where* are not likely to be complete adult phonological forms.	"What?" "Where?"
Late stage 1 MLU = 1.5–2.0 Age = 22–26 months	Combines two words by putting *that* + "X" with a rising intonation	"That doggie?"		"What that?" "Where doggie?"
Early stage 2 MLU = 2.0–2.25 Age = 27–28 months			Child continues to use *What* and *Where* to produce the following combinations: *What* + NP? *Where* + NP? *What* + NP + (doing)? *Where* + NP + (go or going)?	"What kitty doing?" "Where mommy go?"
Late stage 2 MLU = 2.25–2.5 Age = 28–30 months	Continues combining words with a rising intonation	"Doggie go home?"	Produces "What" and "Where" + NP + verb?	"What Daddy kick?"
			Produces: "What" or "Where" + NP + copula (such as "is")?	"Where doggie is?"
			May ask "Why?" as a single word	"Why?"
Early stage 3 MLU = 2.5–2.75 Age = 31–32 months			Toward the end of early stage 3, inverts copula to form comparable to adult	"Where is doggie?"

(continued)

know about producing language. Much of this understanding and producing occurs within the first four or five years of the child's life, and it is all connected. Let's examine a few examples of the language components children must unravel to comprehend what they hear and what they produce.

Table 5.8 Continued

Brown's Stages	Yes/No Questions	Examples	*Wh*-Questions	Examples
Late stage 3 MLU = 2.75–3.0 Age = 33–34 months	Auxiliary verb forms such as *can* and *do* begin to be incorporated with proper inversion of subject and verb.	"Can kitty meow?" "Does kitty like Mommy?" "What is kitty eating?"	May add *Who* to her productions	"Who is that man?"
	Rising intonation *may* still be used without inverting the auxiliary verb.	"Kitty can go bye-bye?"		
Early stage 4 MLU = 3.0–3.5 Age = 35–37 months			*May* add *How* to her productions	"How did she run?"
Late stage 4 MLU = 3.5–3.75 Age = 38–40 months	Continuation of above; more consistent inverting of auxiliary verbs.		Now uses *How* and *When* in her productions	"When is he going?"
Stage 5 and beyond MLU = 3.75–4.5 and above Age = 41–46 months and beyond	Auxiliary inversion is consistent; more modals such as *may*, and *must* are added.	"Are they going away?" "May I have that?"	*Why* questions now appear in combination with other words; may use some tag questions.	"Why is he doing that?" "I want to go outside, OK?"

Cognitive Development: Paving the Way for Understanding and Production

Common sense would certainly suggest that the child cannot receive or produce language that reflects understanding she does not have at the cognitive level. Before the child can embed phrases or clauses to reflect the manipulation of two or more linguistic units, she must be able to cognitively manipulate two or more objects (Ingram, 1975).

The words used in *wh*-questions emerge in the following order: *what, where, who,* and then *when, how,* and *why.* What does this order suggest to you about the order of acquisition of concepts that underlie these words? Why are words such as *when, how,* and *why* acquired late? These last three words relate to the concepts of time and causality, and these concepts are acquired relatively late in cognitive development (Piaget, 1926). Very simply, the child must understand *time* before he can understand or produce *when* questions, and he must understand *cause–effect* before he can comprehend or produce *how* or *why* questions. Before the child has these later *wh*-words, he often responds to *when, how,* and *why* questions as though they are *what, where,* or *who* questions. Tyack and Ingram (1977) suggest that the child with a limited understanding of *wh*-terms uses two strategies in answering *wh*-questions: (1) answer the question as though the *wh*-word is one you already know, or (2) answer the question in a manner consistent with your understanding of the verb. Using the first strategy in responding to the question *"When did Susie eat?"* the child might assume it is a *what* question and respond, "Cracker." Using the second strategy, he might respond in the same way because he associates *cracker* with the verb *eat.*

Piaget (1966) suggested that the child understands the sequencing of events before he understands duration. This too is reflected in his understanding and use of language. The child understands and produces words such as *before* and *after,* that indicate *order,* before he uses words such as *until* or *since,* that indicate *duration.*

These are just a few examples of the obvious connections between what a child understands about the world at a cognitive level and what she is able to understand and produce in language. Look for the cognitive-language connections in the examples that follow. Some are obvious, and others are more subtle, but it may be impossible to find any aspect of receptive or expressive language development that is not directly or indirectly tied to a corresponding development in cognition.

Understanding Active and Passive Sentences

Consider the problems the child encounters as she tries to sort out active and passive sentences. An active sentence is considered **reversible** if either noun can be either the agent or the object. For example, we can say, *"The dog chased the cat,"* or *"The cat chased the dog."* These are reversible active sentences. The child understands the reversible active sentence in stage 1 or 2 (Chapman & Miller, 1975), but she has trouble interpreting reversible passive sentences until she is five years old or older. Why is this a problem?

To interpret an active sentence, the child must learn that the first noun is the agent and the second noun is the object. She encounters an entirely different word order in passive sentences. In the passive sentence *"The cat was chased by the dog,"* the first noun *(cat)* is the object of the verb *chased,* and the second noun *(dog)* is the agent. The child in stage 1 or 2 interprets this sentence in the same way as she interprets active sentences. If she were asked to point to one of two pictures, one showing a dog chasing a cat and the other a cat chasing a dog, she would point to the picture of the cat chasing the dog because she interprets the first noun as the subject and the second noun as the object. The child does not correctly interpret reversible passive sentences until she is beyond stage 5. During the child's early struggles with passive forms, between the ages of three and four years, she will understand passive sentences that include animate objects better than sentences including inanimate objects (Lempert, 1990). Even at five, the child is more likely to correctly interpret reversible passive sentences containing active verbs than those that contain nonactive verbs. That is, *"The boy was bitten by the girl"* would be interpreted more easily than *"The boy was loved by the girl."* The child will probably not completely sort out passive sentences until she is in elementary school.

We should add a cautionary note at this point. The conclusions about understanding active and passive sentences are based on research that required children to act out the sentences they heard. A more recent technique requires that children only look at paired videos, one showing the agent–object relationship reflected in the sentence and the other showing the opposite agent–object relationship (Golinkoff, Hirsh-Pasek, Cauley, & Gordon, 1987). Since acting out sentences is a more intense exercise requiring greater cooperation from the child, it may appear that children gain an understanding of passive and active sentences later than they really do. This new approach, which requires little effort, may eventually demonstrate that this understanding is acquired earlier.

Word Order: Which Comes First, Comprehension or Production?

Because word order is very important in English, experts who study English-speaking children are interested in the word order portion of the acquisition puzzle. Does the child comprehend word order before he produces language containing appropriate word order? The answer is temptingly obvious. There seems little doubt that comprehension of word order would precede production, and early research supported this assumption, but some interesting and contradictory findings have emerged.

Chapman and Miller (1975) studied the comprehension and production of reversible active sentences in stage 1, 2, and 3 children. In the comprehension task, the children were instructed to act out sentences produced by an adult. In the production task, the children were instructed to describe an action produced by an adult. The children in all three stages performed better in the production task than in the comprehension task, leading the authors to conclude that for word order at least, production precedes comprehension. Their conclusions were supported by later research (Gleitman & Wanner, 1982). How can this be?

It may be that we have oversimplified the comprehension–production equation. When the child in normal circumstances responds to the utterances of others, he is responding to more than linguistic information. He interprets the situation and reads all the nonverbal messages he is receiving from the speaker as well as comprehending the language forms he hears. If his caregiver says, "Put your toys in the toy box," while pointing to the toys strewn all over the floor and to the empty toy box, the child sees the toys and the box, hears the tone of his caregiver's voice, observes the caregiver's gestures and facial expression, *and* hears the words of the imperative sentence.

He has been through this routine before and knows that the routine calls for him to pick up the toys and put them in the box. He puts all the information, linguistic and nonlinguistic, together to arrive at a correct interpretation of the total message.

Now consider what occurred in the Chapman and Miller (1975) exercise. The child is instructed to act out a sentence, not unlike the one we have used here, but she is given no other information. She must rely on linguistic information alone. It may be, therefore, that the child first comprehends linguistic messages within situational and nonverbal contexts, then produces language, and then understands language without the supporting situational and nonverbal contexts. Once again, we must be careful not to draw unwarranted conclusions. It may be that the kinds of responses required of children in some of these studies obscure what they really know and what they can really do. Acting out sentences and interpreting sentences being acted out may add levels of complexity that mask the child's true receptive and expressive abilities. Techniques that place fewer demands on the child's attention and that require less physical cooperation, such as the video technique developed by Golinkoff and colleagues (1987), may lead us to different conclusions about how and when the child comprehends and produces word order.

Words Expressing Relations: From Concepts to Production

A **relational** word, as the name suggests, identifies relationships among people, objects, and events. Relational words are used to identify spatial, temporal, quantity, and dimensional relationships. Children's understanding of the concepts that underlie these words and their comprehension of the words that describe the concepts develop during the preschool years. These are difficult concepts, however, and they are not acquired quickly or easily.

Spatial terms include prepositions such as *in, on, under, over, beside, behind,* and *in front of.* By the time the child is two years old, she is using *in* and *on,* but she may be applying a very simple strategy in deciding how to use these prepositions. In general, if she is describing an object in relation to a container, she will use *in.* If she is describing an object in relation to a surface, she will use *on,* but she does not fully understand that *on* can be used to describe an object in relation to a container, and she does not understand *under* until she is about three years old (Clark & Clark, 1977). She continues to have problems with terms such as *beside, next to, behind,* and *in front of* until she is four or five years old (Johnston, 1984). The difficulty with these later developing prepositions is that the child must consider the object she is describing in relation to the spatial orientation of another object. To use the term *behind,* for example, the child must know which is the front and which is the back of the referent object. As common sense would suggest, she will use these prepositions most accurately with referent objects that have clearly defined fronts and backs. She will understand, for example, "Your sock is behind Mommy," more easily than "Your sock is behind the ball," because Mommy has an obvious front and an equally obvious back, but where is the "back" of the ball? When the referent object has no obvious front or back, the adult listener interprets *behind* or *in front of* on the basis of her position in relation to the object. That is, the surface of the ball nearest the listener is the "front," and the opposite surface is the "back." Children first understand these prepositions in relation to their own bodies, then in relation to referent objects with clearly defined fronts and backs, and finally in relation to objects without clearly defined fronts and backs (Conner & Chapman, 1985). This means, therefore, that in the earliest stage of understanding, the child who is directly facing a ball upon hearing the sentence, "Your sock is behind the ball," is likely to turn around and look for the sock behind her own back.

Temporal terms are used to describe relationships based on time. As we mentioned earlier in this section, the child understands terms based on *order* such as *before* and *after* earlier than he understands terms based on *duration* such as *since* and *until*. Although the research has not provided a clear order of acquisition for temporal terms, it does seem clear that the child understands *before* and *after* by the time he is five years old.

Words such as *more* and *less* are **quantity** terms. They are used to identify the amount of something or the number of things in a group. These words are troublesome for the preschooler. When the preschool child is asked to point to the one with "more" or the one with "less," she points to the one with more. When she is asked to point to one of them, she points to the one with more. Some experts have concluded that these undifferentiated responses mean that the child believes *more* and *less* mean the same thing. According to Clark and Clark (1977), the child understands both words to mean "amount." Using this understanding, the child points to the one with the greater "amount," which is, of course, the one with more. Whatever the child's interpretation, she does not understand the difference between *more* and *less* until she moves into the elementary school years, and then she becomes confused about the meanings of words such as *few* and *couple*. Someone asks the child, "Do you understand the difference between 'less' and 'few'?" and she responds, "More or less!" Someone asks the child, "What is the difference between 'couple' and 'few'?" She answers, "When there are more than a couple, use 'few.' When there is more than one but less than a few, use 'couple.' " Although there might be a few disagreements about whether *few* is less than *less* or whether some people use *less* when they should use *few*, the child's response is more or less correct. The point of this hypothetical banter is to remind the reader that these are difficult terms and difficult concepts. It is not surprising that the preschooler does not yet have a solid understanding of quantity concepts and words.

Dimensional terms are used to identify the opposite ends of the limits of a person or object. They include words such as *big/little, tall/short,* and *thick/thin*. More general dimensional terms such as *big/little* are understood before more specific terms such as *tall/short* (Clark & Clark, 1977). That is, the child will first understand that *big* is used to describe something exceptionally tall, wide, or deep. As his understanding of size is refined, he will understand and use more specific terms. If a friend simply described someone as *big*, you would probably request more specific information. You might ask, "Is he tall or fat?" Your friend might then reply, "Oh, he's not fat. He's tall with broad shoulders and a thick chest." Words such as *tall, broad,* and *thick,* which are more specific dimensional terms, are acquired after the more general term, *big*. Within each dimensional pair, the child understands the positive term first. That is, he will understand *big, tall, thick, broad,* and *deep,* before he understands their native counterparts: *little, short, thin, narrow,* and *shallow* (Brewer & Stone, 1975). The positive term in each pair is used to specify the dimension. When we ask about someone's height, we tend to say, "How tall is he?" not "How short is he?" When we ask the waiter about the size of a steak, we are likely to say, "How thick is the steak?" not "How thin is the steak?" We also say, "Bill is six feet tall," not "Bill is six feet short." We say, "The lake is 25 feet deep," not "The lake is 25 feet shallow." Why does the child learn the positive terms in these pairs before the negative terms? It may be that because the positive terms are used more often in the speech of adults, the child uses them earlier simply because he hears them more often, but there is probably a cognitive connection as well. That is, the child understands the concepts that underlie the positive terms before he understands the concepts that underlie the negative terms (Klatsky, Clark, & Macken, 1973).

This discussion has not included all that is now known about the development of comprehension during the preschool years. We have provided examples of concepts, words, and structures that must be understood, and we have tried to emphasize the complex relationships that exist among cognitive development, the comprehension of language, and the production of language. There is much still unknown about the interactions of cognition, language comprehension, and language production, but certainly the simplistic notion that comprehension always precedes production is not valid. The relationship of thinking, understanding language, and the production of language cannot be represented on a linear graph with three colored lines. These three phenomena intersect and interact to such an extent that the lines which seem to separate them are blurred and rendered meaningless. Even as an adult thinker and speaker, you must surely sense that these processes do not work independently. Sometimes in talking aloud about a difficult concept, you suddenly understand the meaning of your own words, and your cognitive grasp of the concept is enhanced. In this case, you have actually operated in a manner that appears backward. The production of language facilitates the comprehension of language, which facilitates cognitive understanding.

And That's Not All, Folks!

The child has been a busy language activist during her preschool years, but she still has more work to do. As she moves into her elementary school years, adolescence, and even into adulthood, her vocabulary will continue to grow, she will refine and elaborate the language structures she has acquired, and she will become a more sophisticated conversationalist. These changes do not occur as quickly as in previous years, and they are not as dramatic, but they are important changes that will make her a more effective language receiver and producer. In the next chapter, we trace language development beyond stage 5.

Review Questions

1. What is meant by obligatory context in relation to grammatical morphemes? What determines obligatory context?
2. What does it mean to say that a child overextends or overgeneralizes a grammatical morpheme? Cite examples.
3. What is the general order of pronoun acquisition? How would you explain this order?
4. In the use of pronouns, what is an *anaphoric* reference? Give three examples of anaphoric references.
5. Define the following terms and provide an example of each: phrase, noun phrase, verb phrase, clause, independent clause, subordinate clause, compound sentence, and complex sentence.
6. What language forms does the stage 2 child use to express negation, ask questions, and make demands or requests?
7. What does it mean to repair in conversation? How does the stage 2 child try to make conversational repairs?
8. How does *fast mapping* contribute to the child's acquisition of word knowledge, and how does the child's acquisition of word knowledge affect overall language competence in stage 2?
9. How does the stage 3 child express negation and questions?
10. Define prepositional, participial, infinitive, and gerund phrases as embedded forms. Provide an example of each.
11. Define the following types of embedded clauses: object complement, *wh-* question, and relative.
12. How does the stage 4 child express negation and questions?
13. What lessons has the stage 4 child learned about the art of conversation?
14. Which grammatical morphemes are mastered by the close of stage 5?
15. Differentiate between contractible and uncontractible forms of the verb *to be.* Why is the stage 5 child still struggling with the issue of contractibility?
16. What problems does the stage 5 child encounter in understanding and using the comparative and superlative forms of adjectives?
17. What is meant by multiple embedding and conjoining? Provide several examples of each.
18. Describe the conversational strengths and weaknesses of the stage 5 child.
19. Compare and contrast *narrative* and *conversation* as forms of communication.
20. What is a *protonarrative?* From what kinds of life experiences are protonarratives drawn?
21. In reference to building narratives, what is *chaining?* What is *centering?*
22. What significant changes occur in the child's narratives between the ages of two and five years?
23. How are cognition, comprehension, and production related?
24. What problems does the child encounter in understanding active and passive sentences?

25. What do you believe is a reasonable answer to the question: "Which comes first in mastering word order, comprehension or production?" Justify your answer.
26. What relationships among people, objects, and events are identified by the use of *relational* words? Discuss common problems the child may encounter in mastering relational words.

References and Suggested Readings

Ames, L. (1966). Children's stories. *Genetic Psychological Monographs, 73,* 307–311.

Anderson, R. (1998). The development of grammatical case distinctions in the use of personal pronouns by Spanish-speaking preschoolers. *Journal of Speech, Language, Hearing Research, 41,* 394–406.

Applebee, A. (1978). *The child's concept of story.* Chicago: University of Chicago Press.

Au, T. (1990). Children's use of information in word learning. *Journal of Child Language, 17,* 393–416.

Bellugi, U. (1965). The development of interrogative structures in children's speech. In K. Riegel (Ed.), *The development of language functions* (Report No. 8). Ann Arbor, MI: University of Michigan Language Development Program.

Bennett-Kaster, T. (1986). Cohesion and predication in child narrative. *Journal of Child Language, 13,* 353–370.

Berko-Gleason, J. (Ed.) (1989). *The development of language* (2nd ed.). Upper Saddle River, NJ: Merrill/Prentice Hall.

Bernstein, D. (1989). Language development: The preschool years. In D. Bernstein & E. Tiegerman (Eds.), *Language and communication disorders in children* (2nd ed.). Upper Saddle River, NJ: Merrill/Prentice Hall.

Beveridge, M., & Marsh, L. (1991). The influence of linguistic context on young children's understanding of homophonic words. *Journal of Child Language, 18,* 459–467.

Bloom, L. (1970). *Language development: Form and function of emerging grammars.* Cambridge, MA: MIT Press.

Bloom, L., & Lahey, M. (1978). *Language development and language disorders.* New York: John Wiley & Sons.

Bloom, L., Lahey, P., Hood, L., Lifter, K., & Fiess, K. (1980). Complex sentences: Acquisition of syntactic connectors and the semantic relations they encode. *Journal of Child Language, 7,* 235–262.

Bloom, L., Miller, P., & Hood, L. (1975). Variation and reduction as aspects of competence in language development. In A. Pick (Ed.), *Minnesota Symposia on Child Psychology,* Vol. 9 (pp. 3–55). Minneapolis, MN: University of Minnesota Press.

Bloom, L., Rocissano, L., & Hood, L. (1976). Adult–child discourse: Developmental interaction between information processing and linguistic interaction. *Cognitive Psychology, 8,* 521–552.

Bloom, L., Tackeff, J., & Lahey, M. (1984). Learning "to" in complement constructions. *Journal of Child Language, 11,* 391–406.

Bretherton, I., Fritz, J., Zahn-Waxler, C., & Ridgeway, D. (1986). Learning to talk about emotions: A functionalist perspective. *Child Development, 57,* 529–548.

Brewer, W., & Stone, J. (1975). Acquisition of spatial antonym pairs. *Journal of Experimental Child Psychology, 19,* 299–307.

Brinton, B., & Fujiki, M. (1984). Development of topic manipulation skills in discourse. *Journal of Speech and Hearing Research, 27,* 350–358.

Brinton, B., & Fujiki, M. (1989). *Conversational management with language-impaired children: Pragmatic assessment and intervention.* Rockville, MD: Aspen.

Broderick, J. (1975). *Modern English linguistics.* New York: Crowell Company.

Brown, R. (1973). *A first language: The early years.* Cambridge, MA: Harvard University Press.

Brown, R., & Bellugi, U. (1964). Three processes in the child's acquisition of syntax. *Harvard Educational Review, 34,* 133–151.

Brown, R., Cazden, C., & Bellugi, U. (1969). The child's grammar from I to III. In J. Hill (Ed.), *Minnesota symposia on child psychology* (Vol. 2). Minneapolis: University of Minnesota Press.

Carey, S. (1978). The child as word learner. In M. Halle, J. Bresnan, & G. Miller (Eds.), *Linguistic theory and psychological reality.* Cambridge, MA: MIT Press.

Carey, S., & Bartlett, E. (1978). Acquiring a single new word. *Papers and Reports on Child Language Development, 15,* 17–29.

Carrell, P. (1981). Children's understanding of indirect requests: Comparing child and adult comprehension. *Journal of Child Language, 8,* 329–345.

Carrow, E. (1973). *Test of auditory comprehension of language.* Austin, TX: Urban Research Group.

Cazden, C. (1968). The acquisition of noun and verb inflection. *Child Development, 39,* 433–438.

Chapman, R. (1978). Comprehension strategies in children. In J. Kavanaugh & W. Strange (Eds.), *Speech and language in the laboratory, school and clinic.* Cambridge, MA: MIT Press.

Chapman, R., & Miller, J. (1975). Word order in early two- and three-word utterances: Does production precede comprehension? *Journal of Speech and Hearing Research, 18,* 355–371.

Chapman, R., Paul, R., & Wanska, S. (1981). Syntactic structures in simple sentences. In J. Miller (Ed.), *Assessing language production in children: Experimental procedures.* Baltimore: University Park Press.

Chapman, R., Streim, N., Crais, E., Salmon, D., Strand, E., & Negri, N. (1992). Child talk: Assumptions of a developmental process model for early language learning. In R. Chapman (Ed.), *Processes in language acquisition and disorders.* St. Louis, MO: Mosby–Year Book.

Chiat, S. (1986). Personal pronouns. In P. Fletcher & M. Garman (Eds.), *Language acquisition* (2nd ed.). New York: Cambridge University Press.

Childers, J., & Tomasello, M. (2002). Two-year-olds learn novel nouns, verbs, and conventional actions from massed or distributed exposures. *Developmental Psychology, 38,* 967–978.

Clark, H., & Clark, E. (1977). *Psychology and language: An introduction to psycholinguistics.* New York: Harcourt Brace Jovanovich.

Clark, E., & Sengul, C. (1978). Strategies in the acquisition of deixis. *Journal of Child Language, 5,* 457–475.

Conner, P., & Chapman, R. (1985). The development of locative comprehension in Spanish. *Journal of Child Language, 12,* 109–123.

Craig, H., & Gallagher, T. (1983). Adult–child discourse: The conversational relevance of pauses. *Journal of Pragmatics, 7,* 347–360.

Crais, E. (1992). Fast mapping: A new look at word learning. In R. Chapman (Ed.), *Processes in language acquisition and disorders.* St. Louis, MO: Mosby–Year Book.

Dale, P., & Crain-Thoreson, C. (1993). Pronoun reversals: Who, when, & why? *Journal of Child Language, 20,* 573–589.

de Villiers, J., & de Villiers, P. (1973). A cross-sectional study of the acquisition of grammatical morphemes in child speech. *Journal of Psycholinguistic Research, 2,* 267–278.

Edmonsten, N., & Thane, N. (1992). Children's use of comprehension strategies in response to relational words: Implications for assessment. *American Journal of Speech-Language Pathology, 1,* 30–35.

Ervin-Tripp, S. (1977). Wait for me roller-skate. In S. Ervin-Tripp & C. Mitchell-Kernan (Eds.), *Child discourse.* New York: Academic Press.

Ervin-Tripp, S. (1979). Children's verbal turn-taking. In E. Ochs & B. Schieffelin (Eds.), *Developmental pragmatics.* New York: Academic Press.

Ervin-Tripp, S., & Gordon, D. (1986). The development of requests. In R. Schiefelbusch (Ed.), *Language competence: Assessment and intervention.* San Diego, CA: College-Hill.

Ervin-Tripp, S., O'Connor, M., & Rosenberg, J. (1987). Language and power in the family. In C. Kramerae & M. Schulz (Eds.), *Language and power.* Urbana: University of Illinois Press.

Forbes, J., & Poulin-DuBois, D. (1997). Representational change in young children's understanding of familiar verb meaning. *Journal of Child Language, 24,* 389–406.

Foster, S. (1986). Learning topic management in the preschool years. *Journal of Child Language, 13,* 231–250.

Gallagher, T. (1977). Revision behaviors in the speech of normal children developing language. *Journal of Speech and Hearing Research, 20,* 303–318.

Gallagher, T. (1981). Contingent query sequences within adult–child discourse. *Journal of Child Language, 8,* 51–62.

Garvey, C., & Berninger, G. (1981). Timing and turn taking in children's conversations. *Discourse Processes, 4,* 27–57.

Gertner, B., Rice, M. L., & Hadley, P. A. (1994). Influence of communicative competence on peer preferences in a preschool classroom. *Journal of Speech and Hearing Research, 37,* 913–923.

Gleitman, L., & Wanner, E. (1982). Language acquisition: The state of the state of the art. In E. Wanner & L. Gleitman (Eds.), *Language acquisition: The state of the art.* Cambridge, MA: Cambridge University Press.

Goldfield, B. (2000). Nouns before verbs in comprehension vs. production:

The view from pragmatics. *Journal of Child Language, 27,* 501–520.

Golinkoff, R., Hirsh-Pasek, K., Cauley, K., & Gordon, L. (1987). The eyes have it: Lexical and syntactic comprehension in a new paradigm. *Journal of Child Language, 14,* 23–45.

Gordon, D., & Ervin-Tripp, S. (1984). The structure of children's requests. In R. Schiefelbusch & J. Pickar (Eds.), *The acquisition of communicative competence.* Baltimore: University Park Press.

Gropen, J., Pinker, S., Hollander, M., & Goldberg, R. (1991). Syntax and semantics in the acquisition of locative verbs. *Journal of Child Language, 19,* 115–151.

Haas, A., & Owens, R. (1985). *Preschoolers' pronoun strategies: You and me make us.* Paper presented at the annual convention of the American Speech–Language–Hearing Association.

Harris, M., Yeeles, C., Chasin, J., & Oakley, Y. (1995). Symmetries and asymmetries in early lexical comprehension and production. *Journal of Child Language, 22,* 1–18.

Hoff-Ginsberg, E. (1990). Maternal speech and the child's development of syntax: A further look. *Journal of Child Language, 17,* 85–89.

Huxley, R. (1970). The development of the correct use of subject personal pronouns in two children. In G. Flores d'Arcais & W. Levelt (Eds.), *Advances in psycholinguistics.* Amsterdam: North-Holland.

Ingram, D. (1971). Transitivity in child language. *Language, 47,* 888–910.

Ingram, D. (1975). The acquisition of fricatives and affricatives in normal and linguistically deviant children. In A. Carramazza & E. Zuriff (Eds.), *The acquisition and breakdown of language.* Baltimore: Johns Hopkins University Press.

James, S. (1990). *Normal language acquisition.* Austin, TX: PRO-ED.

James, S., & Kahn, L. (1982). Grammatical morpheme acquisition: An approximately invariant order? *Journal of Psycholinguistic Research, 11,* 381–388.

James, S., & Seebach, M. (1982). The pragmatic function of children's questions. *Journal of Speech and Hearing Research, 25,* 2–11.

Johnston, J. (1984). Acquisition of locative meanings: "Behind" and "in front of." *Journal of Child Language, 11,* 407–422.

Keenan, E., & Schieffelin, B. (1976). Topic as a discourse notion: A study of topic in the conversation of children and adults. In C. Li (Ed.), *Subject and topic: A new typology of language.* New York: Academic Press.

Kelly, S. (2001). Broadening the units of analysis in communication: Speech and nonverbal behaviors in pragmatic comprehension. *Journal of Child Language, 28,* 325–349.

Klatsky, R., Clark, E., & Macken, M. (1973). Asymmetries in the acquisition of polar adjectives: Linguistic conceptual? *Journal of Experimental Child Psychology, 16,* 32–46.

Klee, T. (1985). Role of inversion in children's question development. *Journal of Speech and Hearing Research, 28,* 225–232.

Klima E., and Bellugi-Klima, U. (1971). Syntactic regularities in the speech of children. In A. Bar-Adon & W. Leopold (Eds.), *Child language: A book of readings.* Upper Saddle River, NJ: Prentice Hall.

Klima, E., & Bellugi, U. (1966). Syntactic regularities in the speech of children. In J. Lyons & R. Wales (Eds.), *Psycholinguistic papers.* Edinburgh: Edinburgh University Press.

Krauss, R., & Glucksberg, S. (1977). Social and nonsocial speech. *Scientific American, 236,* 100–105.

Lemish, D., & Rice, M. (1986). Television as a talking picture book: A prop for language acquisition. *Journal of Child Language, 13,* 251–274.

Lempert, H. (1990). Acquisition of passives: The role of patient animacy, salience, and lexical accessibility. *Journal of Child Language, 17,* 677–696.

McCabe, A., & Peterson, C. (1985). A naturalistic study of the production of causal connectives by children. *Journal of Child Language, 12,* 145–159.

McCormick, L. (1990). Sequences of language and communication development. In L. McCormick & R. Schiefelbusch (Eds.), *Early language intervention: An introduction* (2nd ed.). Upper Saddle River, NJ: Merrill/ Prentice Hall.

McTear, M. (1985). *Children's conversation.* Oxford: Blackwell.

Menyuk, P. (1977). *Language and maturation.* Cambridge, MA: MIT Press.

Miller, J. (1981). *Assessing language production in children: Experimental procedures.* Baltimore: University Park Press.

Miller, P., & Sperry, L. (1988). Early talk about the past: The origins of conversational stories of personal experience. *Journal of Child Language, 15,* 293–315.

Milosky, L. (1990). The role of world knowledge in language comprehension and language intervention. *Topics in Language Disorders, 10,* 1–13.

Mithum, M. (1989). The acquisition of polysynthesis. *Journal of Child Language, 16,* 285–312.

Morgan, J., & Travis, L. (1989). Limits on negative information in language input. *Journal of Child Language, 16,* 531–552.

Mueller, E. (1972). The maintenance of verbal exchanges between young children. *Child Development, 43,* 930–938.

Mueller, E., Bleier, M., Krakow, J., Hegedus, K., & Cournoyer, P. (1977). The development of peer verbal interaction among two-year-old boys. *Child Development, 48,* 284–287.

Naigles, L. (1990). Children use syntax to learn verb meanings. *Journal of Child Language, 17,* 357–374.

Newcombe, N., & Zaslow, M. (1981). Do 2½-year-olds hint? A study of directive forms in the speech of 2½-year-old children to adults. *Discourse Processes, 4,* 239–252.

Owens, R. (1990). Development of communication, language, and speech. In G. Shames, & E. Wiig (Eds.), *Human communication disorders: An introduction* (3rd ed.). Upper Saddle River, NJ: Prentice Hall.

Owens, R. (1995). *Language disorders: A functional approach to assessment and intervention* (2nd ed.). Boston: Allyn & Bacon.

Owens, R. (1996). *Language development: An introduction* (4th ed.). Boston: Allyn & Bacon.

Owens, R. (2001). *Language development: An introduction* (5th ed.). Boston: Allyn & Bacon.

Owens, R. (2005). *Language development: An introduction* (6th ed.), Boston: Allyn & Bacon.

Paul, R. (1981). Analyzing complex sentence development. In J. Miller (Ed.), *Assessing language production in children: Experimental procedures.* Baltimore: University Park Press.

Peterson, C. (1990). The who, when and where of early narratives. *Journal of Child Language, 17,* 433–455.

Piaget, J. (1926). *Language and thought of the child.* London: Routledge & Kegan Paul.

Piaget, J. (1966). Time perception in children. In J. Frazer (Ed.), *The voices of time.* New York: Braziller.

Reich, P. (1986). *Language development.* Upper Saddle River, NJ: Prentice Hall.

Resnick, J., & Goldfield, B. A. (1994). Diary vs. representative checklist assessment of productive vocabulary. *Journal of Child Language, 21,* 465–472.

Rice, M., Buhr, J., & Nemeth, C. (1990). Fast mapping word-learning abilities of language-delayed preschoolers. *Journal of Speech and Hearing Disorders, 55,* 33–42.

Rispoli, M. (2003). Changes in the nature of sentence production during the period of grammatical development. *Journal of Speech, Language, and Hearing Research, 46,* 818–830.

Roth, F., & Spekman, N. (1985, June). *Story grammar analysis of narratives produced by learning disabled and normally achieving students.* Paper presented at the Symposium on Research in Child Language Disorders, Madison, WI.

Ryder, N., & Leinonen, E. (2003). Use of context in question answering by 3-, 4-, and 5-year-old children. *Journal of Psycholinguistic Research, 32,* 397–416.

Sachs, J. (1982). "Don't interrupt!": Preschoolers' entry into ongoing conversations. In C. Johnson & C. Thew (Eds.), *Proceedings of the Second International Congress for the Study of Child Language* (Vol. 1, pp. 344–356). Washington, D.C.: University Press of America.

Samuelson, L., & Smith, L. B. (1998). Memory and attention make smart word learning: An alternative account of Akhtar, Carpenter, Tomasello. *Child Development, 69,* 94–104.

Schober-Peterson, D., & Johnson, C. (1989). Conversational topics of four-year-olds. *Journal of Speech and Hearing Research, 32,* 857–870.

Schober-Peterson, D., & Johnson, C. (1991). Non-dialogue speech during preschool interactions. *Journal of Child Language, 18,* 153–170.

Senecal, M. (1997). The differential effect of story-book reading on preschooler's acquisition of expressive and receptive vocabulary. *Journal of Child Language, 24,* 123–128.

Shatz, M., Wellman, H., & Silber, F. (1983). The acquisition of mental verbs: A systematic investigation of the first reference to mental state. *Cognition, 14,* 301–321.

Shatz, M., & O'Reilly, A. (1990). Conversational or communicative skill? A reassessment of two-year-olds' behavior in miscommunication episodes. *Journal of Child Language, 17,* 131–146.

Shipley, K., Maddox, M., & Driver, J. (1991). Children's development of irregular past tense verb forms. *Language, Speech, and Hearing Services in Schools, 22,* 115–122.

Siedlecki, T., & Bonvillian, J. D. (1998). Homonymy in the lexicons of young children acquiring American Sign Language. *Journal of Psycholinguistic Research, 27,* 47–65.

Stemberger, J. (1993). Vowel dominance in overregularizations. *Journal of Child Language, 20,* 503–521.

Storkel, H. (2001). Learning new words: Phonetactic probability in language development. *Journal of Speech, Lan-*

guage, and Hearing Research, 44, 1321–1337.

Storkel, H., & Morrisette, M. L. (2002). The lexicon and phonology: Interactions in language acquisition. *Language, Speech, and Hearing Services in Schools, 33,* 24–37.

Sutton-Smith, B. (1986). The development of fictional narrative performances. *Topics in Language Disorders, 7*(1), 1–10.

Trantham, C., & Pedersen, J. (1976). *Normal language development.* Baltimore: Williams & Wilkins.

Tyack, D., & Ingram, D. (1977). Children's production and comprehension of questions. *Journal of Child Language, 4,* 211–224.

Van Kleeck, A., Gillam, R. B., Hamilton, L., & McGrath, C. (1997). The relationship between middle-class parent's book sharing discussion and their preschoolers' abstract language development. *Journal of Speech, Language, and Hearing Research, 40,* 1261–1271.

Waterman, P., & Schatz, M. (1982). The acquisition of personal pronouns and proper names by an identical twin pair. *Journal of Speech and Hearing Research, 25,* 149–154.

Weist, R., Wysocka, H., & Lyytinen, P. (1991). A cross-linguistic perspective on the development of temporal systems. *Journal of Child Language, 18,* 67–92.

Wellman, H., & Estes, D. (1987). Children's early use of mental verbs and what they mean. *Discourse Processes, 16,* 141–156.

Wellman, H., & Lempers, J. (1977). The naturalistic communicative abilities of two-year-olds. *Child Development, 48,* 1052–1057.

Wells, G. (1979). Learning and using the auxiliary verb in English. In V. Lee (Ed.), *Language development.* New York: Wiley.

Wells, G. (1985). *Language development in the preschool years.* New York: Cambridge University Press.

Wilkinson, L., Calculator, S., & Dollaghan, C. (1982). Ya wanna trade— just for awhile: Children's requests and responses to peers. *Discourse Processes, 5,* 161–176.

Wootten, J., Merkin, S., Hood, L., & Bloom, L. (1979, March). *Wh- questions: Linguistic evidence to explain the sequence of acquisition.* Paper presented at the biennial meeting of the Society for Research in Child Development, San Francisco.

Xu, F., & Pinker, S. (1995). Weird past tense forms. *Journal of Child Language, 22,* 531–556.

6

Taking Language to School and into Adulthood

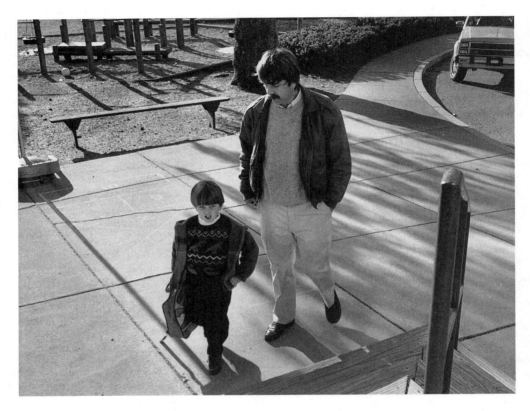

Although much of language acquisition occurs from birth through the preschool years, development continues throughout the school years, especially during the primary grades. It is also true that people continue to add to their language knowledge and their communication competencies into their adult years, perhaps all their lives. In this chapter, we consider the con-tinuation of language acquisition as the child enters school, including the interactive growth of vocabulary and cognition, and developmental changes in syntax, morphology, and pragmatics. We examine the emergence of gender differences in communication, metalinguistic development, and the application of language knowledge to the learning of reading and writing.

Specifically, this chapter is designed to facilitate understanding of the following topics:

- A profile of the five-year-old as a communicator
- The interactive development of cognition and vocabulary, including changes in how words are defined and understood, and the emergence of figurative language forms
- Further developments in syntax, including refinement of passive forms, determining when the principle of minimal distance applies and when it does not apply in the interpretation of sentences, conjoining with conjunctions expressing complex clausal relationships, and creating longer, more elaborate sentences
- Learning that words can function in more than one grammatical category

- Fine-tuning the art of conversation, including responding to stacked repair sequences, more subtle forms of indirect request, and becoming more sensitive to the listener's communication needs
- Narratives: improving storytelling abilities
- The emergence of gender differences in communication
- Dealing with communication demands in the classroom
- Developing metalinguistic skills that enable the child to analyze and understand the language she uses
- Reading and writing: new applications of language
- Language in adolescence and adulthood: changes and challenges

---

The first few years of the child's communicative life have been extraordinarily busy and exciting. Even before she is born, the child is connected to her primary caregivers, literally and figuratively. During the months of her fetal development, her caregivers may sense, or believe they sense, communications from the womb. The child's caregivers may attempt to interpret the meaning of each movement, each kick. Her first communications after birth come in the form of cries and gaze-couplings, but it is not long before she expands her communication system to include coos, giggles, touches, grabs, and first-rate wet kisses. By the end of her first year, she is producing words. Before the end of her second year, she is putting words together. Once she begins combining words, her language development proceeds at a pace that challenges our best efforts to understand and describe what is happening. In the preceding two chapters we have traced the explosion of language development that occurs from birth through the preschool years. In this chapter, we consider the further development of language during the child's school years and beyond.

Bringing My Stuff to School: Pencils, Crayons, and Language

We begin with a profile of the five-year-old child as a communicator. What kind of language and what kind of communication skills does he bring with him to that first day in school, and what do these abilities suggest about what he still needs to learn about language and the use of language? In considering our hypothetical child, it is important to remember that language and language use are both universal and idiosyncratic. That is, there are aspects of language shared by all five-year-old children who speak English, and there are aspects of language shared by all five-year-old children who speak all the languages of the world. At the same time, each child's communication experiences coming into school have been unique, and these experiences have shaped the child's language and his communication skills.

Based on universal aspects of language acquisition, we would expect our five-year-old child to have well-developed receptive and expressive vocabularies, an almost intact speech sound system, fairly sophisticated syntactic abilities, and developing conversational skills. By the time the child enters school, he knows virtually all the words we might consider basic in his language. Although his understandings of words are not fully developed, he has a good idea about what words mean and how they should be used. He is producing complete sentences and is able to transform declarative sentences into question and negative forms, even though he is still learning the nuances of these transformations and still has difficulty with passive sentences. He is able to understand and produce imperative sentences, and, although he is still learning to produce indirect requests, he responds appropriately to indirect requests made of him, assuming they are not too subtle or obscure. The child is still oriented primarily to present time and place, but he is able to use language to talk about something in the past or future, and he is able to talk about things and people that are not in sight. The adult must keep in mind, of course, that *past* and *future* do not mean the same thing to a five-year-old as to an adult, but the child has no difficulty talking about something that happened yesterday, and he may be eager to talk about something exciting that will happen tomorrow or in a few days. If you try to talk to this child about what his life will be like in twenty years, however, be prepared for the blank stare of utter indifference.

If the child's caregivers have included singing, nursery rhymes, and speech-related games such as patty-cake and peekaboo in his early communication experiences, he will come to school ready to engage in language play. If his caregivers have read books to him, he will recognize the difference between writing and drawing, and he will understand that reading and writing are forms of communication related to speech and language. The foundations for teaching the five-year-old child to read and write, therefore, have been laid during the preschool years. Some five-year-old children already know how to read, of course, but they remain exceptions, at least for now. Personally, we anticipate the day when parents will buy their child a subscription to the *Wall Street Journal* during the second trimester of his fetal development. Somehow they will arrange to fax the contents into the womb, and the child will be born ready to read and ready to deal!

And what differences do the differences make? Consider the obvious differences. A five-year-old reared in Dallas, Texas, will not sound like a five-year-old reared in Boston, Massachusetts, and neither of these children will sound like a five-year-old reared in Tokyo, Japan. The child who grows up in a home full of talkative older siblings and adults who constantly engage the child in communicative exchanges is likely to talk more, and perhaps be more interested in language, than the child who is reared by reticent parents who make little effort to facilitate speech and language production. The child who is exposed to vulgar words will use vulgar words. The child who is exposed to complete, correct models of language is more likely to use complete, correct sentences than the child who is exposed to models that are syntactically deficient. We must be careful not to extend this too far, because few children are exposed to only inadequate speech and language models, but as a general rule, we would not expect a child's speech and language abilities to be better than the models to which he is predominantly exposed.

Language Development during the School Years: An Overview

How and where does language development proceed as the child moves through the school years? As we have already noted, the advances in language development after stage 5 are not as dramatic as the changes that occurred through the preschool years, but the changes in language during the school years are of no less importance. Some of the changes are universal and shared by all children. Other changes are the product of the child's unique experiences and often reflect the child's unique interest in language itself. Throughout the school years and throughout the remainder of the child's life, she acquires vocabulary. During the first few years of school, she puts the finishing touches on her speech sound system. The child continues to develop her syntactic and semantic abilities, primarily by expanding and refining the skills she developed during the preschool years. She develops considerably more sophistication in the use of language. She becomes a better conversationalist and learns how to use language more effectively to get things done. She develops an interest in language itself and learns how to use language to analyze and understand language, an ability called **metalinguistic awareness.**

During the school years, she also learns how to read and write, language abilities that will give the child virtually limitless intellectual and creative freedoms. Reading will open vistas absolutely devoid of space and time restrictions. Through the reading of books, the child will be introduced to the thoughts, opinions, and wisdom of the greatest, most influential minds of human history. In writing her own prose and poetry, she may discover means of intellectual and personal expression that are not available to her in speech alone.

The advances in language development we examine in this chapter may not be as explosive as those we observed in the preschool years, but they are important and they are exciting. The changes in language closely parallel other changes the child is experiencing. He is growing up. He is becoming his own person. He is expanding his interests into the greater world beyond his house, beyond his school, beyond his community. It is not an exaggeration to assert that this personal growth depends to a large extent on the child's developing language and communication knowledge and skills.

The Miracle Worker is the story of Helen Keller's struggle to overcome blindness and deafness. In her early years, Keller was a prisoner in a noncommunicative world. Only as she learned to express herself through sign language and to read and write did she grow into the complete, creative, and productive person she was destined to become. The hearing and sighted child does not have to break the bonds of deafness and blindness, but he must still discover how to be a whole person as he grows up, and communication is just as important to him in this discovery process as it was to Keller.

Semantics: Vocabulary and Cognition Still Growing Together

One of the most obvious changes in language that continues throughout the rest of the child's life is the acquisition of new vocabulary. The child not only learns new words but learns to use old words in new ways. The young child understands *crack* as a small fissure in the driveway. As she develops more sophistication with language, she will understand that a person might be referred to as a "crack reporter," and she will understand that *crack* also refers to the sound made by a whip. She will develop more precise definitions for the words she uses, and she will choose from among words with similar meanings the word that best fits the intended communication. As a young child, she uses *big* to describe anything of unusual size. As she matures, she uses words that more precisely differentiate "bigness" such as *tall, deep, wide,* and *broad,* and if she wants to describe someone who is *big* and *tough,* she might use words such as *burly* or *husky.*

The preschool child uses words in a very literal sense. As he matures, he learns to use words figuratively. At three or four years, he might be confused by sentences such as "He's a real animal," or "He comes at you like a Mack truck," but he eventually learns how words are used to create mental images to enhance the specificity or strength of a message. He also comes to understand *puns,* jokes based on words that sound like or remind the listener of other words that do not fit the immediate context. Here is one of our favorite puns: "Did you hear about the guru who went to the dentist but refused novacaine? He wanted to transcend dental medication."

Obviously, vocabulary growth does not continue at the same furious rate we observe during the preschool years, but vocabulary growth does continue throughout a person's life. In fact, the common myth that older people lose vocabulary is simply not true, except in cases of failing health. After the age of seventy, some people are not able to retrieve words as quickly as they once did, but they do not lose words from their vocabularies (Obler, 1989).

Vocabulary Growth: Acquiring, Understanding, and Categorizing New Words

To appreciate vocabulary growth during the school years, one must understand that vocabulary *growth* involves more than the acquisition of new words, although new

Using language to help solve problems and get things done.

words are certainly acquired. Beyond adding words to her vocabulary, however, the child is developing new ways to use words, and she is refining the meanings of the established and new words in her vocabulary. The changes we observe in the child's semantic competencies during the school years can almost certainly be attributed to corresponding maturational changes in her cognitive processing abilities (Emerson & Gekoski, 1976).

As a child moves through the preschool and school years, his vocabulary and word usage tend to mirror his cognitive shift from concrete to more abstract levels of thinking. He learns that words can be placed in categories just as things can be placed in categories. He learns that words can be used in a hierarchical manner such as *big, bigger, biggest*. He learns that words can be used to recall things, people, and events that are not immediate. He learns that words can be used to facilitate the solving of problems.

As one would surmise, vocabulary growth continues throughout a person's lifetime. Through the school years and throughout adulthood, words are added to a speaker's vocabulary. More important, from a language usage point of view, there is greater understanding of words and an increasingly sophisticated understanding about how words relate to one another. By the time the child is becoming a young adult at the conclusion of the high school years, he will understand the meanings of about 80,000 words (Miller & Gildea, 1987). If we take into account the changes in meaning created by the addition of prefixes and suffixes to root words, the total number of words understood greatly exceeds 80,000 (Anglin, 1995).

Factors Influencing Vocabulary Acquisition

As common sense suggests, the primary influence on language development generally and vocabulary growth specifically during the early years of the child's life is spoken language. The power of spoken language in influencing development actually remains unchallenged for most children during the early school years. When the child is about nine or ten years old, however, another powerful influence emerges—written language. Research evidence suggests that children at this age who are highly motivated to read, who read often and read well, acquire significantly larger vocabularies than children who are less interested in reading and whose reading skills are not as well developed (Miller & Gildea, 1987; Nagy, Herman, & Anderson, 1985). There is also evidence that there is a connection between social class and the attachment of meanings to words. Middle class children who live in urban areas have more fully developed meanings than children from lower classes who live in rural areas (Walker, 2001), but there is an interesting twist to this story. Research indicates that the ability to define words is related to academic experience, so some fourth grade children from what is sometimes called the *working class* are more proficient in defining words than their parents, presumably because they actively learn about words and definitions in school (Kurland & Snow, 1997).

The influence of the written word on vocabulary growth is evidenced in another way. As the child moves through the school years, she acquires words that are increasingly less common than base vocabulary words. These words tend to be more abstract and are used to express more complex concepts than earlier words. Not coincidentally, these words are found far more often in written language than they are produced in mundane conversation (Nagy, Diakidoy, & Anderson, 1993).

As to how older children and young adults acquire new words and learn their meanings, at least three primary influences seem to be involved: (1) direct teaching from adult models, usually parents and teachers, (2) the use of clues embedded in the context surrounding unfamiliar words, and (3) the ability to use existing morphological knowledge to figure out the meanings of unknown words (Nippold, 1998).

The Influence of Adult Models

Sometimes the influence in the process of acquiring a new word is obvious. A teacher, parent, or some other language model presents a new word and provides its definition or application (Nagy, Herman, & Anderson, 1985). We all recognize this influence because we have been on both ends of it. When we teach a course in which this book is used, we present words that many students have not used before: *morpheme, phoneme, syntax,* and so forth. We present the word. We define it. We show how it is applied. That is the direct teaching of a word.

When you were young, and perhaps not so young, you probably asked questions such as, "What does *exacerbate* mean?" If you were reared in a typical family, the inevitable and probably unwelcome response was "Look it up!" You may or may not have run to a dictionary, but if you did, you experienced another form of direct vocabulary teaching. In today's world, the question might be the same, but the child might be sent to his computer for a definition search. The technology is different, but the teaching/learning strategy is the same. The child typically begins to use a dictionary when he is about seven or eight years old and in the second grade (Miller & Gildea, 1987). As he proceeds through the school years, he will be called on to use a dictionary, in either traditional book form or in some computer version, more frequently. We should not assume, however, that just because the child looks up the definition of a word, he will understand the definition, especially if the definition is abstract. Miller and Gildea (1987, p. 2) found, for example, that when children in the range of ten to twelve years were asked to find words in the dictionary and then write sentences using those words, they wrote some interesting sentences. One of the words was *erode*, which means "to eat out," as in "My car was eroded by rust." In what we hope was a clear misinterpretation of the definition, one child wrote, "Our family *erodes* (eats out) a lot."

The Influence of Contextual Cues

Adults often use context to decipher the meanings of words they do not know. This skill is learned during the elementary years and is refined during adolescence and adulthood. Using context is another strategy children use to expand their vocabularies and acquire meanings (Nagy et al., 1985; Sternberg, 1987). This strategy is encouraged by teachers throughout the school years (Bennett, 1981; Duffy & Roehler, 1981). Whether or not the child is directed to attend to context, she certainly has many opportunities to use context to expand her understanding of words. Consider the volume of words to which the typical child is exposed when she listens to her parents talk and her teacher teach. Think about the words she hears when she watches movies and television programs, as well as the words she reads in school books and in the books and magazines she reads recreationally. The typical child is awash in hundreds of thousands of words every day. Some she knows, many she does not. If she is a typical child with a typical curiosity to know, she will use the words she knows to figure out those she does not know. That is, she learns words and their meanings by using *contextual cues*.

The Influence of Morphological Knowledge

Children, like adults, also use their understanding of the parts of words, the morphemes that are added to base words, to figure out what words mean (Anglin, 1993; Nagy et al., 1993). When the speaker or reader—again regardless of age—approaches a word he does not know, he will identify the parts of the word he does know to try to determine what the whole word means. If, for example, he is confronted with the word *wholeheartedly,* he might grasp that *heart* is the base of the word and that *heart* is sometimes used to mean something like *spirit*. He knows what *whole* means, and he knows that *-ly* is used to indicate *adverb*. He puts all the pieces together to understand that this word means that whatever the agent is doing, he is doing it *enthusiastically, with his* *entire spirit, with his whole heart.* According to White, Power, and White (1989a, 1989b), this strategy is a powerful influence in the vocabulary acquisition of students when they are reading in school and outside school. The strategy is successfully employed by children as young as six to ten years of age (Anglin, 1993), but it obviously becomes a more powerful influence in the acquisition of words and their meanings as children get older.

Expanding Word Meanings: Strategies for Storage

The child's definitions become more specific and precise as she expands her understandings of words **horizontally** and **vertically** (McNeil, 1970). The horizontal expansion occurs as she adds semantic features to her definitions. When the child first uses the word *doggie,* it might have only two features: animal and four legs. This is why the two-year-old child uses the word *doggie* to name a horse, pig, elephant, and giraffe. These objects are all animals, and they all have four legs. As the child matures, she adds more semantic features to her understanding of *doggie,* such as wagging tail, wet nose, domestic pet, barking sounds, and canine. This horizontal expansion makes the child's definition of *doggie* or *dog* more specific, and it helps her to recognize the similarities and differences between dogs and other animals.

A definition expands vertically as the child learns the various meanings a given word may have. As mentioned earlier, the child will first understand that the word *crack* refers to a fissure or slit, but he gradually adds other meanings for *crack* including "smash," "sever," "chip," "fracture," "bang," "insult," "hit," "leak," and "puncture." Each of these meanings adds to the vertical dimension of the definition of *crack,* and unfortunately as a sign of the present day, the child is likely to add "cocaine" to his definition of *crack.* Horizontal and vertical expansions of definitions occur throughout the preschool years, of course, but they are most noticeable during the school years when the child is using and understanding words in a progressively more adultlike manner.

Defining Words

Most of us understand the word *define* to mean *to determine the boundaries of, to state the meaning of,* or words similar to these. When we define a word, we identify its meaning, but we also limit its meaning so that it cannot be confused with a word that is similar but different in some important respect. Scholars, philosophers, politicians, and linguists can spend hours arguing about what words mean, and because they can, they do. What is most curious about all this can be summarized in one simple question: "How does the child ever figure out what words mean?" Before we can answer that question, we really need to back up a little bit to understand more about the process of defining.

First, we need to appreciate that there is not a single way to define a word. We are all familiar with *dictionary* definition, or what is sometimes called the *Aristotelian* definition. In this kind of definition, the general category of the thing to be defined is established, and the characteristics that differentiate it from other things in the general category are identified. We might say, for example, that an *apple* is a fruit (general category) that is typically red, yellow, or green and grows on apple trees (differentiating characteristics).

Another form of definition is *operational*. For example, to say that a hitter *executed properly* means that he moved the runner. We might define by *comparing* as in "A bat is like a mouse with wings." A definition might be based on *negation,* for example, a person might say, "When I say that she is a *strong* person, I don't mean that she's stubborn" (Makau, 1990). Over the total course of language development, the child must learn dictionary definitions, but she will also learn and use other forms of defining to refine her understanding of word meanings.

As we would expect, definitions offered by preschool and early elementary schoolchildren are incomplete. They lack semantic content. The definitions often reflect their own personal experiences and fail to capture the shared meanings that we associate with adult definitions (Litowitz, 1977). Early definitions tend to be *functional* in nature, which means that they allude to something an object does rather than what the object is. A child at the age of five years, for example, defines most words in this *functional* manner. If he is asked what a *dog* is, he is likely to say something like, "A dog barks." By the time the child is ten years old, more of his definitions will be *categorical,* which is a big step toward *dictionary* or *Aristotelian* definitions. That is, when asked to define *dog,* this child will say, "A dog is an animal" (Al-Issa, 1969).

It is important to emphasize at this point that defining words is not just a semantic exercise. It is also a metalinguistic phenomenon. The semantic part of defining a word involves establishing the general category and identifying the differentiating characteristics—the basic components of a dictionary definition. The metalinguistic part of defining words is the pervasive language awareness that comes with age, maturation, knowledge, developing cognitive skills, and increasingly refined perceptual skills. The more the child knows about life, and the more she knows about language, the more skillfully and completely she will identify the components of the dictionary definition. The metalinguistic influence is clear in the evolution of the child's definitions. We know, for example, that the preschool child's definitions and the early elementary school child's definitions are concrete and personal (Snow, 1990). As he proceeds through the elementary school years and gains more experience with life and language, the child's definitions become more conceptual, more abstract (Swartz & Hall, 1972).

Johnson and Anglin (1995) have found that when defining words, children tend to include correct semantic information before they can put their definitions into correct syntactic form. In addition, as one would expect, children define base words more accurately and completely than they define derived words.

Not until the child approaches adolescence does he begin to define words in an adultlike manner. The adolescent child's definition of a word includes the general category we expect to find in a dictionary definition, and he includes at least some of the differentiating characteristics (Nippold, Hegel, Sohlberg, & Schwarz, 1999).

A Shift from Personal to Shared Definitions

The child's earliest definitions are personal and based on her own unique experiences. Her initial definition of *dog,* for example, may be strongly influenced by her first experiences with a dog. A child whose first dog experiences are with a small, friendly, playful poodle will have a very different definition of *dog* than a child whose first en-counters involve a larger, more ferocious dog. As the child matures through the early school years, her definitions progress from personal, experience-based understand-ings to more socially shared understandings (Litowitz, 1977). She might still be afraid of dogs if her first experiences with dogs were frightening, but she will develop a def-inition of *dog* that will be independent of her personal fear or distrust of dogs.

Shifting from Single-Word to More Elaborate Definitions

Another change noted by Litowitz (1977) is the shift from single-word definitions to definitions based on sentences providing appropriate detail and explanation. The child begins this shift when he is about seven years old and in the second grade (Wehren, DeLisi, & Arnold, 1981), but it continues throughout the school years and during adulthood. As the child moves through the school years toward adulthood, we notice other significant changes in his definitions. When he is about five years old, the child's definitions are typically limited to features related to function and physi-cal description (McGregor, Friedman, Reilly, & Newman, 2002), but as he gets older, he adds the more abstract features we hear in adult definitions. In addition, he learns the multiple meanings of words. At three or four years, his definitions tend to be con-crete and in the moment. As he gets older, he adds figurative elements to his defini-tions. At three, "sugar" is something you put on your cereal, but by the time the child is eight or nine years old, he understands that "sugar" might also mean "a kiss," as in "Give me some sugar!"

Adult definitions are descriptive and explanatory and typically include restric-tions, synonyms, antonyms, and even the word's grammatical category or categories. Obviously, the shift from single-word definitions to comprehensive, detailed defini-tions occurs gradually in an evolutionary manner. Even the adult has more complete and accurate definitions for some words than others. The less knowledge the adult has about a particular word and its referent, the more childlike will be his definition of that word. Quick—make a list of words you might define in three words or fewer! Make another list of words you use all the time for which you have no cogent defini-tions. How about *cogent?* The point here is that our definitions are always evolving, constantly reflecting more elaborate and complete understandings.

Strategies for Organizing Vocabulary

Vocabulary acquisition involves more than adding items to one's lexical list. It also in-volves the sorting of words into categories. We will consider two strategies children use to organize words as they acquire them.

Chunking

The process of placing words into categories based on their semantic relationships is called **chunking.** The child has a cognitive category for animals, for example, and he also has a vocabulary category for animal words, which includes *horse, dog, fish,* and *elephant.* As he matures, he chunks in a more differentiated manner. He retains a cat-egory for animals, but he develops subcategories, so that farm animals includes words such as *horse, cow, chicken,* and *pig,* and jungle animals includes words such as *elephant, monkey,* and *lion.* These vocabulary chunks facilitate remembering. There is evidence that chunking is a more commonly used strategy for recalling words by seventh-grade children than by children in the first grade (Vanevery & Rosenberg, 1970), a change in vocabulary categorization that is consistent with changes Piaget (1963) identified in cognitive development.

An example of language knowledge shaping thinking can be observed in the child's efforts to cope with ambiguities among words in her vocabulary. How does the child differentiate among words that sound the same, such as *dear-deer, bye-by-buy, not-knot,* and *right-write*? Perfetti and Goodman (1970) suggest that she addresses the potential ambiguities among these words by sorting them according to their semantic functions. That is, *dear* functions as a modifier, and *deer* functions as a noun. *Not* is a negative element, and *knot* is a noun. As the child develops knowledge about the semantic functions of words, therefore, she is able to use this language knowledge to sort and categorize words and their referents cognitively according to the semantic roles they fill.

Syntagmatic-Paradigmatic Shift

Another change we see in the child's processing and organization of words occurs in what is called the **syntagmatic-paradigmatic shift** (Ervin, 1961). In a word-association task, the preschool child is likely to respond to a word according to its syntactic role. In responding to "Mommy," for example, he might say, "Kiss." He processes and organizes the stimulus word according to the word that is likely to follow it in a sentence. As he changes his cognitive processing strategies (Emerson & Gekoski, 1976), he responds to words in a paradigmatic manner, based on the semantic features of the word he hears. If he hears "Mommy," he says, "Girl," "Woman," or perhaps "Daddy" as the opposite of "Mommy." The shift from syntagmatic to paradigmatic processing occurs slowly, but the most rapid change is observed between five and nine years (Muma & Zwycewicz-Emory, 1979), and the shift is not complete until adulthood.

These and other changes in cognitive processing account for the growth in vocabulary we observe during the school years and beyond, and they account for the changes we observe in the meanings of the child's words. We are most likely to notice that the child's vocabulary is growing in size, but she also understands words differently as she matures. Her first definitions of words are developed quickly and are superficial, but over the years these definitions are progressively refined (Carey & Bartlett, 1978). As the child moves through school into adulthood, her definitions become increasingly specific and precise until they resemble the kinds of definitions one finds in the dictionary (Wehren, DeLisi, & Arnold, 1981). The child's initial understandings of words are concrete and are related to immediate contexts. These understandings gradually become more abstract until the child has stable, consistent meanings for words that are not dependent on specific contexts.

Cognition: Retrieving Stored Vocabulary Information

As should be abundantly clear by this point in our journey, language cannot be separated from cognition. We see this connection clearly when we consider how vocabulary information is organized, stored, and retrieved. As with every other part of the complex of human behavior we call *oral communication,* the organizational, storage, and retrieval part is very much developmental. The toddler's abilities in this area are primitive. The preschool child's abilities are developing but incomplete. As he moves from childhood to adolescence to adulthood, the child becomes increasingly skilled in using basic strategies for pulling words from his memory (Kail, 1984; Kobasigawa, 1974; Kobasigawa & Mason, 1982). At least three strategies are used in retrieval: using semantic categorical information, using externally provided auditory cues, and using visual cues.

Using Semantic Categorization

We have already considered how the process, chunking, is used by the child to place words into categories based on their semantic relationships. Chunking actually serves two purposes. It is used to *organize* words according to their semantic features as we have already established, but it is also used to *retrieve* words from memory when words are stored in categories based on their semantic features. The demands on the ability to retrieve words increase dramatically as the child's vocabulary grows exponentially over the course of language development. When her vocabulary is limited to fifty words, her word-finding choices are limited and the semantic categories into which the words are stored are limited. In fact, the words and categories are so limited, she will often retrieve the same word from two or more categories to represent several semantic relationships. When an adult retrieves words from a vocabulary of 80,000 or more words, the task is considerably more complicated. The adult needs to find just the right word to express just the right meaning. All children and all adults use chunking in word retrieval, but the *chunks* change as language matures and vocabulary grows.

Using Externally Provided Auditory Cues

We would certainly expect that retrieval is a much easier process when hints are provided, and that is exactly correct. Halperin (1974) found that when children in three age groups (six years, nine years, and twelve years) were asked to recall words organized into several semantic categories that were read aloud to them, they were able to recall more of the words when they were cued for the category first. One of the semantic categories, for example, was *tools.* When the children in all three age groups were asked, "Can you tell me all the tools?" they retrieved more of the tool-related words than when they were not provided the semantic category. It is interesting and important to note that the nine-year-olds and the twelve-year-olds retrieved more words than the youngest children even when they were not cued for semantic category, which might suggest that they were better able than the younger children to recognize and use the semantic categories to organize and store words as they were hearing them.

Using Visual Cues

And what happens when we add visual cues to the retrieval task? Kobasigawa (1974) asked children in three age groups (six years, eight years, and eleven years) to recall twenty-four words represented in pictures. There were eight semantic categories represented and three words in each category. In addition to the twenty-four pictured words, there were eight pictures depicting the semantic categories. As the three pictures in each semantic category were shown and named aloud, the child looked at the semantic category picture and was told that those words were associated with that category. After all twenty-four words had been presented, the examiner gave the category cue pictures to the child and indicated that they could be used, if the child wanted to use them, to assist in remembering the words. Only one-third of the youngest children used the category pictures to help them retrieve the words, but three-fourths of the eight-year-old children and more than 90 percent of the oldest children used the category cue pictures. Not surprisingly, the children who used the category cue pictures recalled more words than the children who did not use them. The older children who used the picture cues retrieved more words per category than the younger children who used the cues, indicating that the older children used this retrieval strategy more effectively than their younger counterparts.

We can conclude from all this that finding words is really a two-part process. Successful word finding depends first on successful word **storage.** If we do not store words in an efficient manner, if we do not store them in meaningful and readily recognizable categories, we will have trouble recalling them when we need them. The second and most obvious part of word finding is **retrieval.** Successful retrieval depends on the efficiency of our storage, but it also depends on our ability to effectively utilize the kinds of retrieval strategies we have identified here—chunking, using auditory cues, and using visual cues. We should note that other factors are involved, of course. We will be able to retrieve a word more easily if it is a word we use often. We will have less difficulty if we are retrieving a word from memory if we have not stored many other words that have the same or similar meaning. Depending on our understanding of the word, we might more readily retrieve a word we have recently learned, especially if we have a particular fondness for it.

From Literal to Figurative: Having Fun with Words

It might seem reasonable to assume that the preschool child uses language only in literal ways, an assumption that would not be true. Young children often use language creatively, but their creativity is usually not intentional. The cute and unusual expressions of the preschool child are often the products of incomplete language knowledge. That is, the child will use the language he has to describe things, people, and events in the absence of more appropriate language he has not yet acquired. When my oldest daughter was about three years old, she ran out of our apartment without benefit of clothing. When I called for her to return, she yelled, "Look, Daddy, my bottom is barefootin'!" She understood that a foot without a shoe is a "barefoot," so she applied this language to other parts of her anatomy including her naked tush! This was not, strictly speaking, figurative language. It was my daughter's honest and direct attempt to describe her public nudity, using the language available to her. (There were no arrests.)

There is evidence that the child as young as five years is able to understand sentences that include figurative language (Nippold & Sullivan, 1987), but he cannot explain these sentences until he is about ten or eleven years old. The most significant developments in the child's understanding and production of figurative language occur during the school years. **Figurative language forms** include metaphors, similies, idioms, and proverbs.

A **metaphor** is a figure of speech involving an implied comparison between two dissimilar things. A **simile** is an explicit comparison. In describing the unseemly eating habits of someone, we might say, *"He eats like a pig,"* which is a simile. The metaphor version would be *"He's a pig."* The preschool child might produce many utterances that sound like metaphors. She might call a man's cap a "head sock," or she might refer to a barn as a "horsie house." The child is using language creatively to describe the cap and the barn because she does not have the words *cap* and *barn* in her vocabulary. The preschool child does not have enough language knowledge to know how to use language figuratively (Hakes, 1982).

Interestingly, as the child's language develops and her vocabulary increases, these apparent metaphors decrease in frequency, especially after the age of six years, probably because she gains enough vocabulary that she does not have to overextend her words to similar but inappropriate referents (Gardner & Winner, 1979). Metaphors increase in frequency again only when the child's vocabulary, language knowledge, and cognitive insights develop enough to allow her to understand the commonalities among dissimilar things that make metaphors and similes effective elements of figurative language. In describing a curious child, we could simply say, *"Juan is a very curious child,"* but if we say, *"Juan is as curious as a hyperactive kitten,"* the image is much stronger. Keeping in mind that Piaget (1963) describes the child's thinking as "concrete" throughout the elementary school years, we would not expect her to produce and process metaphors and similes frequently and effectively until she moves into the formal operations stage of cognitive development, which takes her from the sixth grade through her sophomore year in high school. That is, during the preschool and elementary school years, the child thinks and talks about what is real and immediate. As she moves into her junior high and high school years, she begins to think and talk more abstractly. If she should falter, there is always that helpful English teacher who insists that she identify and understand the "symbolism" in great pieces of literature. Surely, you remember this kind of challenge: *"The Old Man and the Sea* is about an old man who fishes, but what does the fish represent, and who is the old man?"

An **idiom** is a figurative expression peculiar to a particular language or group of people. Idioms cannot be understood literally, and that is why they are so troublesome for people learning the language to which they are indigenous. If someone just learning to speak English requested a favor you could not grant because of institutional rules, you might say, *"I'm sorry, but my hands are tied."* As you might imagine, this would create some confusion for the listener because, under normal circumstances, your hands are rarely tied. The idiom means that there is nothing you can do. The person learning English must learn not only the vocabulary of the language and the rules but also the idioms. Consider the problems one might have trying to literally interpret the following American English idioms in simple sentences:

He was beating around the bush.   It takes two to tango.
I beat you to the punch.   I lost my shirt in that deal.
I'll fix your wagon.   Just keep your pants on.
I put my foot in my mouth.   Did the cat get your tongue?
The cat's out of the bag.   She'll have to face the music.
He'll have to toe the line.   He's still wet behind the ears.
She made money hand over fist.   My back is to the wall.
His nose is out of joint.   I bent over backward for you.
He really flew off the handle.   She's just spitting into the wind.
I'll fly by the seat of my pants.   We'll play it by ear.

The child learning English as his native language does not encounter the problems associated with translating idioms from English into another language, which creates extraordinary and sometimes humorous confusion, but he must still learn how to use and understand idioms.

During his preschool and early elementary school years, the child's interpretations of idioms tend to be literal. When the child in this age range is shown pictures depicting literal and figurative interpretations of idioms, he chooses the literal interpretation first (Nippold & Duthie, 2003). Given the same choices, adolescents and adults are more likely to choose the figurative interpretation first. The child as young as five or six will understand some idioms, but he does not handle all the common idioms of his language until he is about twelve or thirteen years old. Beyond adolescence, he learns some of the more unusual idioms, and he gradually understands the derivations of at least some idioms. As one would expect, not all children acquire and understand idioms at the same pace. There is evidence that idioms are learned more quickly by children who have superior reading and comprehension skills (Nippold, Moran, & Schwartz, 2001), and that certainly makes sense. The more immersed a child is in language and in the processing of language, the more familiar he will be with the figurative nuances that add the layers of meaning characteristic of idioms.

A **proverb, adage,** or **maxim** is a popular, wise saying or a precise statement of truth. Proverbs often provide common sense advice or cautions. See whether you can interpret the meanings of the following proverbs:

You can lead a horse to water, but you can't make him drink.

An ounce of prevention is worth a pound of cure.

A penny saved is a penny earned.

A rolling stone gathers no moss.

The grass is always greener on the other side of the fence.

The squeaky wheel gets the grease.

Time is money.

Haste makes waste.

Don't put the cart before the horse.

You can't have your cake and eat it, too.

A bird in the hand is worth two in the bush.

People who live in glass houses shouldn't throw stones.

A stitch in time saves nine.

There is none so blind as he who will not see.

Now try to imagine how the preschool child would interpret these statements. As with idioms, the young child initially interprets proverbs literally. Proverbs are more difficult for the child to understand than other forms of figurative language, including idioms and metaphors. There are some fairly logical reasons for this difficulty. The syntactic structures of proverbs are often unusual. They sometimes contain unfamiliar words, or familiar words used in unfamiliar ways. The concepts that underlie proverbs are often difficult for the young child to comprehend. Even if you can help the preschool child unravel the language meaning of "There is none so blind as he who will not see," you will probably find it difficult to teach her the proverb's lesson. Truth and wisdom, no matter how precisely or eloquently stated, are difficult matters for mature adults. We should not expect the child to easily grasp the truths in proverbs or understand the language in which they are packaged. Although some common proverbs may be understood by the child during the early elementary school years, she will typically not understand proverbs until she is an adolescent (Billow, 1975).

Even in adulthood, the understanding of some proverbs may be murky and incomplete. Many of us struggle with *You can't have your cake and eat it too.* If one ingests the cake, does he not still have it? Is having the cake in its decorated, uneaten form any more satisfying than having the cake in one's stomach? Of course not, unless, *One's eyes are bigger than one's stomach*, which creates another confusion that is as much anatomic as philosophic.

And then there are proverbs well known to children that turn out not to be true at all. We all grow up hearing that "Sticks and stones may break my bones, but words can never hurt me," but we all know that some words from some people in some circumstances hurt far more than sticks.

Figurative language plays an important role in humor, and we see the same growth in the child's understanding of the language of humor as we see in his understanding of metaphors, idioms, and proverbs. A joke can be a physical prank, but we normally think of a joke as a brief humorous narrative, a funny language form. Humans typically laugh at actions or words that are unexpected or incongruous. Consider the following common riddle: "What is it that a man does standing up, a woman does sitting down, and a dog does with one leg in the air? Shake hands." Sometimes the humor in language is not by design, especially when children are involved, but the humor is still evoked because what is said is unexpected. When a Sunday school teacher asked a child about the "epistles," he said, "The epistles were the wives of the apostles." Another child in talking about Mount Vesuvius said, "Vesuvius is a volcano. You can see the creator smoking there day and night." Another child, a nine-year-old girl, came home from school on the Monday before Easter. She was terribly excited as she told her mother that this was going to be the last week of school. Her mother, knowing that school would be in session for several more months, told her daughter that she must be mistaken. The little girl said, "But, Mommy, it's true. The teacher sent home a note about it. It says that all Brownsburg schools will be closed for Good Friday."

To appreciate the humor in each of these examples, one must understand the incongruities. As we have already established, preschool children tend to interpret language literally, and because they do not understand multiple meanings of words or appreciate that some words that sound alike have different meanings, they are likely to miss the humor in common jokes. Research (Lund & Duchan, 1988; Schultz & Horibe, 1974) indicates that as the child matures and comes to appreciate and understand figurative language, she responds to progressively more sophisticated forms of humor. Prior to her sixth birthday, for example, the child will laugh at slapstick actions, the physical pratfalls and pies-in-the face antics of circus clowns, but she will not understand language-based jokes. Between the ages of six and nine years, she will laugh at jokes based on words that are phonologically similar to other words she knows, as in this example provided by Lund & Duchan:

A diner says, "What is this?"

The waiter responds, "It's bean soup."

The diner says, "I don't care what it's been. What is it now?"

Between the ages of nine and twelve years, the child appreciates the humor in jokes that rely on words with multiple meanings. You may remember this oldie from your own childhood: "What's big and white, has four wheels, and *flies?* A garbage truck." When the child passes his twelfth birthday, he understands humor based on two or more possible meanings within a single sentence, as in this classroom classic:

A teacher asks, "Where was the Declaration of Independence signed?"

The student answers, "At the bottom."

The essence of this joke has been repeated thousands of times in movies and television programs when one character says, "Johnny kissed Susan," and another character, usually overwrought by this development, asks, "Where did he kiss her?" The first character answers, "Right in the living room!" Most jokes adults find funny are based on words with multiple meanings or on sentence structures that can be interpreted in two or more ways. What makes them funny is that the listener anticipates the most obvious meaning and is caught off guard by a different meaning or by an unexpected twist in the way a word is used.

It should be easy to understand, therefore, that the child will understand language-based jokes only to the extent that he knows and understands all the possible meanings of the words contained in these jokes and only to the extent that he understands that a single sentence might have two or more possible underlying meanings.

These understandings develop throughout the school years and even into adulthood. We all know a few adults we think of as naive, innocent, or gullible because they do not seem to know all the possible meanings of the words in punch lines, especially unsavory or potentially offensive meanings.

Syntax and Morphology: Still Expanding and Acquiring

There is so much to understand about the pieces of language and about how to put the pieces together in grammatically acceptable ways that the business of acquiring syntax and morphology is never really complete. One of the fascinations of language is that it is a creative process. Creative processes are never complete because there are always innovations and new adaptations of old productions. This is true in art and music, and in a very real sense, it is true of language. From birth through the preschool years, the child has learned the rudiments of language. During the school years, she improves her language skills by expanding the forms she has already acquired, by increasing her language knowledge, and by learning how to use language creatively.

Figuring Out Passive Sentences

As mentioned in the preceding chapter, the child has considerable difficulty with passive sentences. In active sentences, the first noun is the agent, and the second noun is the object. In passive sentences, the order changes, and this apparently causes the child to be confused. The preschool child understands "The dog chased the cat" but has trouble interpreting "The cat was chased by the dog." Passive sentences remain troublesome throughout most of the child's elementary school years.

Even though the five-year-old child understands some passive sentences, especially those that include action verbs such as *hit* or *eat,* he produces very few passive forms. The passive sentences he does produce tend to be abbreviated forms that exclude the agent. He might say, "Billy was pushed," or "The ball was kicked," rather than "Billy was pushed by Tom," and "The ball was kicked by Tasha."

Horgan (1978) studied the development of **reversible** and **nonreversible passive** sentences in preschool and school-age children. You may recall that a passive sentence is considered reversible if either noun can act as the agent. For example, "The dog was chased by the cat" is a reversible passive because it is also possible to say, "The cat was chased by the dog." The passive sentence "The candy was eaten by the boy" is nonreversible because its opposite version, "The boy was eaten by the candy," is not a viable alternative. Horgan found that her preschool subjects under the age of four years produced more reversible passive sentences than nonreversible forms. Although reversible and nonreversible passive forms were produced by her preschool and school-age subjects, no child produced both forms until about eleven years, and even among the children between eleven and thirteen years, only 50 percent produced both forms.

There is no question that the development of passive sentences is slow. Although preschool children produce some abbreviated passive forms, most children are not producing full passive sentences until the late elementary school ages. Baldie (1976) found that about 80 percent of eight-year-old children produce full passive sentences, and Horgan's (1978) findings suggest that some passive forms do not emerge in productive language until about eleven years.

The Principle of Minimal Distance: Dealing with an Exception

As noted by Slobin (1978) and others who study the development of language, the young child goes out of his way to avoid exceptions. He learns general rules first, and then over time he gradually sorts out and masters the exceptions to the rules. We have noted examples of this strategy in the preceding two chapters. The child learns the rule for regular past tense first and overextends the rule to verbs that require different past tense markers. That is, he says "bak*ed*," "kiss*ed*," and "play*ed*," which require regular past tense, but he also says "go*ed*," "sitt*ed*," and "hitt*ed*," which should be "went," "sat," and "hit." Many of the exceptions to the rules of language are discovered and mastered during the school years.

One intriguing example of learning an exception was studied by Carol Chomsky (1969), who analyzed the problems children have in interpreting sentences that violate the principle of minimal distance. She was specifically interested in sentences containing the verbs *ask, tell,* and *promise.* According to the principle of minimal distance, the preceding noun closest to the verb is treated as the subject of the sentence. This principle certainly holds in most basic sentences such as the following:

The boy hit the ball.

Yoko jumped over the fence.

Mom picks me up after school.

The dog ate my birthday cake.

In each of these sentences and countless others that we all produce every day, the subject immediately precedes the verb. When there is a separation, it is typically only one word, as in "Mom *always* picks me up after school." Chomsky found that the principle of minimal distance, and exceptions to the principle, are demonstrated in sentences that include the verbs *ask, tell,* and *promise.* If the verb *tell* is used, the principle of minimal distance can be consistently applied in sentences such as "Tanya told Joe to cook dinner." In this sentence, *Tanya* and *Joe* precede the infinitive verb *to cook,* but *Joe* is closer to the infinitive verb, and according to the principle of minimal distance, is the subject of this verb. In this sentence the principle works because Tanya is the one doing the telling and Joe is the one doing the cooking.

Consider what happens, however, when we use a verb that violates the principle of minimal distance as in the sentence "Tanya promised Joe to cook dinner." Even though the surface structure of this sentence is the same as in the earlier example, the principle of minimal distance cannot be used in the interpretation. In this sentence

Tanya is doing the promising, but she is also the one who will be doing the cooking, even though *Joe* is closer to the infinitive verb *to cook*.

The verb *tell* consistently adheres to the principle of minimal distance, and the verb *promise* consistently violates the principle. The verb *ask* is especially troublesome because it sometimes adheres to the principle and sometimes violates it. If we say, "Tanya asked Joe to cook dinner," application of the principle of minimal distance will result in a correct interpretation; but if we say, "Tanya asked Joe what to cook for dinner," the principle will not work. In the first case, Joe will be doing the cooking, but in the second case, Tanya will be doing the cooking. What really matters here, of course, is that someone will be cooking dinner, because Tanya and Joe are getting hungry!

The child uses the principle of minimal distance by the time she is about five years old, but learning the exceptions takes time. In reference to the verbs in Chomsky's (1969) study, she will have little trouble with *tell* because it consistently adheres to the principle. She will have only somewhat more trouble with *promise* because, although it violates the principle of minimal distance, it violates the principle consistently. Chomsky found that the child correctly interprets *tell* and *promise* by the time she is nine years old, but she does not master her interpretation of the pesky, inconsistent *ask* until she is about ten.

The child's struggle with the principle of minimal distance relative to *tell, promise,* and *ask* is a revealing example of the overall struggle with rules and their exceptions. He learns general rules relatively early and tends to overapply them. He then learns the exceptions. The greater the inconsistencies and the further the exceptions deviate from the general rules, the longer it takes the child to understand and produce these forms that are the square pegs of language trying to fit into round holes.

Conjoining and Embedding: Becoming More Complex

Making language constructions more complex does not occur by simply pasting words onto the ends of sentences. Increased complexity is the product of combining constructions and by placing new strings of words within already existing constructions. The reader will recognize these as the processes of **conjoining** and **embedding**.

Conjoining with More Complex Conjunctions

Over the course of the school years, the child increases the complexity of his sentences by using more embedded and conjoined forms. He begins to conjoin clauses during the preschool years, usually with the conjunction *and.* During the school years, when his narrative skills are improving, he continues to favor *and* over other conjunctions. In fact, as many as 80 percent of the sentences in the narratives produced by the school-age child begin with *and.* As the child grows older, he relies less on this conjunction. By the time he is an early teenager, *and* initiates about 20 percent of his narrative sentences; when he writes narratives at this age, the percentage drops to about 5 percent (Scott, 1987).

During the school years, he not only conjoins more often but also uses a wider range of conjunctions expressing more complex relationships among the clauses of his sentences. Through the later elementary school years, *because* and *when* are commonly used. *If* and *in order* are produced, but are used less frequently (Scott, 1987). Menyuk (1969) identified the categories of conjunctions the child will eventually acquire to express the more complex clausal relationships he is expressing: *conditional* (*if*), *causal* (*so, because, therefore*), *disjunctive* (*but, or, therefore*), and *temporal* (*before, after, when, then*). There is evidence that the child may use some of these conjunctions before he fully understands them (Hood & Bloom, 1979). Among other concepts, he must understand time and the subtleties of truth as expressed in language before he can understand and use all of these conjunctions meaningfully. Nevertheless, by the time he completes his elementary school years, that understanding is emerging, and he is using most conjunctions appropriately most of the time. However, some thorny issues with some conjunctions persist for a time.

The conjunction *because* is troublesome for the child because she must understand the underlying cause–effect relationship expressed in the conjoined clauses and the temporal relationship between the events described. In the normal thought process, a cause is identified before its effect is considered. For example, if we stand in the rain (cause), we will get wet (effect). If you prick your finger with a pin (cause), your finger will bleed (effect). The preschool child understands cause–effect relationships and can express them in conjoined sentences such as "I fell down the stairs, and I hurt my knee." Notice the difference, however, between this sentence and a version using the conjunction *because:* "I hurt my knee because I fell down the stairs." The cause and effect are now reversed. "I hurt my knee" is the *effect*, but it is mentioned before the *cause* ("I fell down the stairs"). The child who is accustomed to interpreting cause-effect on the basis of order of mention is likely to be confused. Prior to her seventh birthday, the child will use *because, and,* and *then* as though they mean the same thing (Corrigan, 1975). She might say, for example, "I fell down the stairs, *and* I hurt my knee," but she might also say, "I fell down the stairs *because* I hurt my knee." Apparently, the child has less difficulty when she is describing two events that are occurring simultaneously or that overlap in time than when she is describing related but distinctly successive events. That is, she can produce and understand sentences such as "I'm eating ice cream because it tastes good" (simultaneous events), and "I throw the ball because we're playing baseball" (overlapping events), but she has trouble interpreting sentences such as "I have to stay in my room because I told a lie" (distinctly successive events). Not until she is about ten or eleven years old does she fully and consistently comprehend the ordering and causal meanings of *because* (Emerson, 1979).

Other conjunctions pose similar problems for the child. He must understand *contrast* before he can use *but* correctly. He must understand *consequence* before he can use *therefore* appropriately. He must understand *condition* before he can use *if* properly. Wing and Scholnick (1981) have noted that the child at ten years may still have problems with the conjunction *unless* because he does not fully understand disbelief and uncertainty. Conjunctions may seem to be simple words, but the concepts and relationships they denote are clearly not simple. The child must have a cognitive understanding of the concepts underlying conjunctions before he is able to comprehend and produce conjoined sentences that include these conjunctions. As the child moves through his school-age years, his understanding of the concepts and his ability to apply this knowledge to language interpretation and production improve steadily.

Embedding: More Forms and More Often

The same persistent, if occasionally stumbling, improvements we observe in conjoining are observed in embedding during the school years. The preschool child produces relatively few embedded sentences, and when she does, she embeds infinitive phrases, object complements, and relative clauses modifying noun phrases in the object position but not in the subject position. Over the course of the elementary school years, the percentage of sentences with embedded elements grows to about 30 percent (Scott, 1984). Her repertoire of relative pronouns grows to include *whose, whom,* and *in which* (Scott, 1988a). After she passes her seventh birthday, the child will produce sentences in which the relative pronoun is deleted but understood, as in "I just saw a movie [that] you would really enjoy," and she will embed in the subject position or center of a sentence as in "The man *who bought our car* is a teacher" (Menyuk, 1971). As the child matures, she produces more multiple embeddings as well. This is quite noticeable in the narratives of school-age children. The first- or second-grade child seldom includes multiple embeddings in her narratives, whereas they are common in the narratives of the fifth- and sixth-grade child.

Sentences involving subject position or center embedding are initially difficult for the child to interpret because they violate the expected subject–verb–object order. If the child hears "The dog that bit the cat ran away," and applies the subject–verb–object rule, he may conclude that the cat ran away. He may understand the sentence correctly if he relies on his understanding of semantic roles. That is, in the world most children understand, dogs are aggressive toward cats, not the other way around. If that is the child's understanding, he will interpret the sentence correctly even if the subject–verb–object rule is violated. Confusion in center embedding may be avoided if the object of the center embedding is inanimate (Maratsos, 1974). For example, if the child hears "The dog that chewed the shoe ran away," he will correctly conclude that the dog ran away, not the shoe, because dogs are animate and can run, whereas shoes are inanimate and cannot run. If the child cannot depend on his understanding of semantic roles to figure out center embeddings, he might have trouble interpreting these structures because of limitations on his auditory memory (Lewis, 1996). As he grows older and his auditory memory retains more information for longer periods of time, he is able to sort out the possible ambiguities presented by these embeddings. By the time the child is about twelve years old, he will correctly interpret embedded sentences no matter where the embeddings occur, and he will base his interpretations on his grammatical knowledge, not simply on word order or semantic roles (Abrahamsen & Rigrodsky, 1984).

Noun and Verb Phrases: Still Expanding

Do you remember the first time a teacher asked you to write a 500-word essay? You may remember thinking that it must be almost impossible to write 500 words about any topic, or counting the words. If there were not enough words, you may rarely have considered elaborating your thoughts. Your first instinct may have been simply to add words to the sentences you had already created. Surely you remember how this works:

The man walked. (3 words)

The man walked across the street. (6 words)

The haggard, gray-bearded man whose last meal must have been consumed about three weeks before the birth of the New World, walked with short, labored, arthritic steps across the windswept, deserted street to the dark and desolate hole in the wall that twenty years ago was the most exquisite restaurant in the city. (53 words . . . only 447 to go!)

As this example suggests, a sentence can be made longer by adding adjectives and adverbs, and by embedding prepositional phrases and subordinate clauses into the original sentence, which consisted of a basic noun phrase (*The man*) and simple verb phrase (*walked*). The child has been elaborating these phrases throughout the preschool years. As he moves through the school years, he produces longer and more elaborate noun and verb phrases. He refines forms he has been producing. He adds new forms. He learns which language forms must be retained and which forms can be eliminated because they are redundant.

During the early school years, when the child is about five to seven years old, she may still be omitting articles (*a, an, the*) even though she adds other redundant information, such as the infamous double negative. The child might say, for example, "I don't got [the] ball no more." This same child is likely to have problems with using some prepositions, with marking verbs appropriately for tense, and with marking plurality (Menyuk, 1971). As one would expect, cases of plurality and tense changes that violate the regular rules are the most troublesome for school-age children. As the child moves through elementary school, she addresses each of these problems. She learns to retain function words, including the articles. She eliminates redundant negative terms, and she gradually learns the exceptions for verb tense, plurality, and other language forms.

During the school years, the child completes his sorting of pronouns. He learns to separate subject pronouns (*I, we, he, she, they*) from object pronouns (*me, us, him, her, them*), and he learns to use reflexive pronouns such as *myself, herself,* and *themselves.* The school-age child learns to recognize the antecedents of pronouns even when the nouns and pronouns are in different sentences, as in the following example: "Joe's brother was badly hurt in an automobile accident. He [Joe] goes to see him [Joe's brother] in the hospital every day."

As demonstrated in the example in the opening of this section, one of the ways to elaborate noun phrases is to add adjectives. When the child begins to string adjectives together, he must learn the rules for ordering adjectives. Each adjective in a sequence refers to a specific attribute of the noun being modified or described. There are rules for how adjectives are ordered (Whorf, 1956), although we do not have a complete understanding of these rules. We do know, however, that "three, hyperactive, preschool children" *sounds* right, whereas "hyperactive, preschool, three children" does not even sound close. We also know that children as young as three years demonstrate some of the same sequencing rules used by adults (Richards, 1980). During the school years, the child will develop a more complete understanding of the attributes reflected in adjectives and a more complete understanding of how these attributes are related to one another. As these understandings mature, he will learn the remaining rules for sequencing adjectives, even if he is never able to express the rules. Can you explain why *four, wild-eyed, ice cream lovers* is "correct," and *ice-cream, four, wild-eyed lovers* is kinky but "incorrect"? Probably not!

You are probably familiar with the differentiation between a **common noun,** which refers to a general class of people, places, or things, and a **proper noun,** which refers to a specific member of a class. Nouns are also classified as **concrete** (names of real, tangible objects), **abstract** (names of ideas, emotions, concepts), **collective** (names of groups of people or things), **count** (nouns that can be counted or tallied), and **mass** (names of homogeneous, aggregate substances). The child learning language must understand all these categories of nouns, of course, but the distinction between count and mass nouns is especially difficult. During the school years, the child gradually comprehends the difference between these categories and learns which quantifying adjectives can be used with each category (Gathercole, 1985).

Count nouns can be modified by numbers, of course, but they can also be modified by adjectives such as *many* and *few,* as in the following examples:

There are *few* students in class today.

Miguel keeps *many* pencils in his desk.

Mass nouns require different modifiers, such as *little* and *much,* as in the following examples:

There was *little* meat left on his plate.

You put too *much* sugar in my coffee.

Now mix these adjectives by using *few* for *little, many* for *much,* and vice versa. You will quickly discover that you know which adjectives should be used with count nouns and which should be used with mass nouns. The child has usually mastered this understanding by the time he approaches adolescence, although he might still use *much* when *many* is appropriate, as in "Can you believe how much girls were at that party?" While he is trying to figure out which adjectives should be used with which category of nouns, he might use *lots of* in reference to both categories. In fact, if you listen carefully to the speech of adults, you may hear sentences such as the following:

Miguel keeps *lots of* pencils in his desk. (count)

You put *lots of* sugar in my coffee. (mass)

Since one can get lots of mileage out of *lots of,* one may tend to use *lots of* lots of the time!

During the school years, the child learns what adverbs mean and how to use them. As with other categories of words, some adverbs are easier to understand than others. Adverbs of likelihood such as *definitely, probably,* and *possibly* are especially difficult because, although they can be used in the same contexts, they express varying degrees of likelihood. The differences may seem small or nonexistent to the young child, but they are critical. Assume that you are standing with your back to a friend, who tells you to fall straight backward. You ask, "Will you catch me?" You will listen very carefully to the adverb of likelihood in your friend's answer because you know there is a bodily risk difference between "I will *probably* catch you" and "I will *definitely* catch you." During the preschool years, the child does not understand the subtle but vital differences among adverbs of likelihood, but she has a fairly good grasp of the differences by the time she is in the fourth grade. She does not learn these adverbs at the same time, and, as you might guess, she tends to understand *definitely* before she understands *probably* and *possibly* (Hoffner, Cantor, & Badzinski, 1990).

Morphological Modifications

During the school years, the child expands his overall vocabulary by *morphing* or reshaping root words. These modifications are clearly the products of his growing understanding of how words are formed and how the constituent parts of words can be manipulated to change their meanings or to affect how they are used in relation to other words. During the school years, the child's use of inflectional suffixes to indicate things such as plurality, possession, and changes in verb tense matures, but the most dramatic improvement comes in his use of inflectional prefixes, such as adding *non* to *sense* to create the word *nonsense*, or adding *dis* to *respect* to create the word *disrespect*. In both of these examples, the inflected words are opposite the root words in meaning. We also see improvement in his use of derivational suffixes, such as adding *ly* to *slow*, changing the word from an adjective to an adverb, or *ness* to *sad*, changing the word from an adjective to a noun (Nagy, Diakidoy, & Anderson, 1991).

Morphophonemic Alterations

One of the more interesting developments in morphology that occurs during the school years is something called **morphophonemic alterations.** If we analyze the parts of this term, we will understand what it means. *Morph* refers to *morpheme,* which refers to the smallest unit of meaning in language. *Phonemic* refers to *phoneme,* which refers to speech sound. *Alteration* means change. A morphophonemic alteration then refers to a speech sound change that occurs when the shape of the base morpheme is changed. For example, the final sound in the word *public* is the "k" sound, but when *public* becomes *publicity,* that "k" becomes an "s" sound. That is a morphophonemic alteration. In the word *sign,* the letter *g* is silent, but notice what happens when *sign* is morphed into *signature*—the *g* is now pronounced. The child learns to make many of these changes during the elementary school years.

By the time the child is in the first grade, she understands a very basic morphophonemic alteration related to plurality. She knows that when a noun ends with a voiceless consonant, she adds the sound "s" to make it plural (*cat* → *cats*), but when it ends with a voiced consonant, she adds the sound "z" to make it plural (*dog* → *dogs*[z]"). Within another year or two, she will know that some words require vowel + "z" to make a plural (*ditch* → *ditches*[z]").

Yet another type of morphophonemic alteration, vowel shifting, is not mastered until the child is at the end of the school years, when he is perhaps seventeen or eighteen. When the shapes of certain words are changed, their vowels change. For example, in the word *finite*, the first vowel is a long vowel, but when the word is morphed into *infinity*, the corresponding vowel is short. In the word, *profound*, the *ou* is produced like "ow," but when the word is changed to the noun form, *profundity*, the spelling changes, as does the pronunciation of the corresponding vowel—it is now produced like "uh." Some adults struggle with these changes because they do not always follow the rules of common sense.

Gerunds

Early in the elementary school years, at about seven, the child understands how to produce gerunds. A gerund, you may recall from earlier discussions, is a noun form of a verb created by adding -*ing* to the verb. *Running* is the gerund form of *run*, for example, and *fishing* is the gerund form of *fish*. The seven-year-old child also understands the agentive forms of common verbs (Carrow, 1973). The agentive form identifies the person who performs the action of a verb. Someone who *runs*, for example, is a *runner*, and someone who *sings* is a *singer*, but as with other language forms, there are many exceptions. Someone who *cooks* is a *cook*, not a *cooker*, although *cooker* refers to a certain kind of cooking pot. Someone who fishes is a *fisherman*, not a *fisher*. A person who *types* is a *typist*, not a *typer*, but a person who sets type is a *typesetter*.

Creating Adverb Forms

When the child is seven years old, she also understands and is able to produce the adverb forms of common adjectives by adding the bound morpheme -*ly*. By adding this morpheme, the adjective *slow* becomes the adverb *slowly*. The adjective and adverb forms of *slow* are included in the following sentence: "The train moved *slowly* [adverb] down the tracks on a *slow* [adjective] day in August." Many adverbs are created by adding -*ly*, including *quickly*, *rapidly*, and *swiftly*, but notice that the child must learn exceptions here, too. The adjective *fast*, for example, does not have an adverbial form, *fastly*. The adverb form of *fast* is *fast*, and sometimes nouns can function as adverbs as in the following examples:

After watching the movie, Tony went *home*.

Nora moved *yesterday*.

In the first sentence *home* modifies the verb *went* by specifying *where* Tony went. In the second sentence, *yesterday* specifies *when* Nora moved. Still other adverbs, which always function as adverbs, do not end in -*ly*, such as *again*, *often*, *now*, and *never*.

Pragmatic Development: Conversational Skills Continue to Improve

The most dramatic changes in language development during the school years are in the area of pragmatics or the use of language. The child comes to school understanding and producing virtually all basic language forms, but his conversational skills are still pretty rudimentary. As the child moves through the school years and into his adult years, he masters the art of conversation. He becomes more sophisticated in using language to manipulate the behaviors, feelings, and attitudes of other people. He learns how to manipulate people so indirectly with his words that they scarcely know they are being manipulated. He learns the art of narration or the telling of stories. He learns how to adjust his vocabulary and modify his language style to accommodate listeners of varying ages, backgrounds, and genders. Some people make greater progress in pragmatic development than others, of course. Some become effective communicators at an early age, and some adults never become adept conversationalists or storytellers. Some people have excellent pragmatic skills in some speaking situations but are inept in others. Whatever pragmatic competence one ultimately achieves, however, he begins to seriously hone these skills during the school years.

Establishing Relevance and Topic Shading

As the child matures through the preschool and school-age years, she becomes more capable of maintaining a conversational topic, moving from one topic to a related topic, and introducing new topics, but this progress is slow. At three years, the child typically sustains a topic only if she is interested and only if her partner responds directly to the child's utterances. Even at four years, the child has difficulty sustaining a true dialogue (Gelman & Shatz, 1977). As the child grows older, she becomes increasingly sensitive to the issue of **relevance,** which guides the conversations of adults. That is, the more pertinent, useful or timely a topic, the more likely the older conversationalist will sustain that topic.

The preschool child tends to move from one fairly discrete topic to another, sometimes without warning. As she matures, she learns how to **shade** conversations by moving from one topic to a different but related topic. In adult conversations, shading occurs so subtly that it is often difficult to determine, based on the final topic, how the conversational partners got there. The preschool child talks about concrete topics, about things, people, and events in the here and now. By the time the child is eleven or twelve years old, she is able to discuss abstract topics. If you ask a four-year-old to talk about *love,* you are likely to be greeted by a blank stare, but a twelve-year-old would be able to discuss questions such as "What does love mean to you?" or "How does love affect a person's happiness?"

Introducing and Maintaining Topics

How a topic is maintained changes as the child develops. The preschool child typically maintains a topic by repeating some or all of his partner's utterance. The elementary school-age child maintains a conversation by adding new information to the established topic. Adolescents and adults maintain their conversations not only by adding information during their turns but also by shading one topic into another.

Conversational Repairs

In the preceding chapter, we traced the preschool child's attempts at conversational repair. If the listener does not understand what the speaker has said and asks for clarification, the speaker tries to repair the conversational breakdown. The preschool child, even as young as twenty to thirty months (Gallagher, 1977), will respond to requests for clarification, but these early repairs are crude and rarely helpful. At twenty months, the child tries to repair by changing a speech sound in an important word. At twenty-five months, he typically deletes a word. By thirty months, he changes words. The point is, he tries to repair the broken conversation even if he does not know exactly where the failure has occurred. If the preschool child's first attempt to make a repair does not succeed, he will try again, but he finds the process increasingly difficult and will eventually give up (Brinton, Fujiki, Loeb, & Winkler, 1986).

A series of requests and attempted repairs is called a **stacked repair sequence.** The following example illustrates a typical sequence:

SPEAKER: My wife and I are thinking about getting one of those new hybrid cars.
LISTENER: What in the world is a hybrid car?
SPEAKER: A hybrid car operates on two or more power sources.
LISTENER: Are you telling me that there are two or more power sources operating at the same time?
SPEAKER: Well, there are actually two forms of hybrids—a parallel hybrid and a series hybrid.
LISTENER: Now I'm really confused.
SPEAKER: Actually, it's not terribly complicated. In the parallel hybrid of a gas-electric car, both the gasoline engine and the electric motor power the car at the same time, but in a series hybrid using the same two power sources, the gasoline engine turns a generator that charges the batteries, and the batteries power the electric motor, so the gasoline engine never directly powers the car.
LISTENER: So, I assume you save money on a hybrid?
SPEAKER: They are more cost efficient to operate, but the technology makes them more expensive to manufacture, so the initial cost is pretty high.
LISTENER: I think I'll stick with my scooter!

The preschool child typically makes a valiant effort to respond to the first request for clarification, but she has trouble with additional requests. The five-year-old will usually respond to two requests, but if she is asked for a third repair, she will either give an inappropriate response or simply give up. As the child matures through the elementary school years, she is more likely to respond to repeated requests for clarification, but she also learns how to use information in the requests to shape her attempted repairs. In other words, she becomes more skilled at determining exactly where and why the breakdown has occurred, and she responds to that problem. We can expect to see evidence of this pragmatic ability when the child is about nine years old (Owens, 2005, p. 351). Keep in mind, however, as the prior example suggests, that all speakers have their limits in the area of conversational repair. Sometimes the listener is so entirely disconnected from the message the speaker is attempting to convey that all efforts to make the message clear are futile. Listen to conversations between parents and teenage children, and you will hear some classic examples of failed conversational repairs!

Indirect Requests: The Delicate Art of Hinting

As indicated in the preceding chapter, an indirect request is a subtle, more polite form of request than a direct request. If the room is cool because a window is open, you might make a direct request or demand by saying, "Shut the window," or "Please shut the window," but you can accomplish the same request indirectly by saying, "It's a little too cool in here for me," or "Don't you think it's cool in here?" Children learn to understand and use indirect requests gradually over the preschool and school years.

The preschool child tends to be very direct in his expressive language, and he has difficulty understanding subtle language, including indirect requests (Ervin-Tripp, 1977). The four-year-old might respond to "Don't you think it's cool in here?" by saying, "Yes," but he would probably not understand the question as an indirect request to close the window. He needs the more direct "Please shut the window." By the time the child is six years old, he is responding to many forms of indirect requests, including a form as subtle as a loud sigh (Cherry-Wilkinson & Dollaghan, 1979). If, for example, a parent tells the child to pick up her coat, and the child does not respond immediately, the parent might look the child in the eye and produce a clearly audible sigh that nonverbally and indirectly restates the request and signals impatience. The six-year-old child will correctly interpret this kind of indirect request.

As would be expected, some forms of indirect request are more difficult for the preschool and early school-age child to comprehend than others (Carrell, 1981). He understands declarative terms such as *you should, you shouldn't,* or *you must* more easily than he understands their interrogative versions, *should you? shouldn't you?* and *must you?* He understands positive forms more easily than negative forms. One of the obvious problems with negative forms in indirect requests is that what appears on the surface does not match the intention of the message. Assume, for example, that an adult says to a child on a rainy day, "Shouldn't you put on your boots?" This indirect request includes a negative form, but it is calling for positive action. Even the words contained in indirect requests can be troublesome. The child at four and five years has more difficulty understanding indirect requests that include *should* and *must* than requests containing *can* and *will* (Leonard, Wilcox, Fulmer, & Davis, 1978). By the time the child reaches adolescence, he responds to indirect requests as well as adults, although even adults become confused at times by negative and interrogative forms of indirect request (Clark & Chase, 1972).

The child first produces indirect requests during the preschool years, and the number of her indirect requests compared to direct requests increases between three and five years (Garvey, 1975). Throughout this time, however, direct requests are far more frequent than indirect requests, and the child is seven years old before she is fairly proficient in producing indirect requests (Grimm, 1975).

When the child enters school, she becomes increasingly adept at using nonstandard or creative forms of indirect request based on two simple rules: (1) be brief, and (2) be clever enough to avoid appearing demanding (Ervin-Tripp & Gordon, 1986). As the child applies these rules to her use of indirect requests, she begins to shape the manipulative behaviors that bring joy and delight to the lives of all who know and love her through her school years. Even at the tender age of eight years, the child understands the importance of being more polite to adults than to her peers and to people whose favor she is trying to win than to people whose favor she already possesses (Corsaro, 1979; Parsons, 1980). After the age of eight years, the child's indirect requests are more likely to be influenced by her sensitivity to her listener's situation (Ervin-Tripp & Gordon, 1986). She will no longer assume that a request will be filled but will ask in a manner that suggests the listener has a right to exercise a real option. Whereas a younger child might say, "Take me home," or "Can you take me home?" the older child might say, "If it's not too much trouble or too far out of your way, could you take me home?" The older child will also recognize that the need to be polite in making requests increases when she is interrupting her listener or when she is asking the listener to do something that is difficult or inconvenient (Mitchell-Kernan & Keman, 1977). There is a difference, you see, between "Would you mind opening that door for me?" and "Excuse me, I know you're busy, but when you finish painting your house, you wouldn't mind painting mine . . . would you . . . perchance?"

Presuppositional Skills: Considering the Listener's Perspective

As we noted in Chapter 5, the preschool child may appear to be deficient in presuppositional skills when the real problem is a lack of knowledge about the conversational topic. It is difficult for any speaker to provide information to his listener if his own understanding is lacking. The school-age child not only is continuing to improve his language abilities but also is learning more about the things, people, places, and events in his world. The combination of general knowledge, improved cognitive abilities, and greater language competence leads directly to improved presuppositional skills.

Whereas the four-year-old child has difficulty describing blocks of unfamiliar geometric shapes to another four-year-old child when they are separated by a screen (Krauss & Glucksberg, 1977), the school-age child is much more successful in the same task. The school-age child has learned the names for geometric shapes, and he has acquired other words that he can use to describe shapes he does not know. His knowledge of shapes and his increased vocabulary allow him to provide more specific and helpful information to his conversational partner. The school-age child understands the importance of organizing and sequencing information for his conversational partner as evidenced by his ability to explain how a game is played.

He first describes the purpose of the game and clarifies what is required to win. He then delineates the rules and explains the mechanics of playing the game, step by step. The preschool child is unable to structure his explanations in a manner that facilitates his listener's understanding, and he does not grasp the importance of moving from general to more specific information.

Conjuncts and Disjuncts: Applying Reasoning to Language

As children get older, they begin to apply what they are beginning to understand about logic and reasoning directly to their language constructions in the form of what are called *adverbial conjuncts* and *adverbial disjuncts.* To appreciate these language forms, however, we need to understand the forms of logic they express.

Most people who have studied logic even superficially associate basic forms of logic, called *syllogisms,* with Aristotle, the ancient Greek philosopher (384–322 B.C.E.). It is beyond the scope of this book to provide a detailed analysis of all these forms, but a brief examination of what might be considered basic syllogisms will help the reader appreciate how logic and reason are subsumed within the language constructions children are learning as they move through their elementary and high school years and beyond. According to Freeley (1993), there are three major types of syllogisms: *conditional, categorical,* and *disjunctive.* Sternberg (1979) addresses a fourth that is relevant to our discussion: *conjunctive.*

We are all familiar with the *conditional* syllogism even if we do not use its name. This is the basic *if–then* form of logic we all use every day:

If you tickle Peyton's belly, he'll laugh.

Nina tickled Peyton's belly.

He laughed.

In a *categorical* syllogism, we establish what is called a *major premise,* which is a general statement of what we believe is a fact or truth, and we offer a *minor premise,* which is an example of something that presumably fits the major premise.

All mammals are warm-blooded animals.

A bear is a warm-blooded animal.

A bear, therefore, is a mammal.

In a *disjunctive* syllogism, there is a general statement that includes options followed by a statement that refers to one of the options. Following this statement is a conclusion based on logic and reason.

We can either drive my car or we can walk to the restaurant.

The restaurant is an easy walk from here, perhaps three or four blocks.

Because it's so close, and because it's such a beautiful day, let's walk.

Finally, in what might be understood as a fairly arbitrary kind of argument, a *conjunctive* syllogism, a statement is made about two conditions that co-exist even if the reasons for the two conditions are not obvious. This kind of statement is often subsumed within the rules of a game. Consider this football example:

> In football, some players on offense are permitted to go down field on pass plays, and other players must stay within a few yards of the line of scrimmage.
>
> Only running backs, receivers, and the quarterback may go downfield on pass plays.
>
> Therefore, linemen must stay within a few yards of the line of scrimmage on pass plays.

As the child is learning the nuances of conversation, she learns to use language forms that express the types of logical conclusions that are subsumed in these examples. In the process of linking her utterances together, she also learns to use words designed to make her attitude about what she is saying clear to the listener. Speakers use *adverbial disjuncts,* for example, to provide a kind of buffer between their attitudes about what they are saying and the actual content of their messages. When a person says, "To be quite honest with you, you're making a mistake," he is disjoining his attitude of honesty from the surface message of his utterance. It's not a divorce of intentions. It is more a separation of attitude and message that might be intended to soften the message or perhaps to focus attention on the speaker's purpose, apart from or in addition to the communication.

An *adverbial conjunct* is a device that connects, but it can be either concordant or dissonant. If a person says, "He ran around with the wrong crowd. Consequently, he has been in constant trouble with the law," there is concordance, or harmony, between the two statements. The word *consequently* is an example of a concordant adverbial conjunct. If someone says, "Catherine has always studied hard and earned good grades. Jane, in contrast, spends almost no time studying and she is just scraping by," there is dissonance between the two statements, as reflected in the words *in contrast.*

Conjuncts do not develop quickly. They emerge in the child's conversational applications gradually over the course of the school years and into adulthood. As with every other aspect of communication, the ability to understand conjuncts outpaces their actual use (Nippold, Schwarz, & Undlin, 1992). By the time the child is six years old, he is using some adverbial conjuncts, including *now, though, so,* and *then,* but he uses very few disjuncts. By the time he is twelve years old, he has expanded his repertoire of conjuncts to includes words such as *however, therefore,* and *anyway,* and he is using the disjuncts *probably* and *really.* The gap between children and adults in their use of these devices is substantial. Scott (1988b) found that adults use conjuncts at three times the rate used by twelve-year-olds.

The Evolution of Narratives

You may recall the Child Talk Model (Chapman et al., 1992) from Chapter 2, the theory of language development that emphasizes the importance of *context* and *world knowledge* in the acquisition process. In the early stages of language development, there is an immediacy aspect to every part of the child's communicative experiences. She talks about things and people in her immediate environment. She talks about events that are happening right now, in the immediate present. As a communicator, she is powerfully influenced by this context and by what she knows about people, things, events, and concepts—knowledge shared by the caregivers who shape and control the context in which all her language experiences are occurring.

As the child grows older, her communication experiences change dramatically because her life changes dramatically. She finds herself removed more frequently from the carefully fenced environment her caregivers have provided. She interacts more often with people, old and young, who do not share her world knowledge, at least not all of her world knowledge. The context that nurtured her communication development is no longer intact because the fence has been breached. When the child goes to preschool and then to school, she must learn how to talk about herself and about her life experiences to people who do not know her, people who were not part of the context of her development. As she progresses through the school years, she will be called on to talk about people and events far removed from her own time and place. She might talk about flights into space, for example, or about the role George Washington played in the founding of the United States of America, or she might talk about what the world will be like one hundred years from now. In each of these cases, the child will use what some writers now refer to as *decontextualized language*. This term refers to language a person uses when talking about things, people, events, and concepts that are not included in her immediate and personal context (Snow, 1991; Snow & Dickinson, 1991).

We have been tracing the development of one form of decontextualized language—narratives. The process of *decontextualizing* is clearly reflected in the changes that occur in a child's narratives over time. His first narratives are quite contextualized, very much limited to the here and now and populated by the people he knows best. Over time, he will drift farther and farther away from that context in his real life and in his narratives.

As the reader will recall from the preceding chapter, the child began to develop narrative abilities during his preschool years. In the beginning, the child's narratives were not true stories, but they had "storylike" qualities. More important, his first narrative attempts laid a solid foundation for the narrative discourse skills he will develop during his school years. To appreciate what happens relative to narrative discourse development during the school years, we should briefly review the child's narrative attempts between the ages of two and five years.

At the age of two years, the child's narrative-like productions were sets of brief unrelated statements called *heaps*. There was no discernible organization in these primitive narratives. They were, in the most elemental sense, stories about things the child found frightening, upsetting, or shocking in his own life (Ames, 1966). Style was more important than substance (Sutton-Smith, 1986) in these early narrative attempts, and the child relied more on prosody than on information to make his stories work (Scollon & Scollon, 1981).

Between the ages of three and five years, the child began to take the temporal factor into account, so that his narratives had beginnings, middles, and endings, but his stories lacked identifiable plots, and he did not develop cause–effect relationships. Even though the child at the age of three years understood cause–effect and expressed this understanding in his language, he was not able to incorporate causal sequences in his narratives (Kemper & Edwards, 1986).

Obviously, there is a considerable gap between the primitive narratives produced by the preschool child and the kinds of narratives produced by older children and adults. A primitive narrative lacks the elements we typically associate with a story. There is no plot. There is little or no organization. There are no characters, and there is certainly no character development. The story is not pushed from one event to another by causality, by what one person does or says to another or by how one act prompts another act. During the school years, we see all of these story elements emerge in the child's narratives. The single factor that is essential to making more mature narratives possible is *organization*, and that is where we pick up our story about storytelling.

Researchers have studied common stories to discover how they are organized. According to Stein and Glenn (1979), a story consists of a setting and one or more episodes. The **setting** provides information about the main character, and about the time and place in which the story occurs. Each **episode** contains the following elements: (1) an initiating event that causes the main character to do something, (2) an internal response in the form of thoughts or feelings the character has about the initiating event, (3) the main character's plan of action, (4) the main character's attempt to carry out the plan, (5) the consequence of the main character's implemented plan, and (6) the main character's reaction to the end result. You will recognize many of these elements in the stories adults tell about the events in their own lives. Mature speakers understand the importance of the information contained in these elements, and they understand the necessity of framing this information into appropriate narrative structure. When you listen to a narrative and complain about not being able to follow the story, you are almost certainly responding to an organizational problem or to the fact that important information has not been included. At the very least, we must know why the main character is motivated to do what she is going to do. We must know what she is going to do, and we must know the consequences of her actions (Stein, 1979).

By the time the child is seven years old, his stories have plots, even if they are not fully developed plots. A problem, the plan of action for resolving the problem, and the results of the actions implemented are included. There is still not much focus on motives and feelings, and there is not much detail, but the essential elements of the narrative are present. As is true of the adult, the child prefers narratives in which there is a clearly established goal (Stein & Policastro, 1984). That is, a story about a child who struggles to make the baseball team and ends up hitting the winning home run in the championship game is more intriguing to a child than a story titled "A Day in the Life of a Bookkeeper."

After the child passes his eighth birthday, he begins to create narratives with more clearly defined plots (Peterson & McCabe, 1983; Sutton-Smith, 1986). As the child moves through the remainder of the elementary school years and into junior and senior high school, his narratives mature in a number of important ways (Johnston, 1982). Problems are more clearly identified and more neatly resolved. He includes important detail but eliminates superfluous information. He is more careful about establishing the time and place settings of his narratives. He introduces his characters with greater care. He attends to the feelings, thoughts, and motives of his characters, and he includes the organizational elements required of complete narratives.

According to Stein (1982), there are four basic types of narrative discourse: recounts, eventcasts, accounts, and fictionalized stories of people or other animate beings who are trying to reach a goal. In a **recount,** the speaker talks about a past personal experience or about an event she has seen or read about. Recounts are common in the homes of middle- and upper-middle socioeconomic children whose parents often ask the question, "What did you do in school today?" or "Tell us about your trip to the zoo," and they are common in school. The age-old assignment "What I Did during My Summer Vacation" calls for a recount narrative. An **eventcast** is a narrative that describes a future event or something happening now. The child learns to use an eventcast to manipulate the behavior of other people with whom he is interacting. To get his way about what will happen tomorrow, for example, he might say, "Tomorrow, we'll all go to Manuel's house after school. He has a big yard, so we can play football, and then Manuel's mom can give us some milk and cookies like she always does." An **account** is a narrative in which a child spontaneously shares her experiences, usually beginning with "You know what?" The crucial difference between an account and a recount is that an account is initiated by the child, and a recount is initiated by a request from someone else, usually an adult. As you might expect, most children prefer accounts to recounts! A story is the kind of narrative we have been describing. Although it might be reality based, Stein views a story as a **fictionalized narrative** that follows the story form we have already outlined. By the time the child begins school, he is usually well acquainted with all four types of narrative discourse.

Although narratives tend to have the same components, compelling evidence indicates that how children and adults relate personal narratives is dependent on the cultures in which they live (McCabe, 1996). For example, the narratives of Hispanic children center far more on interpersonal relationships, especially family relationships, than on the events of their stories (Rodino, Gimbert, Perez, & McCabe, 1991). Japanese children construct their narratives in a manner reminiscent of haiku, a popular literary form in their culture (Minami & McCabe, 1990). A haiku is a very disciplined literary form based on the principles of minimalism and immediacy. It is the principle of immediacy that is particularly noticeable in the narratives of Japanese children. They connect events by theme rather than present them in temporal order so that the aggregate of events is presented at once.

How narratives are constructed is also affected by more narrowly defined cultures. White middle-class American children, for example, tend to generate narratives that are *topic based.* Their narratives center on single characters or on single events that have clearly defined chronologies. African American girls from working-class families generate very different narratives. Their stories are *topic associating* (Michaels, 1991), which means that they connect two, three, or more different events that share a common theme. Each episode in the narrative might have different characters, and the stories might occur in different places and times.

The contrast presented here between the narrative styles of white American children of both sexes and African American girls should give us pause about what might happen in school. If a classroom teacher is white and knows only the narrative style of white children, she might not respond appropriately to the narratives generated by the African American children in her classroom. She might, as Michaels found (1991), place greater value on the style used by her white students than on the style used by her African American students. From the white teacher's perspective, the topic-associating style might be viewed as *scattered* or *not sufficiently focused* or *undisciplined*. It is, of course, none of these. The topic-associating style used by African American girls is the strategy these children use to make sense of their life experiences, just as the topic-based style is the strategy white children use to make sense of their life experiences. Neither is inferior to the other. Each is *right* within the cultural experiences of the children who use it.

Shifts in Style and Vocabulary: The Emergence of Gender Differences

Are there differences between men and women in terms of how they talk? There are. Are these differences genetically or environmentally determined? Although we do not know for sure, it seems likely that most, if not all, the communicative differences between men and women are the products of environment. That is, boys are probably socialized to talk like men, and girls are socialized to talk like women. As other gaps between the genders close, we may discover that the differences noted in this section will no longer exist. The reality today, however, is that there are differences in the way males and females communicate, resulting in what some experts call *genderlects*. These genderlects include vocabulary differences and striking conversational style differences.

Men and women do not include different words in their vocabularies so much as they use different words with greater frequency (Thorne, Kramerae, & Henely, 1983). Men are more likely than women, for example, to use coarse or crude language and to use profanity in their conversations, whereas women are more likely than men to use polite words such as *please, thank you,* and *you're welcome* (Greif & Berko-Gleason, 1980). Women use words such as *lovely, darling,* and *adorable* more often than men. Whereas a man might call all shades of a color *red,* a woman is more likely to name shades of red. When a woman breaks a plate, she is likely to use an expression such as *"Oh, my goodness!"* or *"Dear me!"* whereas a man is more likely to say, *"#*##@*+=#%!!"* Part of the perception that the female is the gentler sex is probably based on the fact that women use gentler language.

One of the oldest stereotypes about women is that they talk more than men. Wrong! Although there are wide individual variations, of course, men tend to talk

Gender differences in interests and in language emerge early.

more than women (Swacher, 1975). The conversations between men and other men are longer than women's conversations with men or with other women. Women are also more courteous in conversation than men. Men interrupt more often than women, and men are more likely to interrupt women than to interrupt other men (Parlee, 1979). It is interesting, and probably socially revealing, that both sexes are more likely to interrupt a woman than a man (Willis & Williams, 1976). Women are more likely than men to surrender their conversational turns. Women introduce more new topics into conversation than men, but only about a third of the topics introduced by women are sustained in conversation, and nearly all topics introduced by men are sustained (Ehrenreich, 1981).

One of the common stereotypes about men and women in conversation is usually true. Whereas women tend to talk openly about their relationships and feelings, men avoid these topics and prefer to talk about impersonal subjects such as cars, politics, work, and sports.

When do children first become aware of gender differences in language, and when do listeners first notice these differences in the speech of children? By the time children are in the first grade, they are able to determine the gender of a speaker based on the vocabulary used in emotional expressions (Edelsky, 1977). At this same age, the early elementary school years, the language children use begins to reflect the same gender differences we have noted in the language of adult men and women (Craig & Evans,

1991; Haas, 1979). Even before adultlike gender differences are noted, boys and girls talk about different things. Boys as young as four years old talk about sports (Haas). Kindergarten girls talk about subjects related to traditional female roles (Sause, 1976).

Although we do not know the full importance of these findings, research has demonstrated that parents talk differently to their sons and daughters. Both parents, but particularly fathers, influence the development of genderlects in their children (Perlmann & Berko-Gleason, 1994). Mothers imitate their preschool daughters more often than their sons, and they spend more time talking to their daughters (Cherry & Lewis, 1976). Fathers attach nicknames such as *nutcake* and *ding-a-ling* to their sons, but they call their daughters *sweetheart* and *honey* (Berko-Gleason & Greif, 1983). Consistent with gender differences noted among adults, fathers interrupt their daughters more often than their sons (Warren-Leubecker, 1982).

As children grow older, they are less influenced by their caregivers and more influenced by their peers. This shift of influence is apparent in the way children interact with one another and talk to one another. During the school years, children tend to segregate themselves by sex, so that same-sex influences are more profound than influences across sex lines. Not surprisingly, we see the same sex-based differences in children that we see in adults. During the school years, girls seek relationships, whereas boys try to establish authority and independence (Gilligan, 1982; Maltz & Borker, 1982). When school-age girls interact with their same-sex friends, conversation is a focal point, and they are much more likely than boys at this age to talk about their feelings (Aukett, Ritchie, & Mill, 1988; Barth & Kinder, 1988). School-age boys, like men, are more likely than girls to use coarse language, including profanity (Jay, 1992; Martin, 1997).

Gender differences in language are fascinating, not so much because of what they tell us about language as because of what they tell us about the differences between the sexes. We shall return to this topic in Chapter 8, which includes an examination of a wide range of environmentally determined language differences.

The Classroom and Language: New Demands

The child learns most of his language in the comfort of his own home, in interaction with the most caring people in his world. The child acquiring language at home has the advantage of knowing the routine of his family life and knowing the nuances of the nonverbal communicative assists provided by his caregivers. If he does not understand all that is said to him, he can fill in the missing information by taking all the familiar nonverbal context into account. Most of his conversations at home are one on one, so if there is a breakdown and a repair is needed, his partner will usually recognize the need immediately. If not, he is comfortable enough with his partner to ask for help. Home is a safe and comfortable place for learning and using language, but what happens when the child begins school?

The child soon discovers that the language environment at school differs radically from the language environment at home. To a large extent, the difference reflects the overall purpose served by school. To the casual eye, the classroom for the child just beginning school is a fairly benign place where children color, play, sing songs, learn the alphabet, and learn to count, but those are only the byproducts of a much more serious purpose served by our schools. Wilhelm (1994) suggests that schools are the dominant force in the socialization of children, that it is in the schools that students and teachers engage in a kind of "social negotiation," systematically sharing an understanding about the attitudes, values, and knowledge that underlie the major institutions of their society. That's pretty weighty stuff for five- and six-year-old children, but it is an accurate portrayal of what we expect from schools in the new century. Many people talk about getting schools back to the basics of reading, writing, and arithmetic, but that kind of nostalgic view of *school* does not fit the reality of our present world. Teachers should not be expected to be surrogate parents, but that expectation exists. Teachers should not be solely responsible for imparting lessons about morality and ethics, but that expectation exists as well. The language of the classroom is very different from the language of home because it must be.

The Language Forms of the Classroom

According to Cazden (1988), the child entering school encounters three new forms of language. Each serves a different purpose. Each is important. Each must be learned if the child is to succeed in school. They are (1) the language of academic subjects or curriculum, (2) the language of behavior management, and (3) the language by which personal identity is expressed. That these three forms of language are used in the classroom is not a problem. The problem is that they are not clearly identified for children. Their purposes are typically not explained. Their rules are usually not delineated or discussed. All three language forms are used during the first day of school and during every day over the next thirteen years, but in most American classrooms the child is expected to figure them out for himself. It is not surprising that all children are occasionally unsure about how to make these language forms work together in the learning process. It is even less surprising that children who enter school with language skills that fall below age level, who have perceptual deficits, whose intellectual capacities are at the low end of *normal* or lower, who have sensory problems, who have learning disabilities, and who possess emotional problems become terribly frustrated and discouraged. It is not surprising that some of these children drown in the backwash of the tidal wave of confusion created by these often competing language forms, and they give up.

Most of us, if asked to describe the language of the school, would describe something akin to the first language form identified by Cazden (1988)—the language of **academic subjects or curriculum.** Some children have a head start on this language form because they have heard it at home. They will know words such as *book, arithmetic, map, alphabet,* and *sound* because these and comparable words have been used by their caregivers during their preschool years. They will know how to respond to academic questions, and they will know how to formulate these questions because these questions have been subsumed within their communication culture at home. Unfortunately, not all children will have had these experiences before entering school. Still others bring their pencils and crayons to school like all the other children, but they also bring hearing losses, learning disabilities, attention deficits, visual problems, and the like. Still others speak a dialect that does not match the teacher's dialect or that of the majority of children in the classroom. All of these children must work especially hard to learn the academic subjects language form, or they will quickly fall behind (Bashir & Scavuzzo, 1992).

We might find it amusing as adults to remember times when we were faced with the language of **behavior management** in school, but we might also remember the embarrassment and pain associated with learning the rules of this language form. The teacher traditionally uses this language form to establish who is allowed to talk, what one is allowed to say, and how one is allowed to say it. It is clearly a language of *control.* There is no question that this language form is necessary in the classroom, otherwise, chaos would be the order of the day and nothing would be learned by any-one. Consider, however, that many children are not exposed to this language form, or at least aspects of it, until they come to school. All children are exposed to basic ex-pressions in this language, such as these:

"Wait until it's your turn to talk."

"Be quiet and let your sister talk."

"You listen when I'm talking to you."

Other expressions may be less familiar to the child who is just beginning school:

"What you have said is interesting. Is there anything you want to add?"

"Your answer is mostly correct, but what seems to be missing?"

"What you have said is confusing. Could you explain it more clearly?"

Now consider the problems in interpreting these expressions that might be ex-perienced by the child who has reduced language skills or a learning disability or a perceptual or sensory deficit. Keep in mind that communicative exchanges in the classroom are often frenetic, allowing little time for processing and virtually no time for contemplation. Any child with any problem that slows processing will get lost in the exchange, move to the sidelines, and fall further behind academically. If the child cannot master the rules of the language of behavior management, her un-derstanding of the language of subject matter may be irrelevant because she is not an active participant in the verbal processes by which information is imparted, dis-cussed, and analyzed.

The third language form employed in the classroom is used to **express personal identity.** This form might seem to be a minor player in the educational process until you remember how important it was to you when you were in kindergarten or first grade to find just the right item for show-and-tell, or how it made you feel when you were able to share something about your life with a teacher you adored. Cazden (1988) points out that it is only during these sharing experiences that the child can decide for himself what he wants to say and how he will say it. It may be his only opportunity to talk about himself and to hold the communicative stage for several uninterrupted min-utes. We often note that it is during the school years that the child is becoming his own person, establishing his own identity. Part of the process of becoming one's own per-son is learning to use the language necessary for telling others who one is. Children viewed as assertive, self-confident, or self-assured are children who are adept in using this language form. Sadly, notes Michaels (1990), the children who need the most practice in using personal identity language are often denied their opportunities because teachers become impatient when they listen to the personal stories of students who struggle with language because of their disabilities or because they speak a dialect other than the teacher's dialect. If this kind of student does not feel valued when trying to use this language form, he is likely to withdraw from all communicative experiences in the classroom and, as a consequence, fall even further behind his peers academically.

Cultural Diversity in the Classroom

One of the classroom issues to which we must be especially sensitive in this new century is cultural diversity, an issue we will address in more detail in Chapter 8. It is relevant enough in this context, however, to warrant attention. With the dramatic demographic shifts occurring in the United States, no one will be surprised that the language a child uses at home may be quite different from the language she is expected to use in school.

That difference alone is not a problem. In fact, some would argue that from a strictly linguistic perspective, the child is enriched by immersion in two or more languages. The problem is that the language used in the home is often not respected at school (Mehan, 1984). Unfortunately, many children whose cultural experiences, including language, differ from the cultural experiences of the white majority who speak some version of Standard American English are placed in special education classrooms. All dedicated educators would agree that public schools are charged with the responsibility of teaching all children, no matter their cultural backgrounds, no matter their native languages. Unfortunately, the textbooks we use and the courses future teachers take do not adequately address the issue of how we should use the language of instruction (Reid, 1998) and how we should take cultural and language differences into account in making the language of instruction viable for all children.

A Homogeneous Perspective

A common problem in our classrooms is that there is an intended, or perhaps unintended, push toward homogeneity of experience and knowledge. It is understandable that a teacher tends to teach from his own experience. One of the most valuable lessons we have learned about teaching is that a teacher teaches more about who he is than about what he knows. Ideally, of course, a teacher will convey a great deal of what he knows, but if his teaching is a dry, uninspired, depersonalized transmission of tidbits of information, the information will not be retained for long because it does not have the barbed hook of personal expression that makes knowledge *sticky*. Wertsch (1991) notes that during formal instruction, the teaching–learning process tends to exclude the personal experiences of students, even when those personal experiences are germane to the topic. Instead, teachers tend to emphasize the shared knowledge contained in the lesson plan or in the textbook. Teachers recognize the necessity of using decontextualized language in formal instruction, but they often discourage students when they try to communicate from a personal perspective.

If it is true that a teacher teaches best when he teaches who he is as well as what he knows, one could argue that a student will learn best when she learns within the context of her own personal experiences, expanded to include the shared experiences of her classmates and her teacher. Enforced homogeneity may be a correct strategy in some circumstances. It is clearly not a correct strategy in classrooms filled by an increasingly diverse population of students.

Teacher–Student Dialogues: Basic Variations

If you were asked to describe the basic format of instruction in a typical elementary or junior high school classroom, we suspect you would describe what Mehan (1979) calls the **IRE model.** In this version of teacher–student dialogue, the teacher *initiates* (I) a question. The student provides a *response* (R), which the teacher *evaluates* (E). The teacher then asks another question, and the sequence continues until the lesson is completed. Heath (1982) notes that the kind of question most often asked in this model is the *known-information* question, a self-explanatory term. The students have been asked to read specific material. They have been instructed to memorize specific information. The teacher uses the IRE model to determine whether the material has been read, memorized, and understood. Obviously, the IRE model is teacher directed. Student–student interactions are usually not encouraged in this format.

Sometimes, of course, instruction occurs in the context of classroom discussions during which students talk to one another as well as to the teacher. This format is known as **revoicing.** In this format, the teacher might present a problem and ask the class to consider possible solutions. One student offers a solution, which another student criticizes as inadequate. Another student suggests that the proposed solution might work if it is amended in specified ways. Yet another student supports the solution as amended but suggests an additional adjustment. The teacher intervenes when she detects that the process has become stagnant or when she notices a lapse of logic that has not been identified by the other students, but she can keep the responsibility for learning in the students' hands by offering questions that nudge the process forward rather than offering a discussion-ending solution of her own. The teacher listens to what the student says, acknowledges it, and asks a question that will prompt a response from the original speaker or from other students in the class. The teacher *revoices* the topic as necessary and clarifies as necessary, but she is not the unquestioned dispenser of information. She is a learning facilitator in this format.

When the teacher works with small groups of students, he might use an instructional format called **instructional conversation.** Except for attending more carefully to a designated topic, this format can be almost as informal as regular conversation. At the other end of the formality continuum, instructional conversation might be conducted within the confines of predetermined rules and procedures that keep the participants on topic and that require each participant, including the teacher, to fill the *teacher* role as well as the *student* role. This more formal version of instructional conversation serves the purpose of teaching students lessons about behavior management as well as meeting the learning goals established by the teacher.

Finally, in thinking about how classroom instruction is changing in the new century, please revisit the views of Piaget and Vygotsky on cognitive development in Chapter 3. It is rather interesting that the views of these men, both born at the end of the nineteenth century, are resurfacing in the *new* instructional strategies of the twenty-first century. Both men wrote about the importance of the dialogue between child and caregiver/teacher. They stressed the importance of interactive learning within social context, and they stressed the necessity of facilitating the child's independence in the learning process. All of these emphases are resurgent in the new frontier of teaching and learning in classrooms in the new millennium. It's not difficult to imagine Jean Piaget and Lev Vygotsky smiling down on us and saying, "We tried to tell you!"

Metalinguistic Development during the School Years

One of the most significant changes to occur in the child's use of language as he moves from the preschool to the school years is the rapid development of metalinguistic awareness. Before he begins school, the child uses language almost exclusively as a means of communication. Sometimes he talks for the sheer pleasure of hearing his own voice, and sometimes he just plays with sounds and words, but he mostly uses language to communicate. When he enters school, he learns to separate himself from language and to separate language from communication so that he can identify, analyze, study, and think about the elements of language.

Sometimes we have experiences in life that are so intense that we can almost see ourselves from a distance. We call these out-of-body experiences. During these experiences, we see ourselves more objectively and may understand our own behaviors more clearly. In much the same way, the child does not really know what she knows about language until she is able to examine and study language objectively, from a distance. The term **metalinguistic ability** refers to the capacity to use language to analyze, study, and understand language. Metalinguistic ability, or awareness, is the out-of-body experience of language.

The most noticeable and dramatic increase in metalinguistic awareness occurs between the ages of five and eight years (Bernstein, 1989, p. 145). Beginning at this time, but continuing even into adulthood, the child notices and develops an understanding of each of the basic components of language, including phonology, semantics, syntax, and pragmatics. Not surprisingly, the development of metalinguistic awareness is related to cognitive development, intellectual capacity, scholastic achievement, reading skills, and environmental factors, including the child's play experiences and the kind of stimulation he receives from adults (Saywitz & Cherry-Wilkinson, 1982).

The typical adult may not have a sophisticated understanding of the components of language, but every adult has an awareness of each component and has at least a rudimentary understanding of the rules that govern the various dimensions of language. It is a speaker's metalinguistic ability that allows her to make judgments about whether or not a sentence sounds grammatical or about which marker for tense or plurality sounds correct. When a speaker produces language, she does so automatically with little or no conscious attention to the rules she is applying, but when she is asked to make a judgment about a language form, she must consciously attend to the form and apply her knowledge of the rules to determine whether the form is correct. The production of language is a linguistic function. The evaluation of language is a **metalinguistic** function.

Segmentation and Awareness of Speech Sounds

As common sense might suggest, the child can typically separate the words of a sentence before he can separate the syllables and sounds of a word. The process of separating the constituent parts of sentences or words is called *segmentation.* A preschool child can identify the individual words that make up a sentence such as "The spotted dog chased the frightened boy away." He will have considerably more trouble separating the word *spotted* into its syllables, and he will struggle with the individual sounds that make up the word *frightened.* If asked which is the longer word, *bicycle* or *car*, the preschool child is likely to say that *car* is the longer word because he visualizes the referents for these words and knows that cars are longer than bicycles. Awareness of speech sounds as individual entities within words does not typically occur until the early years of elementary school.

We can determine a person's awareness of phonology, or speech sound system, by asking her to count the number of sounds in a word or separate one or more sounds from the word. Some adults have difficulty with these tasks because they associate sounds with their corresponding alphabet symbols. Although our sound system and alphabet are related, there is not always a direct correspondence between what one sees and what one hears. We all know, for example, that some letters are silent. The pronunciation of *caught* does not include sounds for "*g*" or "*h.*" Sometimes sounds are present even when they are not directly represented by letters. The second sound in *quick*, for example is "*w*," and the last sound in *fox* is "*s.*" There are five letters in the word *watch*, but there are only three sounds. Can you identify them? If you cannot identify the sounds now, you should be able to do so after you read the next chapter in this book. Although the child will probably not correctly count the sounds in all words, she does show awareness of phonology by separating and counting speech sounds by the time she is six or seven years old.

It seems likely that the ability to segment words into syllables and sounds is related to learning to read, although we encounter the old "Which comes first, the chicken or the egg?" argument in trying to figure out the relationship. That is, the ability to segment words into their constituent syllable and sound parts probably facilitates reading, but learning to read probably facilitates the ability to segment as well. We do know that children who are accelerated in associating sounds with letters and letters with sounds are typically advanced, in comparison with their less metalinguistically aware peers, in their reading and writing skills (Westby, 1994).

Awareness of Semantics

We typically think of meaning in relation to words, but there is also meaning in sentences that goes beyond the additive meanings of the individual words in sentences. In considering the child's developing awareness of semantics, researchers have considered word meanings and sentence meanings. The child's awareness of word meanings can be evaluated by asking him to define words, to judge words as hard or easy, or as big or little. If the child is asked, for example, whether the word *whale* is big or little, he might say it is big because he is not able to separate the referent from the word. The child who is aware of semantics at the word level understands that the connections between words and the things they represent are arbitrary. Sometimes a little word represents a little thing (e.g., *ant*), but sometimes a big word represents a little thing (e.g., *microorganism*), and sometimes a little word represents a big thing (e.g., *ship*).

The fact that words are arbitrary labels might also mean that one word can have two or more very different meanings. The word *down*, for example, is most commonly understood to mean *in a lower position*, but the word *down* also refers to soft, fluffy feathers. Researchers have used riddles to determine whether children understand the multiple meanings of key words. Consider the following riddle: "Why did the man throw his clock out the window? Because he wanted to see time fly." To understand this riddle, the child must understand that the word *fly* has at least two possible meanings: (1) to move through the air, and (2) to pass quickly. By the time the child is six or seven years old, she is able to separate words from their referents as evidenced by her ability to understand multiple meanings of words and to recognize the arbitrary connection between words and the things they represent. Even though the child will understand many of these expressions during the elementary years, she will be in junior high school before she will be able to explain to someone else the reasons for their meaningfulness (Westby, 1994).

As one might suspect, practice makes a difference in developing definitional skills. Snow (1990) found that the ability of elementary school children to create correct formal definitions was associated with their experience with language, and specifically with their experience in using language to talk about what words mean. That is, definitional skills depend on the opportunity to practice definitions. In this case, practice does not necessarily make perfect, but practice does make better.

Researchers have evaluated awareness of sentence meaning by asking children to evaluate the acceptability of sentences based on their semantic appropriateness. A child who is aware of the rules governing sentence meaning will be able to judge whether a sentence makes sense. For example, he will recognize that the sentence "The dog ate the cookie" is meaningful, whereas the sentence "The paper ate the cookie" is not meaningful because a *dog* is an animal capable of eating, and *paper* is an inanimate object not capable of eating. The child can typically make judgments about the semantic appropriateness of sentences as early as five years, and he can often point out the problem. In the example cited, he might say, " 'The paper ate the cookie' is wrong because paper can't eat."

Awareness of Syntax

The child's metalinguistic awareness of syntax can be assessed by asking her to decide whether sentences are grammatically correct or incorrect. To ensure that the child is making a judgment about a sentence based on a grammatical error, we can ask her to correct the mistake. If she determines that a sentence is incorrect and is able to make the grammatical correction, we may assume she has developed syntactic awareness. By the time the child is six years old, she would be able to determine that the sentence "The dog chased the cat tree up the" is incorrect, and she would be able to produce the correction.

A somewhat more difficult judgment involves the identification of syntactic ambiguities in sentences. For example, "Visiting relatives can be a pain" can be interpreted in two ways: (1) going to visit relatives can be a pain, or (2) having relatives visit can be a pain. The child may be eleven or twelve years old before he has enough metalinguistic awareness to recognize this kind of ambiguity.

Awareness of Pragmatics

Less attention has been given to the development of pragmatic awareness than to other metalinguistic skills. We do know that by the time the child is five or six she is able to make judgments about whether enough information is contained in a message or not. That is, if the child listens to a set of instructions, she will know whether the instructions are adequate or whether more information is needed. At about this same age, the child will recognize glaring contradictions or inconsistencies. She will recognize, for example, that a character in a story cannot be the hero and the villain at the same time. She will understand that a man's saying, "When I was a little girl . . . ," does not make sense even if the sentence is correct according to all the rules of syntax. As early as three years, the child understands that the inclusion of the word *please* makes requests more polite; and by the time she is five years old, she understands that indirect requests are more polite than direct commands.

If there is a communicative failure that requires repair, the preschool child usually faults the listener for the failure, not the speaker. By the time he is eight years old, the child understands that the speaker is sometimes responsible for the failure (Robinson, 1981). In another interesting preschool to school-age comparison, the preschool child tends to answer strange, nonsensical questions without asking for additional information or clarification. For example, in a study by Hughes and Grieve (1980), children were asked questions such as "Is orange taller than purple?" and "Is dirt higher than sand?" The five-year-old children in the study answered these questions as though they were valid. The seven-year-old children indicated in their responses that they did not understand the speaker's communicative intent.

By the time the child reaches adolescence, her pragmatic skills are fairly well developed, at least as they are applied in the most common social experiences she is likely to face (Berko-Gleason, Hay, & Cain, 1988). As evidence of her pragmatic competence, the adolescent child will sometimes purposely violate the pragmatic skills we would categorize as common rules of courtesy. She might purposely snub someone, knowing that this is so inappropriate that it will be noticed and that it has the potential to offend. She might consciously avoid saying, "Thank you," or "You're welcome," as a way of sending a message of defiance or, if we wish to be gracious in our assessment of her intention, an expression of independence. Table 6.1 summarized metalinguistic awareness and abilities in school-age children.

Table 6.1 An Overview of Metalinguistic Awareness and Abilities in School-Age Children

Note: It is well established that the preschool child has some metalinguistic awareness, but her metalinguistic awareness and abilities are not complete until she is about seven or eight years old. Eve Clark (1978) addressed the evolution of metalinguistic abilities in children. The following summarizes her conclusions about the skills mastered during the school years.

- She differentiates basic units of language—i.e., sounds, syllables, words, and sentences.
- She attaches correct inflections to unfamiliar words.
- She recognizes when words are used incorrectly in sentences, and she knows when word order is incorrect.
- She understands how it is possible to construct varying sentence types, and she can convey her understanding to other people.
- She understands the possible meanings framed within these sentence types.
- She knows when utterances are acceptable, based upon who the listener is and/or the setting in which the communication is taking place.
- She knows how to define words in a manner that makes their meanings clear to others.
- She demonstrates an understanding of the language forms used in creating humorous constructions, such as puns and riddles.

Reading and Writing: New Applications of Language

Even though we do not need to immerse ourselves again in all the arguments about the contributions of nature and nurture to the development of language, it is important to emphasize one more time that language expressed through speech is common to all human beings. There is convincing evidence that human beings are born to speak. But are they genetically predisposed to read and write?

The answer to this question lies, to some extent, in two basic facts about human beings as communicators. Anthropologists have never discovered a group of people, no matter how primitive their lifestyle, without a highly developed spoken language. They have found, however, groups of people whose languages have no written forms. In addition, there are many people who speak languages that do have written forms but who are unable to read and write. It is reasonable to conclude, therefore, that a more powerful biological drive exists for humans to speak than to read and write. Although humans are innately endowed with the sensory, perceptual, and cognitive abilities to learn to read and write, environmental factors are more crucial in the emergence of these language capabilities than in the emergence of speech.

Extensive language research conducted over the past several decades has changed our views about how language is acquired, even if this research has not provided closure to all the questions we have posed about how the acquisition process occurs. At the same time that language people have tried to understand how language is acquired by human children, other researchers have tried to understand how reading and writing are learned. They have used their findings to suggest more effective strategies for facilitating literacy development in children, both in their homes and in their schools.

It is often helpful to examine old views in order to appreciate why new understandings emerge from current research findings. A brochure entitled *Current Research on Language Learning,* published by the National Council of Teachers of English (NCTE, 1993), includes summaries of previous and current thinking about the emergence of reading and writing. According to the previous view, the child must learn the smallest parts of language before he can learn to read and write whole texts, a view commonly referred to as "part-to-whole." The teaching/learning strategy that emerged from the "part-to-whole" view involved a progression from teaching and learning the letters of the alphabet, the sounds letters make, simple words, and then the production of short sentences. This strategy invested considerable time in teaching skills that were considered prerequisite to reading and writing. In truth, many children did learn to read and write using the part-to-whole approach, but many other children struggled and failed. The National Council of Teachers of English suggests, in fact, that "such instruction made it difficult for most children to understand the joy and benefit of reading and writing—to make them lifetime readers and writers."

The current view is that learning to read and write is quite similar to learning to talk. Consider, for example, that when caregivers talk to their babies, they are not trying to *teach* them to use spoken language. They certainly do not produce isolated speech sounds in order to teach the phonology of the language. They do not speak single-word utterances in order to teach a vocabulary. They talk to their babies, sometimes in fun sentences and sometimes in babbled productions, in order to make *communicative* contact with them, even if it is a communication that is limited and simplistic. Caregivers tend to accept the child's most primitive productions as languagelike behavior that should be appreciated and celebrated. Children learn to talk then, not by means of direct instruction from language experts, but through the process of hearing language, using language, and sharing language with the significant people in their lives. Current views about reading and writing suggest that children learn these processes in much the same way. That is, they observe the written word. They listen to people read. They read, and they write. In the process of observing and doing reading and writing, they learn to read and write.

Whereas oral language develops rapidly during the preschool years, the child's competence with written language develops much more slowly over a longer period of time. The foundations for reading and writing, however, are established during the child's earliest years. Research indicates that a number of variables contribute to the child's early literacy development, but the single most important factor, particularly in the development of reading, or the command of written language, is the child's home environment (Bernstein, 1989, p. 147). That is, the child who is exposed to the written word early will tend to develop competency in reading more easily than the child who is denied access to written language or print.

Even before babies can talk, they enjoy looking at books and having books or stories read to them. They are able to understand some of the content that is being read to them long before they can read, just as they are able to understand the meanings of some of the words they hear in speech months before they say their first words. Before children understand the content of stories, they enjoy the experience of having

Learning to enjoy books.

people read to them, being held closely, and hearing the soothing voices of loving adults (Fields & Spangler, 1989). The findings from the relevant research about children and their early experiences with the written word consistently lead us to the same conclusion: Reading to children is a successful way to teach them to read, and the influence of these early experiences is not limited to reading. Gordon Wells (1986), after a fifteen-year study of children in England, concluded that the academic success of these children was highly influenced by the frequency with which stories were read to them. Dolores Durkin's (1980) studies showed that the most common factor shared by children who read early is that they are read to frequently. The findings of other research indicate that children learn ways of constructing meaning for print as adults share and discuss stories with them (Altwerger, Diehl-Faxon, & Dockstader-Anderson, 1985; Fisher, 1991; Mason, 1989; Teale, 1988).

Parents and other caregivers can facilitate literacy development by reading stories to their children while encouraging them to follow the pictures, the sense of the story, and the words. As children listen to stories being read, and especially as they actively participate in the experience, they gain control over the language of books. In a very real and meaningful sense, they seem to be able to absorb this language (Doake, 1995). The adult reader can encourage the child to participate in the reading experience by using an invitational and conversational reading style. For example, if the reader pauses at certain highly predictable junctures in a story, the child will likely participate by filling in the gaps. The child might predict the word that is actually written, or he might use a word that closely approximates the target word, but accuracy is not the point. Participation is. Using whatever language the

child has at this point in his communicative development, he gradually repro-
duces, with increasing accuracy, the meaning of the story for himself. At this point,
adults often conclude that the child has memorized the words. While this is undoubtedly true, this is not a minor accomplishment because memorization is part
of the process of constructing the meaning of the story. The emerging *reader* is
demonstrating "readinglike" behavior, an important step in the process of reading
development (Doake, 1995).

As children gain experience with their books and the written language of their
environments, they become increasingly aware that the print on the page actually carries the story. They also begin to connect what they are saying with what they are seeing. At this point, they are beginning to show a metalinguistic awareness of
letter–sound relationships. They are independently discovering and demonstrating
the role of phonics in a contextual, natural setting. Given the language competencies
of preschool children, this can no longer be viewed as simply a preparatory period for
the learning of reading and writing. What is happening at this time in development
goes beyond mere preparation. In their wide-ranging studies of the literacy development of young children, Harste, Woodward, and Burke (1984) found no evidence to
suggest that "children's psycholinguistic and sociolinguistic strategies are qualita-
tively different from the kinds of decisions which more experienced language users
make." They concluded that "the process children engage in is not a pseudo form of
the 'real' process; it is that process" (p. 105).

As young children become increasingly engaged in the reading/language
process, they begin to develop a genuine desire to read. Although reading stories to
children will help facilitate language development, the inherent value of reading goes
beyond language development. To realize this value, children must want to read. Unless they want to read, they will not read enough to become proficient readers, and
unless they become proficient readers, they will not derive the full value of the experience. As melodramatic as it may sound, when parents and other caregivers read stories to young children, they are introducing them to the magic of books. They are
initiating the process that will, if all goes well, awaken in their children the desire to
read. The sharing of high-quality literature with youngsters provides a glimpse of the
excitement, the drama, and the beauty that is contained in books. When adults share
enthusiasm with children for a good story, they provide a model for how to interact
with text. Making the printed page come to life during an animated reading of a story
demonstrates not just the *process* of reading but the *power* of reading as well. As children reenact stories that have been read to them, and as they discuss these stories
with adults, they gradually, and without pressure, construct understandings they
need to become readers (Fields & Spangler, 1995).

The younger children are when they are introduced to the written word, the better their reading competencies will be. As adult literacy programs attest, it is never
too late for a person to learn to read, but at a time when the written word is so pervasive and powerful in the world, the darkness of illiteracy is terribly restrictive and unnecessary. Children who have been immersed in the written word during their early
years at home begin school with significant advantages over children who have had
limited experiences with books. Some of these advantages might vanish when envi-

ronmentally deprived children are given the encouragement and support to use their academic opportunities, but there is little doubt that early experiences with the written word are important for the development of both reading and writing.

From the most traditional perspective, parents send children to school to learn the three *Rs: reading, writing,* and *arithmetic.* (Hmm, perhaps we should have placed a stronger emphasis on spelling.) In any case, parents expect that their sons and daughters will learn how to read and write when they go to school. It is with some alarm then that we note the increasing number of children who are sent to resource rooms for help with reading, and the small percentage of students who are able to read critically by their senior year in high school (Applebee, Langer, & Mullis, 1988). These trends, coupled with the staggering number of illiterate adults in the United States, should cause American educators who are directly concerned with reading and writing to consider whether teaching paradigms for these critical skills are consistent with the natural language/learning strategies used by children (Weaver, 1994).

Prior to the 1970s, most experts in the field of reading viewed reading as a visual-perceptual phenomenon. Reading instruction focused on words and on pronouncing words correctly. Children who were not successful with this exact word-bound model were often considered candidates for special help or for services outside the regular classroom. Children who needed more support with reading were enrolled in programs that focused on correct word pronunciation. In the 1970s and 1980s, reading experts began to explore the relationship between language and reading. Goodman (1986) makes the argument that because speech and writing are both expressions of language, there is no reason to assume that the learning of writing differs fundamentally from the learning of speaking. This point of view led to an understanding that to help children who need special support in learning how to read, teachers must know more about language acquisition and about the functions of language in the early development of young children. According to this view, reading is a language-based activity. This view gave rise to assumptions underlying the two dominant reading instruction approaches currently used in American public schools.

Expressed most simply, one view suggests that reading is *taught.* The other view suggests that reading *develops* as part of the child's natural language development. Those who hold the first view teach reading skills in a direct and systematic manner. Teachers who believe that reading develops within the larger context of language development try to facilitate reading and writing in a manner that is as natural as possible. Some of the differences between these two points of view are reflected in their terminologies. Other differences are reflected in how terms they share in common are used. These differences will be noted in the two models of reading that support these divergent viewpoints: (1) the *transmission model* that supports the view that reading is taught and (2) the *transactional model* that supports the view that literacy develops (Weaver, 1994).

Theoretical Models of Reading

To appreciate how each model explains how reading develops, one must first understand the more global view of each model as it relates to education in general.

Underlying the *transmission model* of education are principles from behavioral psychology. Students are viewed as empty vessels into which knowledge is poured. A curriculum based on this model requires students to practice skills, memorize facts, and accumulate information, typically in a manner that isolates knowledge from the application of the skills learned and the information obtained. In this educational scheme, errors are to be avoided, and near perfection is expected. In principle, what is taught today will be practiced tomorrow, and will be tested for complete and accurate understanding the next day. The commission of errors is penalized to discourage the formation of inappropriate habits. When this model is applied, students often "fail" and are judged to be in need of remedial help (Weaver, 1994).

In the *transactional model,* students are viewed as people who bring significant language competence and a knowledge background to the process of education. The principles underlying this model are derived from what cognitive psychologists and psycholinguists have discovered about human learning, including the development of language. In applying this model, teachers encourage a constructivist view of learning by trying to create rich environmental contexts and situations in which students can learn. Students use their schemas to construct and advance their own knowledge. Taking risks, developing and refining hypotheses, and making errors are treated as essential components in the course of learning. Mastery of processes, such as speaking a language, reading, writing, and spelling, occurs over a period of years, and the learner will probably never reach a level of perfection in any of them (Weaver, 1994).

When applied specifically to reading, the *transmission model* suggests that reading must be taught in much the same way that arithmetic, geography, science, or any other subject is taught. A teacher who uses this model spends time preparing the child for reading, developing "reading readiness." The teacher invests considerable time teaching students to read and testing to determine whether, in fact, students have learned to read. Students invest a great deal of time in practicing reading skills, completing worksheets and laboring in workbooks to hone their skills. There is a strong emphasis on producing words exactly as they are presented in print. Variations, even if they are semantically comparable to the target words, are not accepted and are discouraged. Reading is a separate subject in the curriculum and is even isolated from writing, its close academic cousin. The transmission model explains the development of reading in terms of stages through which all children move at presumably a comparable pace, and the term *development* is used in reference to the stage concept (Weaver, 1994).

The *transactional model* of literacy development presents a very different view of how children learn to read and how teachers can facilitate the development of reading. In this model, there is no dichotomy between readiness to read and learning to read. Literacy development, which includes reading and writing, is viewed as an uninterrupted process. Development is seamless, not divisible into discrete stages. The teacher and students invest their time not in drill work but in actual reading and writing. They talk about what they have read. Students read and write for pragmatic reasons and for the sheer joy of doing so. The competency emphasis is not on articulating exact pronunciations of the words in print but on understanding what words, phrases, sentences, paragraphs, and stories mean. The teacher explains various reading and writing strategies in meaningful context, and she encourages her students to discuss these strategies in this same context. The emphases are always on meaning, pragmatics, and on individual development. In the transactional model, the term *development* is used in reference to the concept that reading and writing literacy emerges in a continuous manner over a period of time (Weaver, 1994).

Underlying the transactional model of reading is the belief that language development and the emergence of literacy cannot be separated. They are interactive partners in the development of communication. Language knowledge certainly prepares children for the development of literacy, and literacy provides children valuable tools in their attempts to understand the language they use, the process we have identified as metalinguistic awareness.

Children's Reading Development

Our discussion of literacy development, including both reading and writing, is based on the transactional model. Keep in mind that within the context of this model, development is not viewed in stages but as a continuous, seamless process. We will identify categories of development, but these categories should not be understood as periods of mastery in which one category is completed before the next category begins. The reader will note instead that there is a great deal of overlapping as we move from category to category, and the emphasis is always on continuous development. Three broad categories will be identified and described in the following paragraphs: (1) *emergent*, (2) *developing*, and (3) *independent*.

Emergent readers are at the beginning of the reading adventure. They have learned that books contain stories, that they can visit these stories as often as they like, that the words will be the same each time they return, and that the pictures accompanying the stories help construct and more fully develop meaning. Emergent readers show progressively more interest in trying to read without assistance from others. They are able to discuss what is happening in a story, and they can predict what is likely to happen next. They are also beginning to recognize certain words in varying contexts. As important as all this is to the development of reading, we need to be very clear about the fact that children at this stage, which typically occurs between 30 and 48 months, are not reading. They are pretending to read (Kaderavek & Sulzby, 2000). We need to remember, however, that pretending is a very good thing in young children because it sets the stage for *representation*, which helps form the very foundation of language—spoken and written. Caregivers should encourage their emergent readers, not just because it is a step toward true reading, but because there is evidence that children whose caregivers actively promote exposure to reading, have greater phonological awareness than children who live in homes that are less reader-friendly (Foy & Mann, 2003).

It is important to choose books for emergent readers with their needs and competencies in mind. The books selected should provide opportunities for these children to enjoy literature even though they cannot yet read independently. The text and illustrations should be clear. The plots should be simple. The language should be repetitive, rhythmic, and natural. Ideally, the illustrations will precede the text that describes the illustrations to assist emergent readers in the process of predicting what the text might say and what is going to happen next in the story. Books suited for these children will possess an invitational tone that will encourage them to participate to the extent they can until they are able to read on their own. Within the context of the transactional model, it is most important that books for emergent readers be designed to guide children toward an understanding of what they are reading, rather than focusing on individual words. From the very beginning of literacy development, children should be made aware that the essence of reading, and indeed the essence of language in all its forms, is meaning (Department of Education, Wellington, 1985).

In the second category we find **developing readers.** These are children who are becoming true readers. At this point in literacy development, children have established the habit of reading for meaning, at least in the sense that they understand that meaning is the reading bottom line. Developing readers are encouraged to use their own life experiences as context for what they read. As they process printed text, they are encouraged to take interpretative risks, to make approximations about what words are or what words mean. Developing readers use the text, illustrations, and their own knowledge of print conventions to sample, to predict, and to confirm printed words. These children also use letter–sound associations, within context, to help confirm their predictions about words. They are encouraged to move beyond unfamiliar words to find lexical content they do recognize, content that may help them figure out what the unfamiliar words are. They are also encouraged to reread and self-correct when the process of interpreting meaning has been interrupted or when the printed words do not seem to make sense. You will recognize, of course, that these are strategies adult readers use when they have difficulty determining the meaning of printed words. What is important to understand is that these are strategies, according to the transactional model, that should be encouraged from the beginning of reading development.

In comparison to books chosen for emergent readers, books chosen for developing readers draw on a wider range of life experiences, and they expand readers' horizons to a significantly enlarged world, complete with more elaborate, mature understandings about how the world works. The vocabulary bases of these books match the rapidly growing vocabularies of the children reading them. They are designed, in fact, to increase readers' vocabularies and to introduce them to more complex and varied language structures. These books, in comparison to the books used by emergent readers, employ a wider variety of cues to help children sample, predict, and monitor what they are reading, and to construct and maintain meaning.

The third category includes **independent readers.** Independent readers read on their own, and they read when they are alone. These children are confident and competent readers who are integrating into the process of reading all the cueing systems available in language. They pay little conscious attention to the details of printed words because their focus is on constructing and maintaining meaning. For independent readers, the printed details are means, not ends. The ends are understanding, interpretation, and meaning. Independent readers are able to read increasingly longer and more structurally complex sentences with meaning. They are able to process a wide variety of prose and poetry. They are also learning to adjust reading rate to accommodate the purposes for which they are reading. One of the most obvious characteristics of independent readers is variety, not just in what they read but in the databases on which they draw to make sense of what they read. To a much greater extent than developing readers, independent readers use knowledge gained from their personal experiences in their homes, schools, and communities, as well as knowledge gleaned from previously read books, movies, and television to understand what they are reading right now. As their reading choices expand, they encounter books that are increasingly challenging in terms of content, format, and style. They read stories about people and places far removed from their own lives in time and space. They read nonfiction as well as fiction. They read essays, poems, novels, plays, and, dare we acknowledge it, even textbooks. As their language becomes more complete, and their reading experiences become more varied, these children experience a knowledge explosion that cannot be fathomed by people who cannot read. The true miracle in this experience is that it all happens inside readers' minds, bounded only by the limits of their imaginations, and all this can take place in the family room or the classroom. The power of books in the hands of readers is truly amazing. As their reading experiences increase in frequency and variety, independent readers learn to enjoy reading. As they learn to enjoy reading, they risk becoming what are called *voracious* readers. You know these people. They are knowledgeable, interesting, creative, and productive.

To this point, we have identified the general evolution of reading development without references to specific ages. We want to digress briefly from this evolutionary perspective to look at Jean Chall's (1983, 1996) model, which links specific aspects of reading development to specific ages. According to Chall's model, there are five stages of reading development preceded by a preparatory stage. The preparatory stage extends from about six months to six years. During this stage, the child is *exposed* to reading in the sense that he looks at books, usually in the company of a caregiver. Early on, he might pretend that he is reading. During the preschool years, he will probably recognize some of the letters of the alphabet and might recognize traffic signs and the names of franchise restaurants. He might know the stop sign more by its color and shape than by the letters in the word *stop*, but he is at least paying attention to the symbols he will soon process in real reading. It is very likely that the preschool child knows McDonald's more by its golden arches than by the letters in the restaurant's name, but again he is beginning to make a connection between symbols and the act of processing symbols, and that is the basis of reading.

In Chall's stage 1, the child is six to seven years old and is receiving *direct instruction* in reading. He learns how letters are connected to sounds. He learns how to *sound out* simple words, typically single-syllable words, and by the end of this stage, he can actually read about 600 words.

In stage 2, he is seven to eight years old. Instruction is still direct. He learns to read simple stories. He is becoming increasingly adept in his decoding skills. He is learning more about the connections between words and meanings, and by the end of the stage, he can read about 3,000 words.

When the child is nine to fourteen years old, he moves into stage 3. He now uses reading as a primary vehicle by which he learns independently. Reading provides the background for class discussions, and he is learning to dissect words more thoroughly to understand the breadth and depth of their meanings.

Stage 4 extends from about fifteen to seventeen years. This stage is essentially an extension of stage 3 during which the emerging young adult becomes more expert in his reading skills and expands his application of these skills to an increasingly large array of topics.

At eighteen years and beyond, the reader is in stage 5—the stage in which he remains during his adults years. The stage 5 reader continues to expand his reading vistas. If he was not a self-motivated reader earlier, he is now becoming one, especially when he finishes school and is no longer motivated by the threat of a failing grade that might be the consequence for not reading assigned material. In or out of school, he reads to understand more fully knowledge he has already attained and to acquire new knowledge. He reads newspapers to be informed. He reads magazines and novels to be entertained. He reads instruction manuals to figure out how to put things together in "102 easy steps." He continues to improve his reading efficiency and ability to comprehend what he is reading, and he reads more rapidly.

Throughout our discussion of language development, we have emphasized that children do not proceed through development at the same pace. We conclude with the same emphasis here. While the general development of reading competencies will be the same for all children, they do not all achieve these competencies at the same ages. Rather than becoming unduly concerned about whether a child is on schedule in terms of literacy development, we should be concerned about doing whatever we can to facilitate development. What we can do is fairly simple. We can support and encourage children who are learning to read and write. We can trust that their natural language abilities, in combination with teaching/learning paradigms that foster natural, language-based reading instruction, will ultimately produce effective and efficient adult readers.

The Development of Writing

Even the casual observer will understand that reading and writing are closely related processes, sharing language as a common bond. Butler and Turbill (1987) note that reading and writing are also functional cousins in that each is an act of composing. More specifically, Butler and Turbill observe, "Readers, using their background of knowledge and experience, compose meaning from text; writers, using their background of knowledge and experience, compose meaning into text" (p. 11).

In a very real sense, then, reading and writing are different facets of a single process. In the development of reading and writing, the knowledge of each process is enhanced by the knowledge gained in the other. This means that the more a person reads, the more she will know about writing, and the more she writes, the more she will know about reading (Fields & Spangler, 1995). From the point of view of Butler and Turbill, the tie that binds reading and writing together is meaning. As the reader processes the printed symbols on the page, she constructs meaning, not by paying attention to every detail, but by sampling only those details she needs for meaning closure. You know from your own experience that if you are reading material with which you are not familiar, you process many more details of the printed symbols than if you are reading material you know well. The reader's knowledge and experience help her gauge how many details are enough in a given reading situation. Alas, sometimes the reader exhausts all the available details and, for want of more, never achieves meaning closure. We have all been there, too.

Writing offers a different challenge. The writer begins with ideas, morsels of meaning, and must decide which symbols in which combination will best represent those ideas. If the writer understands the nuances of this kind of communication, he will also take into account the audience to whom he is directing his packaged morsels of meaning, and he will select the literary style he believes is most appropriate for conveying his message (Department of Education, Wellington, 1985). Consider the differences in symbols and literary styles that might be reflected in the following: writing a diary entry, writing a letter to a lover, writing a letter of inquiry about a job, and writing an essay for a philosophy professor on the relative dangers of optimism and pessimism in humankind's efforts to save the planet.

We should step back for a moment and consider what has been discussed about writing to this point. The opening paragraphs in this section have been devoted to what might be called *real writing*, in contrast to the act of copying letters or words a teacher has written on the chalkboard. It needs to be emphasized that *real writing* is not the same thing as *handwriting practice*. For many years, teachers assumed they were teaching writing when they taught their students how to print their letters and then produce them in cursive, the physical skills included in *penmanship*.

Today, teachers recognize that although the physical skills involved in forming letters are important, the process of writing, real writing, is far more important. Teachers today value writing as a powerful communication tool. They believe their students have the potential to become authors, that they can actually compose meaning into text (Fields & Spangler, 1995). Writing is, as writing experts today remind us, about meaning, and it is about language. The developing child who processes meaning in the speech of others, and who learns how to create meaning in his own oral expressions, eventually extends these meaning–language skills into the processes of reading and writing. Just as she can express meaning in what she says, so can she express meaning in what she writes.

Even though, as we have noted, there is a more powerful biological drive in human beings for the production of speech than for the production of language in written form, there can be little doubt that children have a natural inclination to write. They certainly show evidence of a strong desire to write even before they enter school. Preschoolers are infamous for marking up walls, sidewalks, and newspapers with crayons, chalk, pencils, and pens (Graves, 1983). If speech begins in cooing and babbling, writing certainly begins in the preschool child's scratches and scrawls.

The physical process of moving the fingers and hands to put letters on paper is closely related to drawing in that writing and drawing are both processes of symbolization (Dyson, 1983). Writing and drawing, however, are not the same thing. The child demonstrates that writing and drawing are differentiated processes when he is about three years old (Gibson & Levin, 1975). As soon as the child can hold and manipulate a pencil or crayon and is given an opportunity to experiment with these instruments of expression, he will begin to make marks on any surface that is available. These early marking and scribbling exercises form the foundations of writing. Especially if the young child has been exposed to printed language in books and magazines, he will try to make forms that resemble letters of the alphabet. These early attempts are crude approximations at best. At this point, the child does not know the names of the letters he is trying to form, nor does he understand that printed words represent spoken words, but he is beginning the journey that leads inexorably to written language (Sulzby, 1981).

The first word the typical child learns to write is his own name. Shortly thereafter, he will probably learn to write other words with which he is familiar, including *Mommy, Daddy,* and the names of his siblings. These personally familiar words provide the child with his first understanding that a connection exists between printed symbols and spoken sounds.

Very early in writing development, the child begins to make natural associations between the letters of the alphabet and the speech sounds they most commonly represent. These early sound–letter associations lead to what is called *graphophonemic awareness,* in which *graph* refers to printed symbols (letters) and *phonemic* refers to speech sounds. The child demonstrates graphophonemic awareness when, in a contextual setting, she makes a conscious effort to match letters to sounds (Read, 1981).

It is at this juncture in the development of writing that the child begins to sense a need to spell, and it is at this juncture in our discussion that we need to be reminded that writing and spelling fit within the larger context of language. If it is true, as present-day language experts assert, that language acquisition occurs most efficiently when the child takes risks, when she experiments, develops hypotheses about rules, tests the rules, and revises them as necessary, the child must also risk, experiment, develop and refine rules in written language. Since written language includes spelling, common sense suggests that the child must be allowed, even encouraged, to risk and experiment with spelling. In fact, the typical child is likely to experiment with spelling even if she is not encouraged to do so. Her earliest spelling risks and experiments result in some pretty interesting sequences of letters, often called *invented spellings.* The journey from invented to conventional spelling moves through the following four stages, each of which involves progressively more sophisticated spelling: (1) prephonemic, (2) early phonemic, (3) letter–name, and (4) transitional (Weaver, 1994).

In the **prephonemic** stage, the child is wantonly experimental and blithely uninhibited. When she tries to spell a word, she writes down letters in a manner that is clearly more capricious than calculated. She does seem to understand that longer words require more letters, and she knows that when letters are strung together, they "say" something, but she does not yet understand that there are specific, if not always consistent, relationships between the letters of the alphabet and the sounds of speech.

The changes in the **early phonemic** stage are not dramatic, but they are important because they reflect more sophisticated understanding about spelling and sounds. In this stage, the child often attends only to the first letter of a word. From the child's perspective, this single letter represents the entire word even if other letters are included. The other letters in the child's "written word" typically have no correspondence to the remaining segments of the target word. The child might know, for example, that the letter *D* makes the sound that begins *Daddy,* but she writes *Daddy* as *DBMS.* While the child is most likely to include the letter representing the first sound of a word, she may also include the letter that represents the last sound of the word. The middle of the word is a kind of mystery spelling package in the sense that no one, including the child, knows what letters might be included from one spelling attempt to the next on the same word. We do know that these attempts are not entirely random. For example, early phonemic spellings include consonants and exclude vowels. As the child gains more experience with letters and the sounds they represent, phonemic spellings begin to shade into spellings that more obviously reflect letter–sound relationships.

In the **letter–name** stage, the child is representing vowels as well as consonants. The child is attempting to spell more sounds, but she is most likely to use letters whose names sound like the speech sounds they purportedly represent. Nurtured in a risk-free environment, this understanding that there are relationships between printed symbols and speech sounds, or graphophonemic awareness, enables the child to move to the transitional stage of spelling.

In the **transitional** stage, the child will try a number of spelling strategies. She might use a particular spelling because she *remembers* seeing the word spelled that way in print. She might try to apply rules for spelling she has observed in her own reading. Perhaps she observed that when a word contains a double vowel (e.g., *teeth*), the vowel sound is long, or when a word ends with *e* (e.g., *fine*), the preceding vowel is long. When asked to spell a word she does not know, such as *leaf,* she might assume, based on her knowledge of these rules, that the word should be spelled *leef* or *lefe.* The child might continue to rely on letter–name spellings, so that when asked to spell *sugar,* she might write *shuger.*

A writing sample of a child in the transitional stage of spelling might include productions based on several different spelling strategies, including the examples provided here and others. It would be a very rare child, at this stage of spelling development, who would rely on a single spelling strategy. The typical child is still experimenting. In fact, the development of spelling is facilitated by successful use of an expanding range of spelling strategies (Wilde, 1992). After all, a strategy that works well in one spelling challenge may be of absolutely no help in another.

Given the inconsistencies between the way words are spelled and the way words are spoken, the child who aspires to be a competent speller must have a plethora of spelling strategy options at her disposal. Did we spell *plethora* correctly? The first vowel is not long, so it should not be a double *ee,* and the sound *uh* at the end is probably spelled with an *a,* and. . . . The truth is, many of the strategies used in the transitional stage are used by adult spellers as well. The child learns much of what she will ever know about spelling patterns during the elementary school years, but most people continue to learn how to spell throughout their adult years, or at least until their brains are totally fried by television.

Obviously, much more is involved in writing than forming letters and spelling. Even as these foundational processes continue to develop, the child is learning to express himself through writing, and he is learning the rules of grammar, capitalization, and punctuation that make writing "correct." Whatever limitations others may see in the young child's writing abilities, he is typically unabashed about expressing himself on paper, and the products of these early attempts are often delightful. In the following essay written by a seven-year-old boy, you will notice spelling, punctuation, and capitalization errors but also the simple elegance of the written message:

> spider live in hot dezerd.
> but not oll of them. sum live here.
> sum cude hurt you. they are deadles.
> I saw one before it was not deadles.
> It was a dade-long-legs he was on
> me. they are not fast
> they are not good jumpers at all
> THE END
> of the spiter story

Just as spelling proceeds through stages of development, so does writing. Kroll (1981) suggests that there are four stages or phases in the development of writing: preparation, consolidation, differentiation, and integration. The child is typically a preschooler during the **preparation phase.** He is learning the ground floor basics of writing—how to form letters. His caregivers and teachers provide him models which he imitates. It is a painstaking, but absolutely necessary, phase in writing development that usually continues through kindergarten and first grade.

When the child is about seven years old and in the second grade, he enters the **consolidation phase.** He now writes strings of words, using the same vocabulary and rules of grammar he uses in his speech. When he is in the fifth grade, or about ten years old, the child enters the **differentiation phase.** During this phase, the way he writes becomes *differentiated* from the way he talks. He uses more sophisticated grammar in his writing than in his speaking, a trend that continues for many people throughout their lives. All writers proceed through the first three phases.

Not all will enter the final phase, **integration.** In this phase, the writer develops a *style* that reflects his own personality, makes him unique, and allows him to express varying moods and attitudes in his writing. Less sophisticated writers are fairly regimented in the way they write. They may obey the rules of grammar, and their writing may be clear, but it lacks personal expression. The difference between a writer in the integration phase and one who never enters this phase is comparable to the difference between a concert-level musician and one whose playing is competent but mechanical. Both musicians play all the right notes, but the concert-level musician plays in a manner that is creative and personally expressive. The integration phase writer uses standard words and conventional rules of language, but he uses written language creatively and expressively.

Development in writing has been described at the most mechanical, grammatical level (Perera, 1986). As the child matures, for example, she uses more passive sentences in her writing. At the age of thirteen years, she is producing three times as many passive sentences in her writing as she produced at eight years. The length of her clauses, calculated on a *words-per-clause* basis, increases systematically. The mean length of a written clause at eight years is 6.5 words. That number increases to 8.6 at seventeen years; by adulthood, the writer is creating clauses that average 11.5 words in length. Writers increase the length of their clauses by adding modifiers and by including more words to signal adjustments such as tense changes and modality.

Many of these changes in writing, particularly those associated with developing one's own *style,* continue to evolve as one journeys through adulthood. Many professional writers will look back on their earlier work as being less mature, less expressive than their present work. Just as *life is a journey and not a destination,* so is learning to be an effective writer a journey, not a destination.

Language in Adulthood: Changes and Challenges

There should be no question that the overriding emphasis in this book is on language development in children. That is clearly reflected in the organization of the book, and it is amply demonstrated in the number of pages devoted to that topic. It would be a mistake, however, to assume that when childhood ends, language development ends. Even if *development* in the strictest sense of the word does end at some point in adulthood, changes in oral communication continue throughout a person's lifetime. Some of these changes are positive in the sense that words are added to vocabularies, meanings are refined, pragmatic skills become more sophisticated, and so on. Unfortunately, the process of aging often, although not inevitably, brings deterioration in communication skills as well. We devote this section to a brief review of what we know about language in adulthood, including the enhancement of skills and the possibility of deterioration.

Taking Language from the Classroom to the Workplace

When the child is in junior high school and high school, he is typically eager for this part of his life to be over so he can get started on his *real life.* When he enters college, he may have similar thoughts about getting that phase of his life out of the way so he can put books, papers, exams, and all that other *learning* tedium behind him. Oh, what a poor misguided young person he is. As suggested in countless speeches during innumerable commencement ceremonies at thousands of high schools and colleges across our country, learning does not end when the diploma is pressed into the palm. When a young person enters the workplace, he may be surprised to discover that there are still books and journals to be read. There are new skills to master. There are reports to be written. There are even exams to be taken, but now the stakes are much higher. Failure in the workplace does not mean that someone assigns a grade of F for an assignment that falls short of expectations. It can mean that there is no pay raise, no promotion, or no job. The stakes are definitely higher, and the twenty-one-year-old might find himself yearning for the *old days* when his biggest worry was getting a chemistry experiment finished on time.

We would certainly expect the young college graduate to enter the workplace with intact language abilities, but even this area brings new demands. Every person getting a job for the first time must learn how to use language in a manner that allows her to get along with her superiors and her peers, and that's not always easy because it often means that you have to swallow your pride and temper your temper. You do that by using the language of the workplace—language that is respectful, courteous, not condescending or haughty. The new worker might be required to learn the nuances of talking on the telephone in the business world, a very different style of telephone talking than that used by two friends chatting about the latest gossip. She might have to make the same kind of adjustment in writing letters, memos, and e-mails. The formality of language in the workplace is a challenge for many young people. Not only does this language utilize the higher echelons of a person's vocabulary, but it demands a more exacting application of the rules of grammar.

Think for a moment about the *languages* of certain professions. The young professional will have been exposed to some of the lexicon of his field's language as a college student, but now he is immersed in it, up to his technical jargon eyeballs. Yes, attorneys really do talk like lawyers, and physicians talk like medical doctors, and computer experts talk in that *computerese* that causes many of us who use computers but do not really understand how they work to nod our heads affirmatively when we are really completely bewildered. Elementary school teachers must learn how to convey complete and accurate messages in language forms that match the competency levels of their students. Clergypersons must not just master the special words and phrases of their religions but also learn how to use body language and their voices to grab the attention and touch the hearts and minds of those to whom they speak during religious services. Counselors must learn how to use language to clarify and reflect what their clients are saying while avoiding saying anything that might sound judgmental or accusatory. Actors must learn how to say words they have committed to memory as though they are formulating them and saying them for the first time. Politicians must learn how to respond to questions without answering them and without offending anyone. People who work in the advertising business must learn how to influence people to buy products based on short, usually powerful, written and spoken ads that stretch, but do not break, the truth.

How long could this list of examples be? The underlying point to be made is that whatever language skills a new worker brings to the workplace, she is not done with language learning. She must learn new words and new phrases. In some cases, she must adopt syntactic structures that are conventional in her field. She must learn the styles of speech that are necessary to get along, to get things done, and to get ahead.

Vocabulary: Growing Even in Adulthood

When we talk about language changes in adulthood, it should be clearly understood that we are talking about slow evolutionary changes, not the kinds of dramatic, explosive changes we see during the early years of the child's life. Adults fight the details of language, and you might recognize some of the common battles. Some adults struggle with subject–verb agreement. Others are still trying to sort out when to use *who* and when to use *whom:* "Ali is the man *who* will be writing the letter" versus "Ali is the man to *whom* the letter should be addressed." Another common problem is knowing when to use *good* and when to use *well:* "She is a *good* runner" versus "She runs *well.*" Many adults are not sure about *I* and *me* and will sometimes overuse *I* because they have been told so often that *me* is not appropriate: "You and *I* will be responsible for setting the table" versus "The party was thrown for you and *me.*" Adults sweat the details. They also construct longer, more elaborate clauses, but there are no major pieces of language rules to be acquired and mastered. The most noticeable language acquisitions during adulthood are new words.

Remember that the typical child masters his first meaningful word at about one year. By the time he is three or four years old, he has about 1,000 words in his expressive vocabulary. The typical college graduate has about 22,000 words in his vocabulary. Now, pay attention to this: At the age of sixty-five, the typical adult has about 45,000 words in his expressive vocabulary, a twofold increase in comparison to his vocabulary when he was in his early twenties (Lane & Molyneaux, 1992).

What are the sources of all these new words? Most words acquired during adulthood are the products of new knowledge and work experiences. As mentioned earlier, every profession has its own vocabulary, and while we learn some of that vocabulary while we are being trained, many other terms are added when we begin employment. Consider, too, that many people change careers several times over the course of adulthood. Each career change brings a new jargon and more words to be incorporated into one's vocabulary. Other words absorbed into an adult's vocabulary are derived from hobbies and travel as well as from social, political, and religious activities. The typical adult's life broadens along many dimensions as he gets older. With every new life vista come new words.

Beyond just the acquisition of new words, the adult learns more about what words mean. Definitions of words continue to become more dictionary-like. Word meanings grow vertically as life experiences teach the adult new meanings for long-established words, and they grow horizontally as those same life experiences teach him that a given word often has many meaning applications, especially when one allows for the metaphoric influence. It is, in fact, the metaphoric influence in the horizontal aspect of word meanings that allows adults to understand jokes that fly under the radar of youngsters.

Acquiring the Registers of Adult Speech

Although the child adjusts her style of speech to accommodate changing audiences and social contexts, most of what she learns about this aspect of communication, she learns as an adult. We refer to the various styles of communication people use as **registers.** The adult uses different registers of communication with different groups of people, and she changes registers depending on the circumstances of communication (Lane & Molyneaux, 1992).

One of the most commonly recognized registers is what might be called the courtesy, or politeness, register. This is one of the first registers to be acquired by children, primarily because it is directly taught. In fact, we demand that this register be used by the child whenever we say something like, "What's the magic word?" This register includes more than just words such as *please, thank you,* and *you're welcome,* however. It entails also a communicative demeanor of courtesy that is demonstrated in body language and vocal variations that signal politeness.

As the child moves into adolescence and adulthood, he associates with a variety of groups, and he uses a different register in each one. He uses a different style of communication when he is engaged in sports than when he is in the classroom or in band. If he is a member of the Boy Scouts of America, he learns a register for his interactions with his fellow scouts and his leaders. As an adult, he uses a work register, a family register, a close-friend social register, a stranger social register, and a religious register. The list of registers is as long as the list of groups with which he is affiliated. The list of groups and list of registers changes over the course of a lifetime, so neither is complete until the end.

Cognitive Factors Impacting Language in Adulthood

According to Obler (2001), three cognitive abilities not directly related to language impact language reception and production: processing speed, inhibition, and working memory.

As adults age, there is a decrease in **processing speed,** as one would expect. According to Smith, Wasowicz, and Preston (1987), older adults process speech 20 to 25 percent more slowly than young adults. Older adults are also slower than young adults in their comprehension of speech delivered at a faster than normal rate (Bergman, 1980). The rate at which adults can read with comprehension slows as they get older (Harris, Rogers, & Qualls, 1998), and older adults have more difficulty than young adults when they are asked to quickly generate lists of words that are initiated by a specified letter or that do not include a specified letter (Bryan, Luszcz, & Crawford, 1997). Processing speed alone, of course, tells us nothing about the older person's ability to think, reason, and understand, and speed alone is not a decisive factor in a person's language competence. Whatever it might or might not mean about language ability, the evidence does suggest that processing speed diminishes as the adult moves through his later years.

In the context of cognition, **inhibition** refers to the ability to ignore information that is extraneous or unimportant. Older adults find it increasingly difficult to ignore irrelevant information (Burke, 1997).

Working memory is something like the RAM in your computer. RAM holds programs and files in memory on your computer's desktop until you need to access that information to facilitate the completion of whatever task is the focus of your attention. Working memory allows you to remember information while you are processing a message and/or contemplating your response to the message. The older adult will experience constraints on his working memory, a decline that helps account for problems with comprehension in old age (Qualls, 1998).

In addition to problems with these three cognitive abilities, we should note that cerebral hemispheric changes may impact the way the older adult processes and produces language. It is generally understood that the brain becomes lateralized at about two years. That is, each of the cerebral hemispheres becomes dominant for certain functions. In most people, the left hemisphere becomes dominant for language. At one time, researchers believed that this left-hemispheric dominance for language becomes more pronounced over the course of a person's lifetime. More recent research, however, including studies by Borod and Goodglass (1980) and by Obler, Woodward, and Albert (1984), suggests that there are no substantial changes in hemispheric dominance for language. That is, the left hemisphere is dominant for language in children, and it remains dominant for adults, but the degree of dominance does not change. It is possible, however, that how language is *organized* within the left hemisphere might change over the course of a person's life (Brown & Jaffe, 1975). Organizational changes within the hemisphere could account for the greater automaticity of language production associated with aging (Warren & Warren, 1966).

The Impact of Brain Damage on Adult Language

As long as the adult's health remains good, language abilities remain strong. Whatever natural changes occur in the process of aging, the older adult is able to find ways to compensate for those changes so her communication system remains viable. Unfortunately, the journey to old age is often traversed over rocky roads that adversely affect neurological functions, including cognitive functions. Since oral language is a cognitive-based phenomenon, anything that negatively impacts cognition has the possibility of impacting language. This occurs most dramatically in cases of **aphasia** associated with stroke. It occurs less dramatically, but often with the same outcomes, in conditions that result in **dementia.**

Although most of us automatically associate aphasia with stroke or cerebral vascular accident (CVA), aphasia can result from nonstroke brain injuries as well. The common denominator is the presence of a neurologically based language impairment as the result of damage to the language centers of the left hemisphere, assuming the patient is left-hemispheric dominant for language. There are several major classifications of aphasia based on the language impairments displayed: Broca's, Wernicke's, conduction, anomic, and global. The patient with **Broca's aphasia** understands what is being said to him and is able to speak, but his speech is labored and nonfluent. His messages typically sound like telegrams in the sense that only the most important words are included. **Wernicke's aphasia** is the mirror image of Broca's. In Wernicke's aphasia, comprehension is poor, but speech is relatively good except for some word-selection problems. Sometimes this patient will make common mistakes such as verb tense or plurality errors that have little impact on the intelligibility of her message; other times, she will substitute words or phrases that seem completely irrelevant. The patient with **conduction aphasia** comprehends well and speaks reasonably well, but he has trouble repeating words, phrases, and sentences. The patient with **anomic aphasia,** sometimes called simply *anomia,* can understand what is said, but struggles to recall the names of specific people, places, and things. In **global aphasia,** as the name suggests, there is impairment in both comprehension and production.

Aphasia is not a condition limited to older adults, of course. Young adults and even children suffer strokes, and people of all ages are subject to head injuries that can produce aphasia. Recovery from aphasia, however, is a much different proposition for the typical older adult than it is for the child, adolescent, or young adult. Young children with aphasia, even when it is severe, usually recover completely. Adolescents and young adults also have excellent, if not always complete, recoveries. With older adults, the outlook is not as promising. A minority of older adults experience complete, or nearly complete, recoveries. Many others recover some language function, and others show virtually no recovery, even with intensive therapy.

If damage occurs in the right hemisphere of a person who is left-hemispheric dominant for language, we cannot assume that language will be unaffected. If damage is limited to the right hemisphere, it is probably safe to assume that the basic components of language, including vocabulary, syntax, morphological rules, and phonology, will remain intact, but other aspects of communication may be affected. Right-hemispheric damage might impair a person's ability to convey messages that are emotionally loaded (Bloom, Borod, Obler, & Gerstman, 1992), and it might affect a person's ability to process humor (Brownell, Michel, Powelston, & Gardner, 1983). Prosody is also affected when there is damage in the right hemisphere. Not only is there a reduction in prosodic variation in the person's speech, but he also has trouble processing the communicative intents underlying prosody in the speech of others (Brownell, Gardner, Prather, & Martino, 1995).

The term **dementia** refers to a *deterioration of cognitive functions.* When a person suffers a stroke, the impact on cognitive functions is sudden. The onset of dementia is gradual, and whereas the damage in a stroke occurs in a limited area of the brain, the damage in dementia is more pervasive. Dementia is associated with a number of diseases medical scientists have only recently begun to study in earnest, but one of these is well known to most of us, at least by name: **Alzheimer's disease.**

Some progressive diseases of the central nervous system, such as Parkinson's disease, affect subcortical areas of the brain, structures beneath the brain's surface. Parkinson's disease is the result of deterioration of nerve cells in the area of the midbrain responsible for controlling body movements. Over time, speech may be affected because speech is a voluntary motor activity, but language will remain intact. In Alzheimer's disease the damage occurs in the cortical areas of the brain, the same areas affected by stroke. For this reason, the Alzheimer's patient develops language impairments that strongly resemble the types of aphasia we identified earlier.

The type of aphasia that most closely parallels the language impairment associated with Alzheimer's in its early stages is anomia. That is, the patient has difficulty remembering the names of things. When the Alzheimer's patient is in the middle to late stages of the disease, her language impairment resembles Wernicke's aphasia. Her comprehension is problematic, but her speech is still fluent and usually syntactically correct. Like the Wernicke's patient, however, the Alzheimer's patient sometimes includes words that do not belong or constructions that can only be described as *nonsense words.* In the final stages of the disease, the patient sounds like the global aphasic. She has trouble with comprehension, and her expressive language is either nonexistent or completely inappropriate. If she does talk, she might talk when no one is present, and she might refuse to talk when people try to engage her in conversation. The language she does produce is fairly devoid of meaning and seems to be primarily reflexive in nature.

Problems with reading and writing for the Alzheimer's patient parallel her oral communication problems, although the parallels are not perfect. It is interesting, for example, that in the early stages, the patient can typically read with more understanding than she can listen with understanding. This difference is probably due to the more intense, sustained attention required when one is listening. Writing problems show up quickly with this disease, and writing skills deteriorate rapidly.

And the Beat Goes On . . .

What a magnificent adventure this has been! Children, by virtue of their genetic background, are born to talk, but acquiring language and the abilities to express language through speech and writing is not as simple as acquiring freckles. Language acquisition depends on environmental opportunities and on the child's interactions with the important people in his life. It depends on motor, sensory, perceptual, and cognitive development. It is a complex process that begins before birth, accelerates through the child's first five or six years of life, and continues, only slightly abated, through the remainder of his school years. Even then the learning does not end. As adults, we learn new words. We understand syntactic rules more completely. We learn the multiple meanings of words and the differences between the denotations and connotations of words, which allow us to use words more effectively to convey the exact messages we intend. Language is indeed a wondrous and exciting phenomenon, and we continue to experience the wonder of language as long as we live and speak and listen and read and write.

This marks the end of our journey through the joys and travails of speech and language development, but four chapters remain. Throughout our discussion of language development, we have mentioned the sound system of speech but we have not specifically traced its development. In Chapter 7, we take a closer look at phonology and the acquisition of speech sounds. In Chapter 8, we examine language differences based on geography, culture, and gender. In Chapter 9, we look at bilingual language acquisition. Finally, we review some of the common disorders of speech and language in Chapter 10.

Review Questions

1. How does vocabulary growth parallel Jean Piaget's four stages of cognitive development? That is, what changes in intellectual development seem to account for the acquisition and use of vocabulary over the first fifteen years of the child's life?

2. What is the syntagmatic-paradigmatic shift, and how is it related to vocabulary growth?

3. What is the difference between horizontal and vertical expansion in the development of word meanings?

4. Why do the child's definitions shift from personal to shared, and in what sense do his definitions become more "elaborate" as his language knowledge increases?

5. Define each of the following figurative language forms and provide several examples of each: metaphor, simile, idiom, and proverb.

6. What is the difference between reversible and nonreversible passive sentences? Provide several examples of each type.

7. What is the principle of minimal distance? Why does the child have more difficulty with words that inconsistently violate the principle than with words that consistently violate the principle?

8. Create several conjoined sentences using each of the following categories of conjunctions: conditional, causal, disjunctive, and temporal.

9. Why is *because* a troublesome conjunction for the developing child?

10. What morphological modifications does the child begin to master during the school years?

11. Describe each of the following advancements in conversational skills: shading, stacked repair sequences, and sophisticated versions of indirect request.

12. Describe the major changes that occur in the child's narratives as she moves through the school years.

13. Describe each of the following types of narrative discourse: *recount*, *event-cast*, *account*, and *fictionalized narrative*.

14. When do gender differences in communication begin to emerge? Why do you think these differences exist?

15. What new challenges does the child as communicator experience in the classroom?

16. What does metalinguistic awareness mean? What do we know about metalinguistic development in the following areas: phonology, semantics, syntax, and pragmatics?

17. What can parents do to facilitate literacy development in their children?

18. Compare and contrast the two dominant reading models underlying current reading instruction programs in U.S. public schools: (1) *transmission* model and (2) *transactional* model.

19. Briefly describe the following categories of reading development: (1) *emergent*, (2) *developing*, and (3) *independent*.

20. What is the difference between *writing* and *penmanship*, and why is the difference important?

21. What is *graphophonemic awareness*?

22. Briefly describe the four stages of invented spelling: (1) *prephonemic*, (2) *phonemic*, (3) *letter–name*, and (4) *transitional*.

23. What is the moral of "the spiter story" for adults who teach reading and writing?

24. How might Chall's stages of reading development be related to stages of cognitive and language development?

25. Consider how Kroll's stages of writing development are related to stages of reading, cognitive, and language development.

26. What are some of the characteristics of the language style you will use in the work for which you are being trained? What are examples of the *jargon* used by members of your future profession?

27. Consider the *registers* you use in the groups with which you are affiliated. What are some of the distinguishing characteristics of each of these registers?

28. Assuming you know some "older adults," provide examples from their communication efforts that would reflect the problems Obler identifies in terms of *processing speed, inhibition,* and *working memory.*

29. If you were responsible for providing supportive communication therapy for an Alzheimer's patient, what would you include in your therapy program and why? In planning your therapy, take into account the progressive nature of the disease.

References and Suggested Readings

Abrahamsen, E., & Rigrodsky, S. (1984). Comprehension of complex sentences in children at three levels of cognitive development. *Journal of Psycholinguistic Research, 13,* 333–350.

Al-Issa, I. (1969). The development of word definition in children. *Journal of Genetic Psychology, 114,* 25–28.

Altwerger, B., Diehl-Faxon, J., & Dockstader-Anderson, K. (1985). Read-aloud events as meaning construction. *Language Arts, 62*(5), 476–484.

Ames, L. (1966). Children's stories. *Genetic Psychological Monographs, 73,* 307–311.

Anglin, J. (1985). The child's expressible knowledge of word concepts: What preschoolers can say about the meanings of some nouns and verbs. In K. E. Nelson (Ed.), *Children's language* (Vol. 5, pp. 77–127). Hillsdale, NJ: Erlbaum.

Anglin, J. (1993). Vocabulary development: A morphological analysis. *Monographs of the Society for Research in Child Development, 58*(10), Serial No. 238.

Anglin, J. (1995, April). *Word knowledge and the growth of potentially knowable vocabulary.* Paper presented at the biennial meeting of the Society for Research in Child Development, Indianapolis, IN.

Applebee, A., Langer, J., & Mullis, I. (1988). *Who reads best? Factors related to reading achievement in grades 3, 7, and 11.* Princeton, NJ: National Assessment of Educational Progress, Educational Testing Service.

Aukett, R., Ritchie, J., & Mill, K. (1988). Gender differences in friendship patterns. *Sex Roles, 19,* 57–66.

Baker, L., Scher, D., & Mackler, K. (1997). Home and family influences on motivations for reading. *Educational Psychologist, 32,* 69–82.

Baldie, B. (1976). The acquisition of the passive voice. *Journal of Child Language, 3,* 331–348.

Barth, R., & Kinder, B. (1988). A theoretical analysis of sex differences in same-sex friendship. *Sex Roles, 19,* 349–363.

Bartlett, C. (1982). Learning to write: some cognitive and linguistic components.

In R. Shuy (Ed.), *Linguistics and literacy series* (No. 2). Washington, D.C.: Center of Applied Linguistics.

Bashir, A., & Scavuzzo, A. (1992). Children with language disorders: Natural history and academic success. *Journal of Learning Disabilities, 25*(1), 53–65.

Beaumont, S. (1995). Adolescent girls' conversations with mothers and friends: A matter of style. *Discourse Processes, 20,* 109–132.

Bennett, R. (1981). *Types of literature.* Lexington, MA: Ginn.

Bergman, M. (1980). *Aging and the perception of speech.* Baltimore: University Park Press.

Berko-Gleason, J., & Greif, E. (1983). Men's speech to young children. In B. Thorne, C. Kramerae, & N. Henley (Eds.), *Language, gender, and society.* Rowley, MA: Newbury House.

Berko-Gleason, J., Hay, D., & Cain, L. (1988). Social and affective determinants of language acquisition (pp. 171–186). In M. L. Rice & R. L. Schiefelbusch (Eds.), *The teachability of language.* Baltimore: Brookes.

Bernstein, D. (1989). Language development: The school-age years. In D. Bernstein & E. Tiegerman (Eds.), *Language and communication disorders in children* (2nd ed.). Upper Saddle River, NJ: Merrill/Prentice Hall.

Biemiller, A. (1970). The development of the use of graphic and contextual information as children learn to read. *Reading Research Quarterly, 6,* 75–96.

Billow, R. (1975). A cognitive developmental study of metaphor comprehension. *Developmental Psychology, 11,* 415–423.

Bloom, R., Borod, J., Obler, L., & Gertsman, L. (1992). Impact of emotional content on discourse production in patients with unilateral brain damage. *Brain and Language, 42,* 153–164.

Borod, J., & Goodglass, H. (1980). Hemispheric specialization and development. In L. Obler & M. Albert (Eds.), *Language and communication in the elderly: Clinical, therapeutic, and experimental issues.* Lexington, MA: Heath.

Brinton, B., Fujiki, M., Loeb, D., & Winkler, E. (1986). Development of conversational repair strategies in response to requests for clarification. *Journal of Speech and Hearing Research, 29,* 75–81.

Brown, J., & Jaffe, J. (1975). Hypothesis on cerebral dominance. *Neuropsychologia, 13,* 107–110.

Brownell, H., Gardner, H., Prather, P., and Martino, G. (1995). Language, communication, and the right hemisphere. In H. S. Kirshner (Ed.), *Handbook of neurological speech and language disorders* (pp. 325–349). New York: Dekker.

Brownell, H., Michel, D., Powelston, J., & Gardner, H. (1983). Surprise but not coherence: Sensitivity to verbal humor in right hemisphere patients. *Brain and Language, 18,* 20–27.

Bryan, J., Luszcz, M., & Crawford, J. (1997). Verbal knowledge and speed of information processing as mediators of age differences in verbal fluency performance among older adults. *Psychology and Aging, 12,* 473–478.

Burke, D. (1997). Language, aging, and inhibitory deficits: Evaluation of a theory. *Journal of Gerontology: Psychological Sciences, 52b,* 254–264.

Butler, A., & Turbill, J. (1987). *Towards a reading–writing classroom.* Portsmouth, NH: Heinemann.

Byrne, B., & Fielding-Barnsley, R. (1998). Phonemic awareness and letter knowledge in the child's acquisition of the alphabetic principle. *Journal of Educational Psychology, 81,* 313–321.

Carey, S., & Bartlett, E. (1978). Acquiring a single new word. *Papers and Reports on Child Language Development, 15,* 17–29.

Carrell, P. (1981). Children's understanding of indirect requests: Comparing child and adult comprehension. *Journal of Child Language, 8,* 329–345.

Carrow, E. (1973). *Test of auditory comprehension of language.* Austin, TX: Urban Research Group.

Cazden, C. (1988). *Classroom discourse: The language of teaching and learning.* Portsmouth, NH: Heinemann.

Chall, J. S. (1996). *Stages of reading development* (2nd ed.). New York: McGraw-Hill.

Chapman, R., Streim, N., Crais, E., Salmon, D., Strand, E., & Negri, N. (1992). Child talk: Assumptions of a developmental process model for early language learning. In R. Chapman (Ed.), *Processing language acquisition and disorders.* St. Louis, MO: Mosby–Year Book.

Cherry, L., & Lewis, M. (1976). Mothers and two-year-olds: A study of sex-differentiated aspects of verbal interaction. *Developmental Psychology, 12,* 278–282.

Cherry-Wilkinson, L., & Dollaghan, C. (1979). Peer communication in first grade reading groups. *Theory Into Practice, 18,* 267–274.

Chomsky, C. (1969). The acquisition of syntax in children from 5 to 10. Cambridge, MA: MIT Press.

Clark, H., & Chase, W. (1972). On the process of comparing sentences against pictures. *Cognitive Psychology, 3,* 472–517.

Corrigan, R. (1975). A scalogram analysis of the development of the use and comprehension of "because" in children. *Child Development, 46,* 195–201.

Corsaro, W. (1979). Young children's conception of status and role. *Sociology of Education, 52,* 46–50.

Craig, H., & Evans, J. (1991). Turn exchange behaviors of children with normally developing language: The influence of gender. *Journal of Speech and Hearing Research, 34,* 866–878.

Crais, E. (1990). World knowledge to word knowledge. *Topics in Language Disorders, 10,* 45–62.

Department of Education, Wellington, New Zealand (1985) *Reading in junior classes.* Katonah, NY: Owen.

de Villiers, J., & de Villiers, P. (1978). *Language acquisition.* Cambridge, MA: Harvard University Press.

Doake, D. (1995). *Literacy learning: A revolution in progress.* Bothell, WA: The Wright Group.

Duffy, G., & Roehler, L. (1981). *Building reading skills: Level 4.* Evanston, IL: McDougal, Little.

Durkin, D. (1980). *Teaching young children to read.* Boston: Allyn & Bacon.

Dyson, A. (1983, April). *Early writing as drawing: The developmental gap between speaking and writing.* Paper presented at the American Educational Research Association convention, Montreal, Canada.

Edelsky, C. (1977). Acquisition of an aspect communicative competence: Learning what it means to talk like a baby. In S. Ervin & C. Mitchell-Kernan (Eds.), *Child discourse.* New York: Academic Press.

Ehrenreich, B. (1981). The politics of talking in couples. *Ms., 5,* 43–45, 86–89.

Ely, R. (2005). Language and literacy in the school years. In J. Berko-Gleason (Ed.), *The development of language* (6th ed.) (pp. 396–429). Boston: Allyn & Bacon.

Ely, R., & Berko-Gleason, J. (1995). Socialization across contexts. In P. Fletcher & B. MacWhinney (Eds.), *Handbook of child language* (pp. 251–270). Oxford: Blackwell.

Ely, R., Berko-Gleason, J., & McCabe, A. (1996). "Why didn't you talk to your Mommy, Honey?" Gender differences in talk about past talk. *Research on Language and Social Interaction, 29,* 7–25.

Emerson, H. (1979). Children's comprehension of "because" in reversible and nonreversible sentences. *Journal of Child Language, 6,* 279–300.

Emerson, H., & Gekoski, W. (1976). Interactive and categorical grouping strategies and the syntagmatic-paradigmatic shift. *Child Development, 47,* 1116–1125.

Ervin, S. (1961). Changes with age in the verbal determinants of word-association. *American Journal of Psychology, 74,* 361–372.

Ervin-Tripp, S. (1977). From conversation to syntax. *Papers and Reports in Child Language Development, 13,* 11–21.

Ervin-Tripp, S., & Gordon, D. (1986). The development of requests. In R. Schiefelbusch (Ed.), *Language competence: Assessment and intervention.* San Diego, CA: College-Hill.

Fields, M., & Spangler, K. (1995). *Let's begin reading right: Developmentally appropriate beginning literacy* (3rd ed.). Upper Saddle River, NJ: Prentice Hall.

Fisher, B. (1991). *Joyful learning.* Portsmouth, NH: Heinemann.

Forman, E., & McPhail, J. (1993). Vygotskian perspectives on children's collaborative problem-solving activities. In E. A. Forman, N. Minick, & C. Addison Stone (Eds.), *Contexts for learning: Sociocultural dynamics in children's development* (pp. 213–229). New York: Oxford University Press.

Foy, J., & Mann, V. (2003). Home literacy environment and phonological awareness in preschool children: Differential effects for rhyme and phoneme awareness. *Applied Psycholinguistics, 24,* 59–88.

Freeley, A. (1993). *Argumentation and debate: Critical thinking for reasoned decision making.* Belmont, CA: Wadsworth.

Frith, V. (1985). Beneath the surface of developmental dyslexia. In K. Patterson, J. Marshall, & M. Coltheart (Eds.), *Surface dyslexia: Neuropsychological and cognitive studies of phonological reading.* London: Erlbaum.

Gallagher, T. (1977). Revision behaviors in the speech of normal children developing language. *Journal of Speech and Hearing Research, 20,* 303–318.

Gardner, H., & Winner, E. (1979). The child is father to the metaphor. *Psychology Today, 12,* 81–91.

Garvey, C. (1975). Requests and responses in children's speech. *Journal of Child Language, 2,* 41–63.

Gathercole, V. (1985). "Me has too much hard questions": The acquisition of the linguistic mass-count distinction in "much" and "many." *Journal of Child Language, 12,* 395–415.

Gelman, R., & Shatz, M. (1977). Appropriate speech adjustments: The operation of conversational constraints on talk to 2-year-olds. In M. Lewis & L. Rosenblum (Eds.), *Interaction, conversation, and the development of language.* New York: Academic Press.

Gerber, A. (1981). Problems in the processing and use of language in education. In A. Gerber & D. Bryen (Eds.), *Language and learning dis-*

abilities. Baltimore: University Park Press.

Gibson, E., & Levin, H. (1975). *The psychology of reading.* Cambridge, MA: MIT Press.

Gilligan, C. (1982). *In a different voice: Psychological theory and women's development.* Cambridge, MA: Harvard University Press.

Goodman, K. (1976). Behind the eye: What happens in reading. In H. Singer & R. Ruddell (Eds.), *Theoretical models and processes of reading* (2nd ed.). Newark, DE: International Reading Association.

Goodman, K. (1986). *What's whole in whole language?* Richmond Hill, Canada: Scholastic-TAB Publications.

Graves, D. (1979). What children show us about revision. *Journal of Language Arts, 56,* 312–319.

Graves, D. (1983). *Writing: Teachers & children at work.* Portsmouth, NH: Heinemann.

Greif, E., & Berko-Gleason, J. (1980). Hi, thanks, and goodbye: Some more routine information. *Language and Society, 9,* 159–166.

Grimm, H. (1975, September). *Analysis of short-term dialogues in 5–7 year olds: Encoding of intentions and modifications of speech acts as a function of negative feedback loops.* Paper presented at the Third International Child Language Symposium, London, England.

Gundloch, R. (1981). On the nature and development of children's writing. In C. Frederiksen & J. Dominic (Eds.), *Writing: The nature, development, and teaching of written communication* (Vol. 2). Hillsdale, NJ: Erlbaum.

Haas, A. (1979). The acquisition of genderlect. *Annals of the New York Academy of Sciences, 327,* 101–113.

Hakes, D. (1980). *The development of metalinguistic abilities in children.* Berlin: Springer.

Hakes, D. (1982). The development of metalinguistic abilities: What develops? In S. Kuczaj (Ed.), *Language development: Vol. 2. Language, thought and culture.* Hillsdale, NJ: Erlbaum.

Halperin, M. (1974). Developmental changes in the recall and recognition of categorized word lists. *Child Development, 45,* 144–151.

Harris, J., Rogers, W., & Qualls, C. (1998). Written language comprehension in younger and older adults. *Journal of Speech, Language, and Hearing Research, 41,* 603–617.

Harste, J., Woodward, V., & Burke, C. (1984). *Language stories and literacy lessons.* Portsmouth, NH: Heinemann.

Heath, S. (1982). Toward an ethnohistory of writing in American education. In M. Whiteman (Ed.), *Writing: The nature, development and teaching of written composition* (Vol. 1). Hillsdale, NJ: Erlbaum.

Heath, S. (1986a). Separating "things of the imagination" from life: Learning to read and write. In W. Teale & E. Sulzby (Eds.), *Emergent literacy.* Norwood, NJ: Ablex.

Heath, S. (1986b). Taking a cross-cultural look at narratives. *Topics in Language Disorders, 7*(1), 84–94.

Heath, S. (1982). Questioning at home and at school: A comparative study. In G. D. Spindler (Ed.), *Doing the ethnography of schooling.* New York: Holt, Rinehart & Winston.

Heath, S. (1983). *Ways with words: Language, life, and work in communities and classrooms.* Cambridge: Cambridge University Press.

Hoffner, C., Cantor, J., & Badzinski, D. (1990). Children's understanding of adverbs denoting degree of likelihood. *Journal of Child Language, 17,* 217–231.

Hood, L., & Bloom, L. (1979). What, when, and how about why: A longitudinal study of early expressions of causality. *Monographs of the Society for Research in Child Development, 44.*

Horgan, D. (1978). The development of the full passive. *Journal of Child Language, 5,* 65–80.

Hughes, M., & Grieve, R. (1980). On asking children bizarre questions. *First Language, 1,* 149–160.

Jay, T. (1992). *Cursing in America.* Philadelphia: Benjamins.

Johnston, J. (1982). Narratives: A new look at communication problems in older language disordered children. *Language, Speech and Hearing Services in Schools, 13,* 144–155.

Johnson, C., & Anglin, J. (1995). Qualitative developments in the content and form of children's definitions. *Journal of Speech and Hearing Research, 38,* 612–629.

Kaderavek, J., & Sulzby, E. (2000). Narrative production by children with and without specific language impairment: Oral narratives and emergent readings. *Journal of Speech, Language, and Hearing Research, 43,* 34–49.

Kail, R. (1984). *The development of memory in children* (2nd ed.). New York: Freeman.

Kamhi, A., & Catts, H. (1986). Toward an understanding of developmental language and reading disorders. *Journal of Speech and Hearing Disorders, 51,* 337–347.

Kemper, S. (1984). The development of narrative skills: Explanations and entertainments. In S. Kuczaj (Ed.), *Discourse development: Progress in cognitive development research,* New York: Springer.

Kemper, S., & Edwards, L. (1986). Children's expression of causality and their construction of narratives. *Topics in Language Disorders, 7,* 11–20.

Klecan-Acker, J., & Kelty, K. (1990). An investigation of the oral narratives of normal and language-learning disabled children. *Journal of Childhood Communication Disorders, 13,* 207–216.

Kobasigawa, A. (1974). Utilization of retrieval cues by children in recall. *Child Development, 45,* 127–134.

Kobasigawa, A. (1997). Retrieval strategies in the development of memory. In R. Kail & J. W. Hagen (Eds.), *Perspectives in the development of memory and cognition* (pp. 177–201). Hillsdale, NJ: Erlbaum.

Kobasigawa, A., & Mason, P. L. (1982). Use of multiple cues by children in memory retrieval situations. *Journal of General Psychology, 107,* 195–201.

Krauss, R., & Glucksberg, S. (1977). Social and nonsocial speech. *Scientific American, 236,* 100–105.

Kroll, B. (1981). Developmental relationships between speaking and writing. In B. Kroll & R. Vann (Eds.), *Exploring speaking–writing relationships: Connections and contrasts.* Urbana, IL: National Council of Teachers of English.

Kurland, B., & Snow, C. (1997). Longitudinal measurement of growth in definitional skill. *Journal of Child Language, 24,* 603–625.

Lane, V., & Molyneaux, D. (1992). *The dynamics of communicative development.* Upper Saddle River, NJ: Prentice Hall.

Leonard, L., Wilcox, J., Fulmer, K., & Davis, A. (1978). Understanding indirect requests: An investigation of children's comprehension of pragmatic meanings. *Journal of Speech and Hearing Research, 21,* 528–537.

Lewis, R. (1996). Interference in short-term memory: The magical number two (or three) in sentence processing. *Journal of Psycholinguistic Research, 25,* 93–121.

Litowitz, B. (1977). Learning to make definitions. *Journal of Child Language, 4,* 289–304.

Lund, N., & Duchan, J. (1988). *Assessing children's language in naturalistic contexts.* Upper Saddle River, NJ: Prentice Hall.

Makau, J. (1990). *Reasoning and communication: Thinking critically about arguments.* Belmont, CA: Wadsworth.

Maltz, D., & Borker, R. (1982). A cultural approach to male–female miscommunication. In J. J. Gumperz (Ed.), *Language and social identity.* Cambridge: Cambridge University Press.

Maratsos, M. (1974). When is a high thing the big one? *Developmental Psychology, 10,* 367–375.

Marsh, G., Friedman, M., Welch, V., & Desberg, P. (1981). A cognitive-developmental theory of reading acquisition. In G. McKinnon & T. Weller (Eds.), *Reading research: Advances in theory and practice,* New York: Academic Press.

Martin, R. (1997). "Girls don't talk about garages!": Perceptions of conversations in same- and cross-sex friendships. *Personal Relationships, 4,* 115–130.

Mason, J. (1989). *Reading & writing connections.* Boston: Allyn & Bacon.

Mattingly, J. (1972). Reading the linguistic process and linguistic awareness. In J. Kavanagh & J. Mattingly (Eds.), *Language by ear and by eye.* Cambridge, MA: MIT Press.

McCabe, A. (1996). *Chameleon readers: Teaching children to appreciate all kinds of good stories.* New York: McGraw-Hill.

McGregor, K., Friedman, R., Reilly, R., & Newman, R. (2002). Semantic representation and naming in young children. *Journal of Speech, Language, and Hearing Research, 45,* 332–346.

McNeil, D. (1970). *The acquisition of language: The study of developmental psycholinguistics.* New York: Harper & Row.

Mehan, H. (1979). *Learning lessons.* Cambridge, MA: Harvard University press.

Mehan, H. (1984). Language and schooling. *Sociology of Education, 57,* 174–183.

Menyuk, P. (1969). *Sentences children use.* Cambridge, MA: MIT Press.

Menyuk, P. (1971). *The acquisition and development of language.* Upper Saddle River, NJ: Prentice-Hall.

Michaels, S. (1981). "Sharing time": Children's narrative styles and differential access to literacy. *Language and Society, 10,* 423–442.

Michaels, S. (1991). The dismantling of narrative. In A. McCabe & C. Peterson (Eds.), *Developing narrative structure* (pp. 303–352) Norwood, NJ: Ablex.

Miller, G., & Gildea, P. (1987). How children learn words. *Scientific American, 257,* 94–99.

Miller, L. (1990). The roles of language and learning in the development of literacy. *Topics in Language Disorders, 10,* 1–23.

Minami, M., & McCabe, A. (1991). Haiku as a discourse regulation device: A stanza analysis of Japanese children's personal narratives. *Language and Society, 20,* 577–599.

Minami, M., & McCabe, A. (1995). Rice balls and bear hunts: Japanese and North American family narrative patterns. *Journal of Child Language, 22,* 423–445.

Mitchell-Kernan, C., & Kernan, K. (1977). Pragmatics of directive choice among children. In C. Mitchell-Kernan & S. Ervin-Tripp (Eds.), *Child discourse.* New York: Academic Press.

Muma, J., & Zwycewicz-Emory, C. (1979). Contextual priority: Verbal shift at seven? *Journal of Child Language, 6,* 301–311.

Nagy, W., Diakidoy, I., & Anderson, R. (1991). *The development of knowledge of derivational suffixes.* Technical Report N. 536, Center for the Study of Reading. Champaign: University of Illinois at Urbana-Champaign.

Nagy, W., Diakidoy, I., & Anderson, R. (1993). The acquisition of morphology: Learning the contribution of suffixes to the meanings of derivatives. *Journal of Reading Behavior, 25,* 155–170.

Nagy, W., Herman, P., & Anderson, R. (1985). Learning words from context. *Reading Research Quarterly, 22,* 233–253.

NCTE (1993). *Current research on language learning.* Committee on School Practices and Programs. Urbana, IL: National Council of Teachers of English.

Nelson, N. (1985). Teacher talk and children listening—Fostering a better match. In C. Simon (Ed.), *Communication skills and classroom success: Assessment of language-learning disabled children.* San Diego, CA: College-Hill.

Nelson, N. (1986). Individual processing in classroom settings. *Topics in Language Disorders, 6,* 13–27.

Nippold, M. (1998). *Later language development: The school-age and adolescent years.* Austin, TX: PRO-ED.

Nippold, M., Allen, M., & Kirsch, D. (2001). Proverb comprehension as a function of reading proficiency in preadolescents. *Language, Speech, and Hearing Services in Schools, 32,* 90–100.

Nippold, M., & Duthie, J. (2003). Mental imagery and idiom comprehension: A comparison of school-age children and adults. *Journal of Speech, Language, and Hearing Research, 46,* 788–799.

Nippold, M., & Haq, F. (1996). Proverb comprehension in youth: The role of concreteness and familiarity. *Journal of Speech and Hearing Research, 39*(1), 166–176.

Nippold, M., Hegel, S., Sohlberg, M., Schwarz, I. (1999). Defining abstract entities: Development in preadolescents, adolescents, and young adults. *Journal of Speech, Language, and Hearing Research, 42,* 473–481.

Nippold, M., & Martin, S. (1989). Idiom interpretation in isolation versus context: A developmental study with adolescents. *Journal of Speech and Hearing Research, 32,* 59–66.

Nippold, M., Martin, S., & Erskine, B. (1988). Proverb comprehension in context: A developmental study with children and adolescents. *Journal of Speech and Hearing Research, 31,* 19–28.

Nippold, M., Schwarz, I., & Undlin, R. (1992). Use and understanding of adverbial conjuncts. *Journal of Speech and Hearing Research, 35,* 108–118.

Nippold, M., & Sullivan, M. (1987). Verbal and perceptual analogical reasoning and proportional metaphor comprehension in young children. *Journal of Speech and Hearing Research, 30,* 367–376.

Nippold, M., Taylor, C., & Baker, J. (1995). Idiom understanding in Australian youth: A cross-cultural comparison. *Journal of Speech, Language, and Hearing Research, 39*, 442–447.

Nippold, M., Uhden, L., Schwarz, I. (1997). Proverb explanation through the lifespan: A developmental study of adolescents and adults. *Journal of Speech, Language, and Hearing Research, 40*, 245–253.

Nold, E. (1981). Revising. In C. Frederiksen & J. Dominic (Eds.), *Writing: The nature, development, and teaching of written communication* (Vol. 2). Hillsdale, NJ: Erlbaum.

Obler, L. (1989). Language through the life-span. In J. Berko-Gleason (Ed.), *The development of language* (2nd ed.). Upper Saddle River, NJ: Merrill/Prentice Hall.

Obler, L. (2001). Development and loss: Changes in the adult years. In J. Berko-Gleason (Ed.), *The development of language* (5th ed., pp. 455–471). Boston: Allyn & Bacon.

Obler, L., Woodward, S., & Albert, M. (1984). Lateralization in aging? *Neuropsychologia, 22*, 235–240.

Owens, R. (2005). *Language development: An introduction* (6th ed.). Boston: Allyn & Bacon.

Parlee, M. (1979). Conversational politics. *Psychology Today, 5*, 48–56.

Parsons, C. (1980). *The effect of speaker age and listener compliance and noncompliance on the politeness of children's request directives.* Unpublished doctoral dissertation, Southern Illinois University, Carbondale.

Perera, K. (1986). Language acquisition and writing. In P. Fletcher & M. Garman (Eds.), *Language acquisition* (2nd ed.). New York: Cambridge University Press.

Perfetti, C., & Goodman, D. (1970). Semantic constraint on the decoding of ambiguous words. *Journal of Experimental Psychology, 86*, 420–427.

Perlmann, R., & Berko-Gleason, J. (1994). The neglected role of fathers in children's communicative development. *Seminars in Speech and Language, 14*, 314–324.

Peterson, C. (1990). The who, when, and where of early narratives. *Journal of Child Language, 17*, 433–455.

Peterson, C., & McCabe, A. (1983). *Developmental psycholinguistics: Three ways of looking at a child's narrative.* New York: Plenum.

Piaget, J. (1963). *The origins of intelligence in children.* New York: Norton.

Qualls, C. (1998). *Figurative language comprehension in younger and older African Americans.* Unpublished doctoral dissertation, City University of New York.

Qualls, C., & Harris, J. (1999). Effects of familiarity on idiom comprehension in African American and European American fifth graders. *Language, Speech, and Hearing Services in Schools, 30*, 141–151.

Read, C. (1981). Writing is not the inverse of reading for young children. In C. Frederiksen & J. Dominic (Eds.), *Writing: The nature, development, and teaching of written communication.* Hillsdale, NJ: Erlbaum.

Reid, D. (1998). Scaffolding: A broader view. *Journal of Learning Disabilities, 31*, 386–396.

Reid, D. (2000). Discourse in classrooms. In K. R. Fahey & D. K. Reid (Eds.), *Language development, differences, and disorders.* Austin, TX: PRO-ED.

Richards, M. (1980). Adjective ordering in the language of young children: An experimental investigation. *Journal of Child Language, 6*, 253–277.

Robinson, E. (1981). The child's understanding of inadequate messages and communication failures: A problem of ignorance or egocentrism? In W. P. Dickson (Ed.), *Children's oral communication skills*. New York: Academic Press.

Rodino, A., Gimbert, C., Perez, C., & McCabe, A. (1991). *Getting your point across: Contrastive sequencing in low-income African-American and Latino children's personal narratives*. Paper presented at the Sixteenth Annual Boston University Conference on Language Development, Boston.

Rumelhart, D. (1977). Toward an interactive model of reading. In S. Dornic (Ed.), *Attention and performance* (Vol. 1). Hillsdale, NJ: Erlbaum.

Sause, E. (1976). Computer content analysis of sex differences in the language of children. *Journal of Pycholinguistic Research, 5*, 311–324.

Saywitz, K., & Cherry-Wilkinson, L. (1982). Age-related differences in metalinguistic awareness. In S. Kuczaj (Ed.), *Language development: Vol. 2. Language, thought and culture*. Hillsdale, NJ: Eribaum.

Scollon, R., & Scollon, S. (1981). *Narrative, literacy and face in interethnic communication*. Norwood, NJ: Ablex.

Scott, C. (1984). Adverbial connectivity in conversations of children 6 to 12. *Journal of Child Language, 11*, 423–452.

Scott, C. (1987). *Summarizing text: Context effects in language disordered children*. Paper presented at the First International Symposium, Specific Language Disorders in Children, University of Reading, England.

Scott, C. (1988a). Producing complex sentences. *Topics in Language Disorders, 8*(2), 44–62.

Scott, C. (1988b). Spoken and written syntax. In M. A. Nippold (Ed.), *Later language development: Ages nine through nineteen* (pp. 49–95). Austin, TX: PRO-ED.

Shultz, T., & Horibe, F. (1974). The development of the appreciation of verbal jokes. *Developmental Psychology, 10*, 13–20.

Slobin, D. (1978). Cognitive prerequisites for the development of grammar. In L. Bloom & M. Lahey (Eds.), *Readings in language development*. New York: Wiley.

Smith, B., Wasowicz, J., & Preston, J. (1987). Temporal characteristics of the speech of normal elderly adults. *Journal of Speech and Hearing Research, 30*, 522–529.

Snow, C. (1990). The development of definitional skill. *Journal of Child Language, 17*, 697–710.

Snow, C. (1991). The theoretical basis for relationships between language and literacy development. *Journal of Research in Childhood Education, 6*, 5–10.

Snow, C., Burns, M., & Griffin, P. (Eds.). (1998). *Preventing reading difficulties in young children*. Washington, D.C.: National Academy Press.

Snow, C., & Dickinson, D. (1991). Skills that aren't basic in a new conception of literacy. In A. Purves & E. Jennings (Eds.), *Literate systems and individual lives. Perspectives on literacy and schooling*. Albany, NY: SUNY Press.

Spector, C. (1990). Linguistic humor comprehension of normal and language-impaired adolescents. *Journal of Speech and Hearing Disorders, 55*, 533–541.

Stanovich, K. (1980). Toward an interactive-compensatory model of individual differences in the development of reading fluency. *Reading Research Quarterly, 16*, 32–71.

Stein, N. (1979). How children understand stories. In L. Katz (Ed.), *Current topics in early childhood education* (Vol. 2). Norwood, NJ: Ablex.

Stein, N. (1982). What's in a story: Interpreting the interpretations of story grammars. *Discourse Processes,* 319–335.

Stein, N., & Glenn, C. (1979). An analysis of story comprehension in elementary school children. In R. Freedle (Ed.), *New directions in discourse processing.* Norwood, NJ: Ablex.

Stein, N., & Policastro, M. (1984). The concept of story: A comparison between children's and teachers' viewpoints. In H. Mandl, N. Stein, & T. Trabasso (Eds.), *Learning and comprehension of text.* Hillsdale, NJ: Erlbaum.

Stein, N., & Albro, E. (1997). Building complexity and coherence: Children's use of goal-structured knowledge in telling stories. In M. Banberg (Ed.), *Narrative development: Six approaches* (pp. 5–44). Mahwah, NJ: Erlbaum.

Sternberg, R. (1979). Developmental patterns in the encoding and combination of logical connectives. *Journal of Experimental Child Psychology, 28,* 469–468.

Sternberg, R. (1987). Most vocabulary is learned from context. In M. G. McKeown & M. E. Curtis (Eds.), *The nature of vocabulary acquisition* (pp. 89–105). Hillsdale, NJ: Erlbaum.

Strong, C. & Shaver, J. (1991). Stability and cohesion in the speech narratives of language-impaired and normally developing children. *Journal of Speech and Hearing Research, 34,* 95–111.

Sulzby, E. (1981). *Kindergartners begin to read their own compositions.* Final report to the Research Foundation of the National Council of Teachers of English. Urbana, IL: Research Foundation of the National Council of Teachers of English.

Sutter, J., & Johnson, C. (1990). School-age children's metalinguistic awareness of grammaticality in verb form. *Journal of Speech and Hearing Disorders, 33,* 84–95.

Sutton-Smith, B. (1986). The development of fictional narrative performances. *Topics in Language Disorders, 7,* 1–10.

Swacher, M. (1975). The sex of the speaker as a sociolinguistic variable. In B. Thorne & N. Henley (Eds.), *Language and sex: Difference and dominance.* Rowley, MA: Newbury House.

Swartz, K., & Hall, A. (1972). Development of relational concepts and word definition in children five through eleven. *Child Development, 43,* 239–244.

Tannen, D. (1994). *Gender and discourse.* New York: Oxford University Press.

Teale, W. (1988). Developmentally appropriate assessment of reading and writing in the early childhood classroom. *Elementary School Journal, 89*(2), 173–183.

Thorne, B., Kramerae, C., & Henley, N. (Eds.) (1983). *Language, gender, and society.* Rowley, MA: Newbury House.

Torrey, J. (1979). Reading that comes naturally: The early reader. In T. Waller & G. MacKinnon (Eds.), *Reading research: Advances in theory and practice.* New York: Academic Press.

Vanevery, H., & Rosenberg, S. (1970). Semantics, phrase structure and age as variables in sentence recall. *Child Development, 41,* 853–859.

Van Kleeck, A. (1990). Emergent literacy: Learning about print before learning to read. *Topics in Language Disorders, 10,* 25–45.

Vellutino, F. (1979) Alternative conceptualization of dyslexia: Evidence in support of a verbal-deficit hypothesis. *Harvard Educational Review, 47,* 334–354.

Vellutino, F. (1974). *Dyslexia: Theory and research.* Cambridge, MA: MIT Press.

Walker, S. (2001). Cognitive, linguistic, and social aspects of adults' noun definitions. *Journal of Psycholinguistic Research, 30,* 147–161.

Warren, R., & Warren, R. (1966). A comparison of speech perception in childhood, maturity, and old age by means of the verbal transformation effect. *Journal of Verbal Learning and Verbal Behavior, 5,* 142–146.

Warren-Leubecker, A. (1982). *Sex differences in speech to children.* Unpublished master's thesis, Georgia Institute of Technology, Atlanta.

Weaver, C. (1994). *Reading process and practice: From sociopsycholinguistics to whole language.* Portsmouth, NH: Heinemann.

Wehren, A., DeLisi, R., & Arnold, M. (1981). The development of noun definition. *Journal of Child Language, 8,* 165–175.

Wells, G. (1986). *The meaning makers: Children learning language and using language to learn.* Portsmouth, NH: Heinemann.

Wertsch, J. (1991). *Voices of the mind: A sociocultural approach to mediated action.* Cambridge, MA: Harvard University Press.

Westby, C. (1994). The effects of culture on genre, structure and style of oral and written texts. In G. P. Wallach & K. G. Butler (Eds.), *Language learning disabilities in school-age children and adolescents* (pp. 180–213). Boston: Allyn & Bacon.

White, T., Power, M., & White, S. (1989). Morphological analysis: Implications for teaching and understanding vocabulary growth. *Reading Research Quarterly, 24,* 283–304.

Whorf, B. (1956). *Language, thought, and reality.* New York: Wiley.

Wilde, S. (1992). *You kan red this! Spelling and punctuation for whole language classrooms, K–6.* Portsmouth, NH: Heinemann.

Wilhelm, R. (1994). Exploring the practice –rhetoric gap: Current curriculum for African-American history month in some Texas elementary schools. *Journal of Curriculum and Supervision, 9,* 217–233.

Willis, F., & Williams, S. (1976). Simultaneous talking in conversation and the sex of speakers. *Perceptual and Motor Skills, 43,* 1067–1070.

Wing, C., & Schoinick, E. (1981). Children's comprehension of pragmatic concepts expressed in "because," "although," "if " and "unless." *Journal of Child Language, 8,* 347–365.

Wolf, M., & Dickenson, D. (1989). From oral to written language: Transitions in the school years. In J. Berko-Gleason (Ed.), *The development of language* (2nd ed.). Upper Saddle River, NJ: Merrill/Prentice Hall.

7

The Building Blocks of Speech

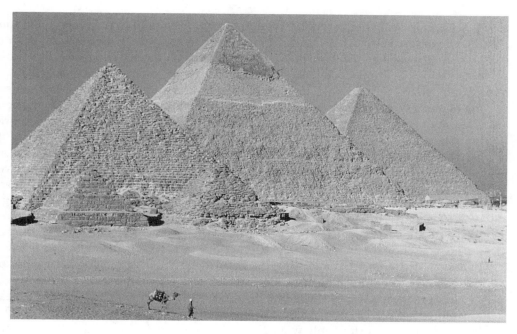

The preceding chapters have focused primarily on language development, but we have made frequent references to speech, and we have made occasional references to speech sounds. We want to emphasize that for the normally hearing, normally developing child, the speech sound system does not exist apart from language, and we want to stress that the child is acquiring the sound system and learning its underlying rules at the same time that she is acquiring language.

You must be reminded, however, as we noted in the opening chapter, that *speech* is not a synonym for *language* and

that speech can exist apart from language, as it does when a mynah bird "talks," and language can surely exist apart from speech as it does when the deaf person communicates through sign language. Because speech is related to language, but in some ways separate from language, and because the speech sound system is mastered according to a different developmental schedule than language, we have chosen to devote a separate chapter to the speech component of the larger communication system. Specifically, this chapter is designed to facilitate understanding of the following topics:

307

- How speech sounds are described
- The influence of co-articulation when sounds are sequenced into syllables, words, and phrases

- An overview of phonological development
- Theories of phonological development

When I was in high school, I lived in Egypt for two years. Although I had some extraordinary experiences during that time and saw many remnants of a remarkable ancient civilization, nothing impressed me as much as the great pyramids outside Cairo. From a distance, the surfaces of the pyramids appear relatively smooth, almost seamless. A closer view reveals structures of enormous size consisting of many huge blocks piled on top of one another in precise patterns. In the years since my visit to the pyramids, I have looked at modern buildings, especially brick buildings, with an eye not only to the total structure but to all the small pieces, the bricks, that together make the building complete.

We can think about human speech in much the same way. As senders and receivers of speech, we pay attention to the final product, the message, but even a simple sentence is actually a structure consisting of many small pieces. A sentence is a string of words, of course, but the words themselves are strings of speech sounds or **phonemes,** which are the building blocks, the bricks, of speech. And when someone speaks, there are no markers at the beginnings and endings of words. An utterance consists of a long, uninterrupted string of sounds. Only our knowledge of the language being spoken and our perceptual abilities allow us to know which segments of the string are words.

In a practical sense, we have little reason to pay attention to the sounds of speech any more than we should pay attention to individual bricks in a building. Individual bricks become important only when they fall out or break, threatening the structural integrity of a wall. In much the same way, we usually pay attention to specific sounds of speech only when they are missing or misarticulated in ways that affect our ability to understand the words of which they are members.

One cannot fully appreciate human speech, however, unless one understands the sound system from which specific phonemes are drawn to make up spoken words. We call the study of speech sounds and the rules that determine how sounds can be sequenced into syllables and words **phonology,** and that is the focus of this chapter. We take a look at how speech sounds are described and classified and how sounds interact with one another when they are joined to form syllables, words, and phrases, and we consider some of the major theories that attempt to explain how children acquire their sound systems as language is emerging.

Describing Speech Sounds

We begin by distinguishing between sound differences that matter and sound differences that do not matter. A phoneme is often described as a distinctive speech sound. That is, a phoneme is a speech sound that is recognized as a specific sound and is distinctly different from all other speech sounds. Consider the words *seat* and *seed*. These two words, when spoken, are exactly the same except for one small, but important, difference. Each word consists of three sounds. The first sound in each word is *s*. The second sound in each word is the long vowel, *e*. Now notice the last sound in each word. Say each of these sounds aloud and feel what is happening in your speech mechanism during each production. Both the *t* and *d* are produced with the front portion of the tongue pressed against the alveolar ridge, and in both productions, the tongue is quickly released to complete the sound. The only difference between *t* and *d* and, in the example used, the only difference between *seat* and *seed* is that when the *d* is produced, the vocal folds vibrate and when the *t* is produced, the vocal folds do not vibrate. The difference between vocal fold vibration and no vibration, therefore, is a difference that makes a difference. It is a difference that can differentiate one phoneme from another.

Not all differences matter, however. In American English, for example, it does not matter if you produce the word *cat* with a release of air following the *t* or with no released air. The listener will hear both productions as *cat* and will perceive the final sound as "t." The term **aspiration** describes a production in which there is a release of air following a sound like "t." Although aspiration is a distinctive sound difference in some languages, it is a nondistinctive speech sound difference in English. That is, it is a difference that does not make a difference. A nondistinctive speech sound change is called an **allophone.** In the "cat" example, the aspirated "t" and the unaspirated "t" are allophones of the *t* phoneme. Think of the phoneme as a sound family. Allophones are members of the family. Each allophone is a little different from every other allophone, but allophones are so similar to one another in all important respects that they are recognized as members of the same family. After we examine the three approaches used to describe phonological productions, we will consider how allophones are created. All of this information is preliminary to a brief overview of phonological acquisition and a summary of major theoretical views about how the sound system of language emerges.

Traditional Phonetics

The most basic approach for describing consonant speech sounds is the threefold classification system used in traditional phonetics. Each consonant is identified according to place of articulation, manner of articulation, and voicing. **Place of articulation** identifies where in the oral cavity the essential articulatory contact or movement is being made. There are three major places of articulation: the *lips* for sounds such as "b," "p," "m," "w," "f," and "v"; the *teeth* and the *alveolar ridge* for sounds such as "th," "t,", "d," "s," "z," "n," and "l"; and the *hard* and *soft* regions of the *palate* for sounds such as "sh," "zh," "ch," "dg," "y," "r," "k," "g," and "ng." A fourth place of articulation, *glottal*, is included to accommodate the "h" that is the square peg of speech sounds searching for a round hole. *Glottal* refers to the *glottis*, which is the variable space between the vocal folds. When "h" is produced, the speaker simply forces a short burst of air through the glottis.

Manner of articulation describes how a consonant sound is produced. The term *plosive* or *stop* is used to describe a consonant produced by stopping the flow of air out of the mouth and then suddenly releasing it. It may be helpful to remember that a plosive sound is produced in a somewhat explosive manner. The plosive sounds in English are "p," "b," "t," "d," "k," and "g."

A *fricative* sound is produced by forcing air through a narrow constriction, producing a frictionlike sound. The following sounds are fricatives: "f," "v," "s," "z," "th," "sh," and "zh." The "h" is also considered a fricative in traditional phonetics, even though one would be hard-pressed to identify where the constriction is. This is another dimension of the "h" as a square peg still in search of its round hole.

An *affricate* is a unique sound that combines plosive and fricative qualities. There are two affricates in English, "ch" and "dg." The "ch" sound is actually a "t" and a "sh" pushed together into a single sound that retains qualities of both original sounds. In the same way, "dg" combines "d" and "zh."

A *nasal* consonant is produced with nasal resonance. The only consonants in English that should be produced with nasal resonance are "m," "n," and "ng." All others should be produced with oral resonance only.

A consonant is considered *lateral* if its production involves directing the flow of air out of the mouth along the sides of the tongue. There is only one lateral consonant in English, and it is easy to remember because it is the first and last sound in *lateral,* the "l" sound.

Glides, such as "w" and "y," are also called *semivowels,* and both names are helpful in understanding how they are produced. They are called *glides* because their productions involve movement. They are called *semivowels* because they are somewhat vowel-like in the sense that they involve a relatively free and continuous flow of air through the oral cavity, unlike other consonants, which involve varying degrees of constriction or closure. Once again, the "h" is a classification problem. As is true of the glides, the "h" does not have the constriction or closure of other consonants, but neither does it have the continuous flow of air characteristic of glides. The "h" just cannot decide what it wants to be!

Voicing is simple. A consonant either involves vocal fold vibration or it does not. The majority of consonants are *voiced.* Those consonants that are *voiceless* are partners with voiced consonants. We call these voiced and voiceless partners *cognate pairs.* A cognate pair consists of two consonants produced in the same place and in the same manner but differing in voicing. For example, "p" and "b" are both produced with the two lips and both are produced in a plosive manner, but "p" is voiceless and "b" is voiced. They are a cognate pair. Cognate pairs account for sixteen of the twenty-four consonants we use in English. The eight consonants that are not members of cognate pairs are all voiced—except for that incorrigible "h," which is voiceless.

Classifying vowels in traditional phonetics is more difficult than classifying consonants, primarily because vowels are so variable in their production. Consider the vowel "e" as in the word *bee.* The "e" is classified as a high, front vowel. That is, the tongue is positioned at the front of the mouth in a relatively high position, but with very little effort, you will discover that you can produce the "e" with the tongue in almost any position. In fact, with a little dexterity, you can produce an "e" with your tongue protruding from your mouth. How and where vowels are produced depends on the sounds that precede and follow them, and vowels can adapt to virtually any phonetic environment. The traditional phonetics classification for vowels, therefore, is a general guide based on the production of these sounds in isolation.

A threefold classification is also used to classify vowels: height of tongue (i.e., high and low), location of primary resonance (i.e., front, central, and back), and tension of the tongue (i.e., tense or lax). **High vowels** have narrow resonating spaces. **Low vowels** have wider resonating spaces. Examples of high vowels include the "e" in *bee* and the "u" in *shoe*. Low vowels include "a" in *cat*, and "a" in *father*. The "e" in *bee* and the "a" in *cat* are **front vowels**. The "u" in *shoe* and the "a" in *father* are **back vowels**. The vowel "u" in *cut* is a **central vowel**. **Tense vowels** include the "e" in *bee* and the "u" in *shoe*. **Lax vowels** include the "i" in *bit* and the "u" in *cut*.

Throughout this discussion of the description of speech sounds using traditional phonetics, you may have noticed that the classification of speech sounds is based on certain basic contrasts. For example, in cognate pairs we contrast voiced and voiceless sounds. We contrast nasal sounds with all other consonants that are oral. Plosives are contrasted with fricatives on the basis of how they are produced, plosives by stopping the airstream completely before release, and fricatives by forcing air through a narrow constriction. With the vowels, we contrast high and low, front and back, tense and lax. The idea of classifying speech sounds by contrast eventually led to a more elaborate system of describing speech sounds known as the **distinctive feature approach.**

Distinctive Features

Many of the distinctive features are replications of contrasts we have already identified in traditional phonetics: *voicing, nasality,* and *lateral* for consonants and *high, low, back,* and *tense* for vowels. The remaining features make smaller distinctions among speech sounds, especially the consonants, than are made in traditional phonetic analysis. The two most basic features, *consonantal* and *vocalic,* are designed to make the most basic contrast among speech sounds. A sound is *consonantal* if it is produced with constriction or closure somewhere in the oral cavity. A sound is *vocalic* if it is produced without constriction or closure, and if air flows relatively unimpeded through the oral cavity. These two features effectively contrast consonants and vowels, but they also help us to understand that some sounds, such as "l" and "r," have characteristics of both features, and other sounds, such as "w," "y," and "h," do not clearly possess the characteristics of either feature. The feature *continuant* makes an important differentiation among sounds that involve constriction or closure. That is, some of these sounds involve more constriction or closure than others. Sounds such as "p," "b," "t," and "ch," for example, involve a great deal of closure and are not marked for the continuant feature. Sounds such as "f," "th," "s," and "sh" are marked for this feature because, while they involve constriction, they involve less constriction than other consonants.

The feature *coronal,* referring to the front portion of the tongue, separates sounds that depend on the front part of the tongue from sounds that either use the middle or back portion of the tongue, or do not use the tongue at all. Sounds such as "s," "t," "l," and "n" are marked for the coronal feature. Sounds such as "m," "p," and "b" are not coronal because they do not involve the tongue at all, and sounds such as "k," "g," and "ng," are not coronal because they use the back portion of the tongue.

The feature *anterior* makes a "place of articulation" distinction. Any sound produced on the alveolar ridge or forward is considered an anterior sound. Sounds such as "t," "d," "n," and "l" are considered anterior because they are produced with the tongue on the alveolar ridge. Sounds such as "p," "b," "m," and "f" are also marked for the anterior feature because they are produced in front of the alveolar ridge, but "ng," "k," and "g" are not marked for this feature because they are produced behind the alveolar ridge.

The last of the consonant features, *strident,* separates some fricatives from others. A fricative is strident if the vibrating air produced by the primary constriction point hits a second constriction point, usually the upper lip or upper teeth, to produce even more turbulence. The sounds "s," "z," "sh," and "zh" are strident. The affricates, "ch" and "dg," are also strident because they include "sh" and "zh" qualities in their productions. The other fricatives, including "f," "v," and "th," are not strident because they are produced so far forward that there are no structures to create the additional turbulence characteristic of stridency.

As already noted, the distinctive features used to describe vowels are the same contrasts used to describe vowels in traditional phonetics with one possible exception, *rounding.* A vowel is considered round if it is produced with natural lip rounding. The round vowels include the "u" in *blue,* the "oo" in *look,* the "o" in *goat,* and the "aw" in *law.*

Phonological Processes

The distinctive features approach to phonology built on and extended traditional phonetics by making finer distinctions among consonant phonemes than were possible with the threefold classification of place, manner, and voicing. The *phonological processes* approach, which dominates present theoretical and intervention discussions of phonology, represents a further extension. In addition to the concepts and terms already introduced by phonetics and distinctive features, the phonological approach gives attention to the effects of syllabic structure, to the sequencing of sounds, and to the effects sounds have on one another in the production of words and phrases. It should also be noted that while traditional phonetics and distinctive features are used to describe standard speech sounds so that we can better understand phonological errors, the phonological approach is designed specifically to describe productions that vary from standard targets.

The concept of phonological processes was introduced by Stampe in 1969 and became the subject of his doctoral dissertation completed in 1973. Phonological processes have been described in a variety of ways, but if we cut through most of the discussion and debate, we come down to this: *Phonological processes are rules children use to make productions that fit into their phonological understandings and abilities.* In most cases, these rules appear to *simplify* adult forms, although those who take a phonological processes approach are careful to point out that these rules *describe* rather than *explain* children's productions. It is tempting to conclude, for example, that faced with the task of producing an adult form consisting of four or five syllables, two or three sequences of consonants, and several sounds he cannot yet articulate accurately, the child makes decisions to reduce the word to one or two syllables, reduce the sequences to single sounds or eliminate them entirely, and omit or substitute for the sounds he cannot articulate. It is tempting to conclude, as Stampe first suggested, that the child uses a *mental operation* to transform the adult target into something he can produce, but the truth is we cannot know what cognitive manipulations, at what levels of consciousness, determine what the child produces. However processes are ultimately explained, it is clear that the child's phonological productions are not random or capricious. He does apply rules, called *processes,* in a fairly consistent and logical manner. For example, he might reduce all multisyllabic words by deleting the unstressed syllable or syllables. He might reduce all consonant sequences to single phonemes. He might always delete a single consonant in the final position if the consonant is a member of a cognate pair.

It is not within the scope of this book to include a detailed description of all common phonological processes, but the inclusion of a few examples may help the reader grasp what these rules contribute to our understanding of children's phonological productions. Actually, a few have already been mentioned. If a child reduces multisyllabic words by deleting unstressed syllables, the rule she is applying is called **syllable reduction** or **weak syllable deletion.** Reducing the number of segments in a sequence or cluster of consonants is called **consonant sequence reduction.** The child might use this process on the word *street* to make it *teet.* If she deletes the final consonants of words such as *dog, cat,* and *house* to produce *do___ , ca___ ,* and *hou___ ,* she is using a process called **postvocalic singleton consonant deletion.**

Some processes are considerably more complicated. For example, the child might produce *foon* for *spoon,* using a process called **coalescence.** He replaces two adjacent phonemes, "s" and "p" with a single phoneme, "f," that retains the fricative quality of "s" and the labial quality of "p." Rather than reducing the number of sounds in a word, the child might actually add sounds, using a process called **epenthesis.** The word *blue,* for example, might become *balue,* or *fork* might become *fwork.* The child might take voicing out of consonants at the ends of words, producing *dok* instead of *dog* or *bat* instead of *bad.* This process is known as **postvocalic devoicing.** If the child adds voicing to sounds at the beginning of words, it is called **prevocalic voicing.** Sometimes the child will include all the sounds in a word but will transpose a couple of the sounds. This process, called **metathesis,** is applied when the child says *aminal* for *animal* or *ephelant* for *elephant.*

The processes included here are only examples. Hodson and Paden (1991) describe nearly forty processes, not including idiosyncratic rules, which are processes unique to individual children. We will probably never have a complete list of processes precisely because children are very inventive in their phonological strategies. Just when we think we have heard them all, we will find a child who uses a rule we have never heard before.

With all three phonological descriptions in mind, consider how each would be used to describe what a child does when she makes "errors" on speech sounds. Using the traditional phonetics point of view, if the child says *bu___* for *bus,* we simply say that she has an "s" problem. A distinctive features specialist might speculate that the "s" is deleted because the child has not yet mastered the strident feature. The phonological processes specialist, taking into account other productions in which final consonants are deleted, might conclude that the problem has nothing to do with "s" specifically, or even with the strident feature. The child says *bu___* for *bus* because she applies the process postvocalic singleton consonant deletion to all words that end with consonants.

Each of these approaches to describing phonological productions leads to a somewhat different interpretation about how phonology develops. The traditional phonetic view suggests that phonemes develop as whole entities. The distinctive features view suggests that the child masters features. When he has all the features for which the "s" sound is marked, for example, he will produce "s." The phonological processes view suggests that the child masters the adult phonological system by gradually suppressing his rules or processes in favor of adult rules. The two-year-old, for example, applies the rule postvocalic singleton consonant deletion to all words ending in consonants, but by the time he is four or five years old, he has suppressed that rule in favor of the adult rule that says that some words do, in fact, end in consonants.

Before we consider specific theories of phonological development, we need to further set the stage by addressing two additional topics. The first, *co-articulation,* is concerned with how speech sounds interact with one another in connected speech. The second, *landmarks of phonological development,* is a description of the real-time acquisition of the speech sound system, independent of the debate about why what happens happens when it happens. The *why-what-when* questions are the prickly issues incorporated into theories of phonological development.

Co-Articulation: The Mix of Sounds in the Making of Speech

If you had never experienced speech, you might assume that a child learns individual speech sounds before she combines them, in much the same way as children learn the alphabet as the foundation for learning to spell, read, and write. If you listen to children who are just beginning to acquire speech, however, you will not hear them practicing sounds in isolation. Even their earliest utterances involve combinations of sounds. These combinations, even in simple syllables or words, involve complicated interactive adjustments of the speech mechanism.

In the opening of this chapter, speech sounds were compared to bricks in a wall. As is true of most analogies, the brick comparison has limitations. It is true that any given word consists of a finite number of sounds just as a wall, no matter how large, consists of a finite number of bricks. In the case of a brick wall, however, each brick retains its individual identity. It looks and feels the same whether it is in the wall or separate from the wall. When speech sounds are joined into words, they lose some of their individual characteristics. They blend together and influence one another so that the final product is something other than the sum of the sounds. We call the influence sounds have on one another in context **co-articulation.**

Many years ago, Hockett (1955) wrote an interesting description of co-articulation that is helpful in understanding the process, but, like the brick analogy, it has limitations. He explained it this way:

> Imagine a row of Easter eggs carried along a moving belt; the eggs are of various sizes, and variously colored, but not boiled. At a certain point, the belt carries the row of eggs between the two rollers of a wringer, which quite effectively smash them and rub them more or less into each other. The flow of eggs before the wringer represents the series of impulses from the phoneme source. The mess that emerges from the wringer represents the output of the speech transmitter. (p. 210)

Hockett's analogy captures the idea that sounds are merged together in a manner that blurs their separate identities, but it also gives the impression that this process is random and not governed by rules. Although there is still much we do not understand about co-articulation, we do know that it is an orderly and lawful process, and therefore, predictable.

We know, for example, that co-articulation works in a forward and a backward manner. That is, an early-appearing sound sometimes affects how a following sound will be produced, and sometimes a later-appearing sound will affect how an earlier sound is produced. When an early sound affects a later sound, it is called **retentive co-articulation.** In producing the word *new,* you cannot avoid producing the "ew" with nasality because of the influence of "n." That is, nasality is retained on the "ew." If you put the nasal sound after a vowel, the same influence will occur in the other direction. When you produce the word *aim,* the vowel is nasalized because you are anticipating the nasal sound, "m." This is called **anticipatory co-articulation.**

Feel what happens to your lips on the production of the two "s"'s as you say the word *seesaw.* Now say the sound "s" in isolation a few times. Repeat *seesaw* a few more times and sense the lip adjustment again. What is happening here? The sounds influencing the "s" productions are the vowels "ee" and "aw." The "ee" is a front vowel produced with the lips slightly spread, so the "s" in the first syllable is produced with the lips in a slightly spread position. The "aw" is a back vowel produced with lip rounding, so the "s" in the second syllable is produced with the lips rounded. These are examples of anticipatory co-articulation. What is truly amazing is that you have no idea you are making these adjustments, and if we asked you how you knew to make them, you could not provide an answer.

Consider what happens when you put two or more consonants together in a cluster or blend as in the words *cluster* and *blend.* In both words, you actually begin to produce the "l" before you release the first sound. Try to produce the beginning of each word in slow motion. In *cluster,* you are using the back of the tongue for "k" at the same time you are moving the front of the tongue to the alveolar ridge for "l." In saying *blend,* you contact the alveolar ridge for the "l" before you release the bilabial closure for "b."

We may not be able to explain *how* we co-articulate, but we should be able to understand *why.* Co-articulation allows us to speak in the most efficient manner possible within the limits of our speech mechanisms. We retain nasality as we move from the "n" to the "ew" in *new,* for example, because we cannot close the velopharyngeal mechanism quickly enough to eliminate nasal resonance on the vowel. We produce the "ai" in *aim* with nasal resonance because we cannot wait for the "m" to begin before we open the velopharyngeal port. Just as a drawbridge begins to open long before a ship arrives because it takes time to accomplish the opening, so the velopharyngeal port begins to open before the nasal sound arrives because it is a slow adjustment.

Articulation follows the path of least resistance, which means that the speaker is constantly adjusting according to the challenges presented by the sounds combined in a word or phrase. The adjustments sometimes result in compromises. In saying the word *little,* for example, the "t" is usually produced as a "d" because every other sound in the word is voiced, and it's too much trouble to turn off the larynx for one sound, and the "d" is produced with lateral emission rather than frontal emission because it is surrounded by "l" 's, which are laterals. When we say *windmill,* we leave out the "d" entirely because the adjustment from nasal alveolar "n" to nonnasal alveolar "d" to another nasal, "m," is just too difficult. We compromise in this case by just saying "winmill," a much easier production than "windmill." Because we all co-articulate according to the same rules, these adjustments and compromises have no effect on the ability of people to understand one another. In fact, if we concisely articulated every sound in every word, we would sound a little strange. Speech that sounds too perfect is not normal!

The Landmarks of Phonological Development

Since we have been down the developmental road with cognition and language already, a few simple reminders about ages and stages should suffice here. Children do not progress through the stages of phonological development on a predetermined schedule. In fact, there is considerable age variation at each stage, but the order of development will be the same for all children. No one knows exactly how many stages there are in phonological development any more than we can say with certainty how many stages there are in cognitive development or in language development. We describe development in stages as an academic convenience, recognizing that there will be overlapping of behaviors at every juncture. With these reminders in mind (which is where reminders belong), we will consider the development of phonology in four general stages.

Phonology before Language: Laying the Foundation for a Speech Sound System

Even the most uninformed person knows that human babies are not mute at birth. In fact, the visual and auditory impression most of us have about the newborn is that he or she enters the world screaming. This is not always true, of course, but if the neonate does not cry with his first breath, he does not wait long before he tests his noise-making equipment.

During her first year, the infant produces a wide range of vocalizations. The first of these vocalizations are reflexive, or unlearned. They include cries, coughs, gurgles, and hiccups. It is generally understood that the child's first cries and certainly the other reflexive noises she produces are automatic responses reflecting the child's general physical condition. When she is hungry, uncomfortable, or in pain, she will cry. If something is threatening to invade her larynx, she will cough. If she swallows too much air with mother's milk, she will burp. If she is perfectly content with the state of her world, she will be silent.

By the time the infant is two or three months old, we begin to hear vocalizations we call *cooing*. These are vowel-like productions the child produces when he is contented. Some children quickly add consonant-like sounds to their vocalizations to produce a behavior commonly called *babbling*. At this point, the child might produce vowel-like productions at times and productions that sound like consonant–vowel syllables at others. The "vowels" resemble adult back vowels as in *shoe* or *look,* and the "consonants" resemble adult back consonants such as "k" or "g." It must be emphasized, however, that these are not true speech sounds because they are not purposive and they are not used, either alone or in combination, to convey specific meanings.

By the time child approaches his fifth or sixth month, he is engaging in what is commonly referred to as *vocal play.* He has not abandoned vowel-like productions, and he continues to produce what appear to be consonant–vowel syllables, but he has added a number of other vocalizations that certainly impress adult listeners as playful. These include squeals, grunts, screams, growls, and the always popular "raspberries." Some children seem to fixate on one particular kind of noise for a few days before moving on to another noise and then sometimes returning to an old favorite for a time.

The child's earliest syllable-like forms are not produced with adult-like prosody. They are produced at a slower rate, and whatever intonational patterns are superimposed are irregular in nature. By the time the child is about eight or nine months old, the prosody superimposed on these syllable-like forms sounds more adultlike. That is, the overall rate has increased, and adults believe they hear stresses and meaningful intonational patterns. The fact that the child is superimposing all of this on reduplicated consonant–vowel forms resulting in productions such as "mamama" or "dadada" leads many adults to erroneously conclude that the child is producing meaningful words at this stage. Although it is not impossible for a child to produce meaningful words at nine months, it is highly unlikely. The test for *meaningful* is that productions be purposive, consistent, and used to convey specific meanings. At this stage in phonological and language development, productions, while not random, tend to be more playful than communicatively purposive, and they are not aimed at particular semantic targets. The sounds the child is producing do not have the consistency of adult phonemes, but they most closely resemble the plosive, nasal, and glide consonants, and lax vowels of adult phonology. As the child enters the last quarter of her first year, she tends to produce the velar sounds ("k" and "g") less frequently and alveolar sounds ("t," "d," "n") more frequently. Although we hear more labial sounds such as "p," "b," "m," and "w" at this point, the alveolar sounds are still more common.

During the last two months of the first year, the child produces *variegated babbling.* Most productions are still consonant–vowel forms, but, as the term suggests, we hear fewer reduplicated forms, and we hear a wider variety of consonants and vowels in more complicated productions such as "gubadee" or, for those with musical connections to the 1960s, "doowadidee!" Even though the child is expanding his consonant-like inventory, the sounds we most often hear continue to most closely resemble the plosives, nasals, and glides of adult phonology. The child will occasionally produce sounds that resemble fricatives, affricates, and even liquids (l, r), but he does not venture down these phoneme avenues very often.

Although there is considerable disagreement about how phonology develops in a general sense, as we will see when we sample common theories of phonological development, experts generally agree that what happens during the first year of phonological development is largely the result of physical maturation in combination with the human instinct to talk. The best evidence of this is that children from widely varying language and cultural backgrounds sound remarkably similar during this first stage of phonological development.

Before we leave this first stage of phonological development, we should briefly address a central controversy regarding the relationship between *babbling* and *true speech.* The controversy was sparked by two very different interpretations of this relationship. The first view, *babbling drift,* is probably most closely associated with Mowrer (1952). According to this view, the vocalizations the child produces that most closely resemble the speech productions of his caregivers are selectively reinforced by his caregivers so that the child's emerging phonological system is gradually shaped to fit the phonological system of his caregivers' language. That is, the child's babblings *drift* into adult speech.

Opposing this view is the *discontinuity theory* most closely associated with Jakobson (1968). According to Jakobson, babbling and true speech are two entirely separate stages of development. Whatever relationship they might have to one another is almost coincidental. During babbling, the child produces a wide variety of sounds common to many of the world's languages. When the child begins to produce meaningful speech, she stops babbling. She might even experience a period of silence before she begins to acquire the true sounds of her native language. The acquisition of true speech sounds, according to this view, is a slow and deliberate process.

Both of these views have problems. If the babbling drift theory were correct, we would expect that children from varying language backgrounds would sound different from one another by the end of the first year because their babblings would be differentially reinforced. That is, a Japanese child's Japanese-like sounds would be reinforced. A Russian child's Russian-like sounds would be reinforced. An Australian child's English-like sounds would be reinforced, and because of the phonological differences among these languages, these three children would sound different. But they do not. If the discontinuity theory were true, we would expect that there would be dramatic differences between the sounds we hear in babbling and the sounds we hear in early speech productions, and we would expect that babbling would have a definite ending and true speech a clearly defined beginning. Neither of these expectations is supported by research. Most children continue to babble for several months after they produce their first true words, and the sounds we hear in true words are remarkably similar to the sounds we hear in babbling.

If neither view is correct, what do we conclude? We conclude that even if we do not fully understand the purposes served by babbling relative to the emergence of speech, the facts of development speak for themselves. That is, the child does not stop babbling one day and begin to produce true words the next. For several months covering the end of the first year and the beginning of the second, babbling and true speech co-occur. To make matters even more interesting, as noted in an earlier chapter of this book, the child will produce what are called *protowords* or *vocables* during the transition period between babbling and true speech. A protoword is a word in the sense that it is used consistently with clear communicative intent. It does have phonemic and semantic consistency, but it is not an adult word, and it may not even be an attempt at an adult word. The child might call his high chair a *baki*, for example. If he uses this production consistently in reference to the same object, it is a protoword, and it is just as meaningful as *high chair*. The transition then from babbling to true speech is just that, a transition. It is not the end of Act I and the beginning of Act II. Perhaps the most important conclusion we can reach about babbling itself is that, based on the evidence we have gathered and examined so far, phonological development begins during babbling, before the child begins to produce his first true words (Lowe, 1994, p. 37).

Phonology in the Child's First Meaningful Words

While the child continues to babble and while he is producing protowords, he is also trying to produce words based on the models provided by his caregivers. His first attempts are far from perfect, of course, but given his limited neurophysiological abilities and his limited language competence at the beginning of his second year of life, he does pretty well. His first words are typically single-syllable productions or reduplicated forms. He might say, "Hi," "Bye," "Mama," or "Wawa." Consonant–vowel–consonant forms, such as "hot," do occur, but infrequently.

The most common manners reflected in the phonology of first words are plosive, nasal, and glide. Not surprisingly, these are the same manners we observed during the latter half of the first year, the manners we hear most often in babbling. The most common places of articulation reflected in the early phonology of meaningful speech are labial and alveolar, although the child will also produce some palatals and velars. Again, these are the same places of articulation we observe in babbled sounds.

When we examined first words from a language point of view, we suggested that the child often chooses her first words based on the personal importance of their referents, as well as their semantic properties and grammatical functions. To this list of selective factors we can also add phonological characteristics. That is, if the language and personal factors are equal, the child will select words that contain phonological segments that are included in her speech sound system, and she will avoid words that contain phonological information she does not yet possess. This means that given a choice between the targets *dog* and *miniature Schnauzer,* the young child will attempt to say *dog* because its phonological makeup is more consistent with her developing sound system than the phonological makeup of *miniature Schnauzer.*

Once the child acquires her first few words, vocabulary development occurs quickly. By the time she is eighteen months old, the typical child will have about fifty words in her productive vocabulary, but do not forget the caution about age. It would not be unusual for a child to be using fifty words as early as thirteen or fourteen months, and it would not be at all unusual for a child to be producing her first fifty words as late as her second birthday.

Putting the Phonological Pieces Together

Most phonological development occurs in the period between eighteen months and four years, during which there are significant advances in language development. The inventory of consonant sounds that has been limited primarily to plosives, nasals, and glides now expands to accommodate all phoneme classes, although this does not mean that all phonemes are correctly produced all the time. Syllable structures become more complex as the child sequences consonants both within syllables and across syllables, and he produces more true multisyllabic words, not just reduplicated forms.

To this point, the child has demonstrated little understanding of phonemes as individual sound segments, and he has not shown much evidence that he uses the same phonological rules used by adults. Early in development, he seems to contrast words, not phonemes. The rules he uses are processes, rules that often simplify adult forms, based on his current knowledge and his present abilities. As the child's phonological knowledge expands, and as his articulatory abilities improve, he uses a phonological system that increasingly resembles the adult system. He contrasts phonemes, not just whole words, and he knows how to generalize phonological rules from one phonetic context to another related phonetic context.

By the time the child is four years old, he has either suppressed or is well on the way to suppressing the phonological processes he has been using. He is producing the majority of consonants correctly, and is using the remainder correctly at least on occasion, and he is demonstrating an understanding of all phonemic contrasts. Phonological development is not complete by the time the child is four years old, but most of the acquisition is complete, and he is ready to begin tying up the loose ends of his speech sound system.

The Finishing Touches: Completing Phonological Development

Between the ages of four and eight years, the child finishes phonological development. Those phonemes she has been producing correctly but inconsistently now become increasingly correct. If there are any sounds she has not been producing at all, perhaps the liquids, they now begin to emerge, and by the end of this final stage, these sounds are mastered. When the child learns to read and write, her metalinguistic awareness increases. As she associates sounds with the letters of the alphabet, her understanding of speech sounds as individual segments solidifies. Because of the inconsistencies in our language between written symbols and the speech sounds they represent, the child may always struggle with some pronunciations and some spellings, but by the time she reaches the end of her elementary school years, she will grasp the obvious written and spoken connections well enough that she will be able to encounter new words in either oral or printed form and make a pretty good guess about how printed words should be pronounced or how spoken words should be spelled.

Theories of Phonological Development

Since the speech sound systems of languages can be described in different ways, it is not surprising that there are varying theories about how phonological systems develop in children. In this section, we will look at a sample of the views that experts have expressed over the last fifty years.

The Phoneme-by-Phoneme View of Development

The first systematic studies of phonemic acquisition were conducted by Wellman, Case, Mengert, and Bradbury (1931), Poole (1934), and Templin (1957). These studies were designed to establish norms for phonemic acquisition by assessing the phonemic abilities of large numbers of children within a broad age range. Although the specific methodologies of these studies varied, there was a fairly consistent general design. That is, attempts were made to include a reasonable distribution of subjects by socioeconomic level, although Templin weighted her sample toward the lower end of the socioeconomic continuum and included only children from urban areas.

In each study, children with hearing problems and language delay were excluded. Responses were typically elicited by asking the subjects to name pictures or objects. In the Wellman and Templin studies, if a subject did not produce a word spontaneously, a model was presented and an imitated response was accepted. Poole accepted only spontaneous productions. In all three studies, sounds were elicited in the word-initial, word-medial, and word-final positions, depending on the positions in which a particular sound is produced. For example, "ng" was elicited in only the word-medial and word-final positions because it does not occur in the word-initial position in English. Each of these large, cross-sectional studies established a criterion for age of mastery. In the Wellman and Templin studies, a sound was considered mastered if it was correctly produced in all appropriate word positions by 75 percent of the subjects at a given age level. In Poole's study, a sound was considered mastered if it was correctly produced in all appropriate word positions by 100 percent of the subjects at a given age level.

In spite of methodological differences and different mastery criteria, the results of these studies were remarkably consistent, as indicated in Table 7.1. The (–) indicates

Table 7.1 Summary of Phonemic Development Studies

Phonemes	Age of Mastery		
	Wellman et al. (1931) 75% criterion for mastery	Poole (1934) 100% criterion for mastery	Templin (1957) 75% criterion for mastery
p	4	3.5	3
b	3	3.5	4
t	5	4.5	6
d	5	4.5	4
k	4	4.5	4
g	4	4.5	4
f	3	5.5	3
v	5	6.5	6
voiceless th	–	7.5	6
voiced th	–	6.5	7
s	5	7.5	4.5
z	5	7.5	7
sh	–	6.5	4.5
zh	–	6.5	7
h	3	3.5	3
voiceless w	–	7.5	–
ch	5	–	4.5
dg	6	–	7
m	3	3.5	3
n	3	4.5	3
ng	–	4.5	3
w	3	3.5	3
y	4	4.5	3.5
l	4	6.5	6
r	5	7.5	4

that this sound either was not tested or was not mastered by the requisite number of subjects.

Templin (1957) compared her results with the findings of the two preceding studies. She noted that among the seventeen sounds included in all three studies, there was a spread in age of mastery of one year or less on eleven sounds, and a spread of two or more years on only six sounds. Considering the differences in subject populations, the element of chance that always enters this kind of research, and the differences in experimental designs, this is significant agreement.

Few surprises arose from these data. The sounds we would expect to emerge early because they appear in children's initial words are apparently mastered early. Among children's first words are productions such as *mama, papa, wawa,* and *no,* and the consonants in these productions are mastered, according to Templin's data, by three years. Sounds we would consider difficult are late to emerge, including "r," "l," "s," "z," voiced and voiceless "th," "sh," "zh," "ch," "dg." It is also interesting that the greatest differences in age of acquisition among the three studies occur on many of these sounds. Additional examination of the findings reveals that plosives are acquired fairly early and continuing sounds are acquired later and that the voiced sounds in cognate pairs tend to be mastered later than their voiceless partners.

Even though these data seem to provide general normative guidelines concerning the mastery of phonemes, they should be viewed with caution. Sander (1972), after reviewing and reanalyzing the data from the Wellman et al. (1931) and Templin (1957) studies, suggests that the ages of mastery derived from these findings should not be understood as representing average ages of mastery. Sander argues that because of the stringent criterion levels used in these early cross-sectional studies, the ages of mastery represent the upper limits for phonemic acquisition.

According to Sander (1972), we should distinguish between the age of customary production and mastery. **Customary production** is correct production of a phoneme in two of three word positions by 50 percent of the subjects at a given age level. **Mastery** is correct production of a phoneme in all appropriate word positions by 90 percent of the subjects at a specified age level. This distinction results in very different interpretations of phonetic acquisition by age levels. Using Sander's reanalyzed data, for example, "g" is produced correctly in at least two word positions by 50 percent of two-year-old children, but it is not produced correctly in all three positions by 90 percent of children until the age of four years. The phoneme "b" is customarily produced by children younger than two years but is not mastered until four years. The distinction between customary production and mastery is useful because it acknowledges that there are individual variations among children while still allowing a sense of what we can expect in phonemic acquisition by age levels.

Consider what we can conclude about phonemic acquisition based on the findings of large, cross-sectional studies, specifically the studies mentioned here. We can conclude that there is a tendency for some sounds to emerge before others, but we must be careful not to assume that there is a specific order of mastery. As we have already noted, wide individual differences exist among children, which are reflected, to some extent, even in the data provided by these researchers. For example, most of Templin's subjects were producing "r" by four years, but some of Poole's subjects did not produce "r" correctly until seven and a half years. All of Poole's subjects were producing "t" correctly by four and a half years, while most of Templin's subjects were six before they mastered the "t." This latter difference is an excellent example, however, of how even a small methodological variation can affect results. As Sander (1972) notes, Templin (1957) found a late age of mastery for "t" because her younger subjects did not produce a voiceless "t" in the word-medial position. She did not take into account the fact that in American English, when "t" occurs in the word-medial position and follows a stressed vowel, it is typically produced with voicing. This means that any speaker is likely to say a word such as *"dating"* as though it were *"dading."* An unrealistic expectation, therefore, undoubtedly resulted in a spuriously high age of mastery.

It is also prudent to note that longitudinal, or diary, data on phonemic acquisition in individual children and the results of studies of small groups of children attest that the individual variability in phonemic acquisition is so great that establishing reliable norms is difficult at best. We should use ages of customary production and mastery, therefore, only as general guidelines for understanding phonemic acquisition and for making determinations about how an individual child is progressing in his own phonemic development.

Finally, we must consider the perspective maintained by those who conducted the early cross-sectional studies of phonemic development. They took the view that children acquire phonemes as whole units. Acquisition, therefore, is an all-or-nothing proposition. This means that if a child is producing voiceless "th" for "s," he is given no credit for what he obviously knows about the target sound. He knows that "s" is a fricative, that it is voiceless, and that it is produced in the anterior portion of the mouth. His production is just slightly off target in terms of place of production. Instead of having the tongue tip against the alveolar ridge, he has moved it forward between the teeth. There is the assumption in the phoneme-by-phoneme view of acquisition that unless the target sound is produced in a completely correct manner, the phoneme does not exist in the child's sound system. Considering that the voiceless "th" for "s" substitution reflects more knowledge of the target sound than ignorance, this seems a harsh assumption. As you will see, more recent theories give the child credit for understanding the pieces of the phonemic jigsaw puzzle, not just the complete puzzle.

The Behaviorist Theory

One of the most popular theories of phonological acquisition during the 1950s and 1960s was the *behaviorist theory*, originally formulated by Mowrer (1952) but later adapted by other influential phonologists (Olmsted, 1966; Winitz, 1969). This theory emphasizes selective reinforcement and the role of the child's caregiver in the acquisition process.

Mowrer suggests that there are fairly discrete steps through which the child's vocalizations are gradually shaped as they become more and more similar to the speech patterns of her adult models. In the beginning, the child identifies with the primary caregiver, usually the mother, and attends to her speech patterns during pleasurable activities such as feeding, bathing, and fondling. As the child associates the mother's speech patterns with the pleasures of these nurturing activities, the mother's speech patterns themselves become secondary reinforcers. Because the infant's speechlike productions resemble the mother's speech patterns in certain basic respects, they also develop secondary reinforcing traits. The mother, other adults, and the child herself will selectively reinforce those utterances produced by the child that are the most adultlike until the child's phonological system includes just those sounds that are germane to her language.

Even though this theory is appealing because it emphasizes the role of the mother, and most of us would like to believe that mothers—or other caregivers—play a major role in all aspects of child development, it is not a widely accepted theory today. Critics point out that we do not have evidence supporting the dominant role of reinforcement in the acquisition process, and we do not have evidence that mothers, or other caregivers, selectively reinforce the adultlike productions in their children's speech. Most important, the behaviorist theory suggests that children learn phonology in much the same way animals are conditioned to learn tricks, a view not consistent with the present belief that children are not passive and manipulated creatures but are very active in phonological acquisition. That is, they explore, discover, create, apply, retain, and throw away until all the pieces are finally in place.

Structuralist Theory

The *structuralist theory* was formulated by Jakobson in 1941 and was translated into English in 1968. While this theory and the behaviorist theory both focus on the relationship between babbling and the emergence of meaningful speech, they are contrasts in at least one important respect. The behaviorist theory suggests that babbling is continuous with meaningful speech in the sense that babbling drifts into meaningful speech. The structuralist theory is based on the discontinuity view that suggests that babbling and meaningful speech are two clearly separate periods of speech production. During babbling, the child's productions are random, transitory, and extremely diverse, reflecting sounds heard in many of the world's languages. Furthermore, the sounds in babbling do not emerge in any particular or meaningful order. When meaningful speech begins, the child loses his ability to produce an unlimited variety of sounds. His sound inventory is dramatically reduced, and true speech sounds emerge slowly, in a predictable order, until the phonological system of the child's native language is complete.

Phonological development in meaningful speech follows a predictable, universal, and innately determined order, based in large part, on fundamental contrasts among speech sounds. In the beginning, the child's productions reflect mastery of major contrasts, such as vowel versus consonant and oral versus nasal. As development proceeds, the child makes narrower contrasts, filling the gaps between the larger contrasts. When she has mastered all the contrasts inherent in the phonological system of her language, she will produce all the sounds included in that system.

Longitudinal studies of phonological acquisition and the large-scale studies completed by Wellman et al. (1931), Poole (1934), Templin (1957), and Sander (1972) suggest an order of acquisition of phonemes that is consistent with Jakobson's assertions about an order of contrasts. For example, these studies confirm, as suggested by Jakobson's claims, that children acquire plosives and nasals before they acquire fricatives, affricates, and liquids and that front consonants emerge before back consonants. Critics point out, however, that we have no evidence supporting Jakobson's assertion that this order is universal. More importantly and contrary to the basic premise of the structuralist theory, we know that the emergence of sounds in babbling is not irregular or random. We know that babbling and true speech are not two distinct and unrelated periods of vocalization, that children babble for several months after they begin to produce meaningful words.

Natural Phonology Theory

According to the *natural phonology theory* (Donegan & Stampe, 1979; Stampe, 1969, 1973), the child does not actually *acquire* a phonological system. Rather, he suppresses processes that do not occur in the phonological system of his language. Stampe, like Jakobson, asserts that phonological development is universal. Jakobson saw universality in the contrasts the child must master in order to acquire his sound system. Stampe argues that all children are born with the same set of phonological processes, rules by which "phonological oppositions" are modified to reflect the natural "restrictions of the human speech capacity." The child's challenge, as he puts his phonological system together, is to discover the processes that must be suppressed in his language. The English-speaking child, for example, must suppress **consonant sequence reduction, postvocalic consonant devoicing,** and **liquid gliding** because in English phonology, consonant sequences must be complete, postvocalic consonants are sometimes voiced, and there is a phonemic difference between a liquid and a glide.

Some of the criticisms leveled at the natural phonology theory focus on Stampe's most basic theoretical tenet that phonological processes are "mental operations." Since we cannot identify the cognitive functions associated with the use of phonological processes or with their suppression, it is difficult to determine how one can prove or disprove Stampe's assertion. A more common criticism of this theory concerns Stampe's assumption that children perceive words and their segmental components the same way adults do, and that whatever differences there are between the speech forms of children and the speech forms of adults reflect production constraints, not perceptual limitations, on the part of children. Data to support this assumption about the perceptual abilities of children during the phonological acquisition period are not available, yet the assumption is key to the theory's viability.

Prosodic Theory

In at least one important respect, the *prosodic theory* (Waterson, 1971, 1981) stands in stark contrast to the natural phonology theory. Whereas Stampe assumes that children's perceptual abilities are complete and accurate at the beginning of true speech production, Waterson believes that the child's perceptual abilities, like his production abilities, are incomplete and emerging when language development is beginning. Furthermore, she believes that words, rather than speech sounds, should be viewed as the most basic phonological structures. Accordingly, she describes words in terms of their suprasegmental features as well as their segmental features. According to this view, the child attends to and perceives the salient characteristics of words. These salient characteristics might include segmental features such as nasality, voicing, and manner class, but they also include prosodic or suprasegmental features such as intonational patterns and stress. In the early stages of phonological development, the child struggles to match adult models in terms of segmental and surprasegmental features. The child's phonological system matures as a consequence of mastering information in both parts of the system, that part concerned with phonemes and that part concerned with the prosodic characteristics superimposed on sounds sequenced into syllables, words, and phrases.

Because the prosodic theory takes a wider view of phonological development than other theories, it provides a reasonable explanation for the great variability of phonological productions by context. That is, if a child's productions are influenced not only by her attention to phonemic characteristics but also by her attention to elements of prosody, we would expect wide variations in production because the combination of segmental and suprasegmental features will vary widely from one linguistic context to another. Unfortunately, this theory deals only with the earliest stages of phonological development, and although it accounts for intrapersonal variability, it does not account for the common patterns of phonological development we observe in children as a group.

Cognitive Theory

As is true of the prosodic theory, the *cognitive theory*, or the similar *interactionist-discovery* or *problem-solving theory*, focuses on the early stages of word acquisition (Ferguson, 1978, 1986; Macken & Ferguson, 1983; Menn, 1976, 1983). Both the prosodic theory and the cognitive theory suggest that during the early stages of production, the child addresses words rather than the sound segments of words, and both theories emphasize individual variations in phonological development. The cognitive theory is, in part at least, a reaction to the assertion in other theories that phonological development occurs in a universal, highly predictable, linear manner, and to the failure of other theories to account for individual variability in phonological development.

The cognitive theory suggests that although all children face the same challenges in mastering the phonological systems of their languages, and although they all devise strategies for meeting these challenges, they do not all develop the same strategies. While proponents of this theory concede that there are some universal or nearly universal patterns in phonological development, they believe these tendencies are the products of the uniform development of children's auditory and speech systems.

The primary focus of the cognitive theory is on what happens as each child confronts the challenges he perceives in the words he hears. Each child notices phonological patterns in his developing vocabulary. These patterns may reflect understandings of what adults know as distinctive features or syllabic shapes. The child then formulates phonological rules he applies to new words that contain the sound features he knows or the syllabic shapes with which he is familiar. Different children will recognize different patterns and develop different rules, but they will choose words to add to their vocabularies that are characterized by the patterns they recognize, and they tend to reject words characterized by patterns they do not recognize. As development proceeds, the child continues to develop new hypotheses about how the phonological system works. If these hypotheses seem viable within his communicative experiences, he retains them. If a given hypothesis is not viable, he will revise it and test it again.

This process presumably continues until the child's hypotheses are consistent with those that underlie the rules of the adult phonological system. Along the way, he will generalize when generalizations are not appropriate according to adult usage, he will reduce long words by deleting syllables, and he may even appear to regress because he will replace words he acquired as whole units with words designed according to his rules. He might, for example, produce a word such as *blue* with both sounds of the prevocalic cluster intact, only to reduce the word to *bue* a few months later. While this might seem to be a clear regression, it may be that the child is applying a newly formulated phonological rule regarding prevocalic clusters, which is that two-segment clusters should be reduced to one segment, and if one of the two segments is a liquid, that is the segment that will be deleted.

Although the cognitive theory appeals to those who believe the child is an active agent in phonological development, it may go too far in its emphasis on individual exploration and hypothesis building and testing. Critics suggest that this theory does not adequately account for limits on learning imposed by the physical and psychological maturation of the child. It does not address later phonological development, and it gives too little attention to the universal patterns of phonological acquisition noted in large-scale studies.

Biological Theory

As the name implies, the biological theory (Locke, 1980, 1983; Locke & Pearson, 1992) suggests that phonological development, especially its early stages, can be explained on the basis of biological forces. All children, regardless of the language environments in which they are reared, are born with the same basic perceptual abilities and tendencies. All children are innately predisposed to produce the same articulatory motor acts.

Vocalizations during babbling, for example, are the products of these innate abilities and tendencies, and for this reason, the babblings of children from widely varying language environments sound the same. Because the sounds heard in late babbling and the phonological patterns in early words are remarkably similar, Locke argues that the phonological patterns observed in early words are also universal. When the child begins to produce true words, the influence of her language on her phonological system begins, but this influence is minimal until the child's vocabulary begins to expand dramatically at about eighteen months. At this point, in what Locke sees as the third of three major stages of phonological development, the biological forces that have been primarily responsible for development begin to interact with cognitive factors, eventually driving the child to complete the phonological system of her native language.

Most theorists are reasonably comfortable with the notion that biological forces influence the earliest stages of speech development, and most would probably accept the idea that there are some universal phonological patterns during these early stages. Critics of the biological theory suggest, however, that Locke places too much emphasis on the innateness of the acquisition process and gives too little attention to the variability of development that has been well documented in the research literature, including evidence that a child's native language might influence productions during the first year (de Boysson–Bardies & Vihman, 1991).

What Do We Make of All This?

The differences that exist among theories of phonological development bring us back to the old nature-versus-nurture debate. Is phonological development a universal experience and primarily the product of biological forces, as suggested by the structuralist theory and the biological theory, or is it primarily the product of environment, as suggested by the behaviorist theory? What is the role of the child in phonological acquisition? Is he a fairly passive experiencer, as suggested by the behaviorist theory and the natural phonology theory, or is he an active and creative participant in the process, as suggested by the cognitive theory or its close cousin, the interactionist-discovery theory? We find that some theories successfully account for individual differences that exist among children who are acquiring their sound systems but fail to account for universal tendencies, and other theories focus on general or universal patterns without giving adequate attention to individual variations in phonological acquisition.

As is almost always true in this kind of debate, we will eventually find that the answer lies somewhere in the middle of the argument's extremes. The *self-organizing theory* (Lindblom, 1992) seems to represent a step in that direction. This theory takes both biological factors and language environment into account. It begins with the assumption that the phonological systems of all languages have been gradually shaped to accommodate the perceptual needs of listeners and the productive needs of speakers. That is, speakers need phonological features that make production manageable, and listeners need phonological features that make sounds and words easy to discriminate. When the needs of both speaker and listener are met, we are given phonological systems that contain segments common to most languages and segments that are unique to languages that have exceptionally large phonemic repertoires. Part of phonological development, from this point of view, involves the discovery of universal patterns, but the development of a particular language's phonological system will not be complete until the child also discovers the patterns unique to that language.

Whatever we might conclude about the value of any of the theories briefly described in this section, we can certainly agree that the process of phonological acquisition is far more complex than envisioned by Wellman, Poole, and Templin. We can also agree that we are still searching for a theory that addresses all relevant aspects of development. Such a theory will address the cognitive and perceptual aspects of oral communication as well as the productive aspects. It will account for how developing cognitive and perceptual abilities are related to the neuromuscular requirements for speech. It will certainly attempt to reconcile universal patterns of phonological development with individual variations in acquisition tied to language environment and to children's active role in the process of discovering phonological patterns. Such a theory will address how children formulate hypotheses about how these patterns work and should be applied to newly acquired words, how they test their hypotheses in real-life communication challenges, and use their communicative experiences to help build the phonological systems of their languages.

Someone once observed that the more you know, the more you know what you don't know, and that is certainly true in our attempts to understand speech and language, even in an area like phonology, which at one time seemed so simple. Seventy-five to fifty years ago, researchers such as Wellman, Poole, and Templin thought all we needed to do was count the bricks—the sounds of speech—but the more we have learned about phonology, the more complex we have discovered it to be. It is impossible to separate what the child produces from what he hears. It is impossible to separate what the child performs from what she understands, and it is impossible to separate what she knows and understands from the physical processes that generate speech sounds. Although we are learning more about these intricately interconnected relationships every day, we must accept that a complete understanding of the development of phonology lies somewhere in the future.

Review Questions

1. Define the following terms: *phonology, phoneme,* and *allophone.*
2. What are the three means by which consonants are classified in traditional phonetics?
3. How are vowels classified in traditional phonetics?
4. What is a cognate pair? Identify three cognate pairs among English consonants.
5. What does it mean to say that the distinctive features approach to phonology extends traditional phonetics and that the phonological processes approach to phonology extends the distinctive features approach?
6. What is a phonological process?
7. What is co-articulation? What is the difference between anticipatory and retentive co-articulation?
8. What accounts for changes in the child's vocalizations over the course of her first year?
9. Differentiate the following terms: *cooing, babbling,* and *variegated babbling.*
10. Briefly explain the babbling drift theory and the discontinuity theory. Why has each, as a sole explanation of the relationship between babbling and true speech, been dismissed?
11. What are protowords? What does the existence of protowords suggest about the relationship between babbling and true speech?
12. What are the most common manners and the most common places of articulation of the sounds used by the child in his first true words?
13. How does the metalinguistic awareness facilitated by learning to read and write help the child better understand her phonological system?
14. Briefly describe each of the following views of phonological development: phoneme-by-phoneme, behaviorist

theory, structuralist theory, natural phonology theory, prosodic theory, cognitive theory, and biological theory.

15. How does the nature-versus-nurture argument fit into the varying theories of phonological development?

16. In what sense is the self-organizing theory a compromise between the nature and nurture extremes?

17. Identify the essential issues that should be addressed by a viable and comprehensive theory of phonological development.

References and Suggested Readings

Bauman-Waengler, J. (2004). *Articulatory and phonological impairments: A clinical focus* (2nd ed.). Boston: Allyn & Bacon.

Bernthal, J., & Bankson, N. (2004). *Articulation and phonological disorders* (5th ed.). Boston: Allyn & Bacon.

Blache, S. (1978). *The acquisition of distinctive features.* Baltimore: University Park Press.

Blache, S. (1982). Minimal word-pairs and distinctive feature training. In M. Crary (Ed.), *Phonological intervention, concepts and procedures* (pp. 66–96). San Diego, CA: College-Hill.

de Boysson–Bardies, B., & Vihmann, M. (1991). Adaptation to language. *Language, 61,* 297–319.

Chomsky, N., & Halle, M. (1968). *The sound patterns of English.* New York: Harper & Row.

Donegan, P., & Stampe, D. (1979). The study of natural phonology. In D. A. Dinnsen (Ed.), *Current approaches to phonological theory* (pp. 126–173). Bloomington: Indiana University Press.

Eisenson, J. (1985). *Voice and diction: A program for improvement* (5th ed.). New York: Macmillan.

Ferguson, C. (1978). Learning to pronounce: The earliest stages of phonological development in the child. In F. D. Minifie & L. L. Lloyd (Eds.), *Communicative competence and cognitive abilities.* Baltimore: University Park Press.

Ferguson, C. (1986). Discovering sound units and constructing sound systems: It's child's play. In J. S. Perkell & D. H. Klatt (Eds.), *Invariance and variability of speech processes.* Hillsdale, NJ: Erlbaum.

Ferguson, C., Menn, L., & Stoel-Gammon, C. (Eds.). (1992). *Phonological development: Models, research, implications.* Timonium, MD: York Press.

Hockett, C. (1955). A manual of phonology. In *International Journal of American Linguistics (Memoir II).* Baltimore: Waverly.

Hodson, B., & Paden, E. (1983). *Targeting intelligible speech.* San Diego, CA: College-Hill.

Hodson, B., & Paden, E. (1991). *Targeting intelligible speech* (2nd ed.). Austin, TX: PRO-ED.

Hoffman, P. (1990). Spelling, phonology, and the speech-language pathologist: A whole language perspective. *Language, Speech, Hearing Services in Schools, 21,* 238–243.

Ingram, D., Christensen, D., Veach, S., & Webster, B. (1980). The acquisition of word-initial fricatives and affricates in English by children between 2 and 6 years. In G. Yeni-Komshian, J. Kavanaugh, & C. Ferguson (Eds.), *Child phonology: Vol. 2. Production.* New York: Academic Press.

Jakobson, R. (1968). *Child language, aphasia, and phonological universals* (A. R. Keiler, Trans.). The Hague: Mouton.

Katz, W., Kripke, C., & Tallal, R. (1991). Anticipatory coarticulation in the speech of adults and young children: Acoustic, perceptual and video data. *Journal of Speech and Hearing Research, 34,* 1222–1249.

Lindblom, B. (1992). Phonological units as adaptive emergents of lexical development. In C. A. Ferguson, L. Menn, & C. Stoel-Gammon (Eds.), *Phonological development: Models, research, implications.* Parkton, MD: York.

Lleo, C. (1990). Homonymy and reduplication: On the extended availability of two strategies in phonological acquisition. *Journal of Child Language, 17,* 267–278.

Locke, J. (1980). The prediction of child speech errors: Implications for a theory of acquisition. In G. Yeni-Komshian, J. F. Kavanaugh, & C. A. Ferguson (Eds.), *Child phonology (Vol. 1).* New York: Academic Press.

Locke, J. (1983). *Phonological acquisition and change.* New York: Academic Press.

Locke, J., & Pearson, D. (1992). Vocal learning and emergence of phonological capacity: A neurobiological approach. In C. A. Ferguson, L. Menn, & C. Stoel-Gammon (Eds.), *Phonological development: Models, research, implications.* Parkton, MD: York.

Lowe, R. (1994). *Phonology, assessment and intervention applications in speech pathology.* Baltimore: Williams & Wilkens.

Macken, M., & Ferguson, C. (1983). Cognitive aspects of phonological development: Model, evidence and issues. In K. E. Nelson (Ed.), *Children's language* (Vol. 4, pp. 256–282). Hillsdale, NJ: Erlbaum.

Menn, L. (1976). Evidence for an interactionist-discovery theory of child phonology. *Papers and Reports on Child Language Development, 12,* 169–177.

Menn, L. (1983). Development of articulatory, phonetic, and phonological capabilities. In B. Butterworth (Ed.), *Language production* (Vol. 2.) London: Academic Press.

Mowrer, O. (1952). Speech development in the young child: The autism theory of speech development and some clinical applications. *Journal of Speech and Hearing Disorders, 17,* 263–268.

Ohde, R., & Sharf, D. (1992). *Phonetic analysis of normal and abnormal speech.* Upper Saddle River, NJ: Merrill/Prentice Hall.

Olmsted, D. (1966). A theory of the child's learning of phonology. *Language, 42,* 531–535.

Paul, R., & Jennings, P. (1992). Phonological behavior in toddlers with slow expressive language development. *Journal of Speech and Hearing Research, 35,* 99–107.

Poole, I. (1934). Genetic development of articulation of consonant sounds in English. *Elementary English Review, 11,* 159–161.

Prather, E., Hedrick, D., & Kern, C. (1975). Articulation development in children aged two to four years.

Journal of Speech and Hearing Disorders, 40, 179–191.

Sander, E. (1972). When are speech sounds learned? *Journal of Speech and Hearing Disorders, 37,* 55–63.

Spencer, A. (1996). *Phonology, theory and description.* Cambridge, MA: Blackwell.

Stampe, D. (1969). The acquisition of phonetic representation. In *Papers from the fifth regional meeting of the Chicago Linguistic Society* (pp. 433–444). Chicago: Chicago Linguistic Society.

Stampe, D. (1973). *A dissertation on natural phonology.* Unpublished doctoral dissertation, University of Chicago.

Stoel-Gammon, C., & Dunn, C. (1985). *Normal and disordered phonology in children.* Baltimore: University Park Press.

Templin, M. (1957). Certain language skills in children: Their development and interrelationships. *Institute of Child Welfare Monographs* (Vol. 26). Minneapolis: University of Minnesota Press.

Vihman, M. (1996). *Phonological development: The origins of language in the child.* Cambridge, MA: Blackwell.

Waterson, N. (1971). Child phonology: A prosodic view. *Journal of Linguistics, 7,* 179–211.

Waterson, N. (1981). A tentative developmental model of phonological representation. In T. Myers, J. Laver, & J. Anderson (Eds.), *The cognitive representation of speech.* Amsterdam: North-Holland.

Wellman, B., Case, I., Mengert, E., & Bradbury, D. (1931). *Speech sounds of young children.* University of Iowa Studies in Child Welfare. Iowa City: University of Iowa Press.

Winitz, H. (1969). *Articulatory acquisition and behavior.* Upper Saddle River, NJ: Prentice Hall.

8

Language Diversity:
Regional, Social/Cultural,
and Gender Differences

Throughout this book, we have stressed that language is a universal human phenomenon. People are all born with the same genetic predispositions for language use, and although people have different experiences with their speech and language models, most are exposed to adequate samples of speech and language and have normal interactive relationships with their models. We do not have to travel very far outside our homes or neigh-

borhoods, however, to discover that there are some significant differences in language. In some cases, of course, people speak different languages, but even within a single language, there are differences.

In this chapter, we consider differences within a national language, differences called *dialects*. We examine some of the characteristics of major dialects and consider how they have evolved. We also consider differences in language that are the products of gender. Specifically, this chapter is designed to facilitate understanding of the following topics:

- Variables that influence the acquisition of language and language behaviors

- Meanings of key terms such as dialect, accent, standard dialect, and nonstandard dialect

- Lexical characteristics of several easily recognizable regional dialects

- History and continuing evolution of three social/cultural dialects of American English: African American English Hispanic English, and Asian English

- Cultural diversity in U.S. public schools

- Gender differences in language

Although children are born to talk, they are not born to speak a particular language or to speak a particular variation of a language. If a child is born in Paris to French-speaking parents, he will speak French. If a child is born to Korean parents but adopted shortly after her birth by English-speaking parents who live in Peoria, Illinois, she will speak English, and she will speak the same kind of English modeled for her by her adoptive parents. A black child reared by white parents will speak the dialect of his parents, not African American English, and a white child growing up in a predominantly black community will speak the dialect to which she has been exposed. We have purposely belabored the message here in the hope that it will be clearly understood and not soon forgotten. That is, the language one speaks and the variation of the language one speaks are not products of biology. They are products of environment.

According to Taylor (1990, p. 132), seven major variables influence the acquisition of language and language behaviors: (1) race and ethnicity; (2) social class, education, and occupation; (3) region; (4) gender; (5) situation or context; (6) peer group association or identification; and (7) first language community or culture. It should be obvious that these factors operate in an interactive manner to determine the language one speaks, and it should be equally obvious that the language one uses in one situation with one group of people may differ from the language one uses in another situation with a different group of people. This might mean, for example, that the Vietnamese child who emigrated to the United States with his family speaks Vietnamese to his parents but speaks English to his U.S. friends. It might also mean that a black child uses African American English when conversing with her family but uses Standard American English at school, and it might mean that a white child attending a predominantly black school uses African American English when talking with her black friends even though she speaks Standard American English at home.

What Is a Dialect?

It should be apparent that the issue of language variation is fraught with sensitivities. We must take care to approach this topic with thoughtful and considerate respect, beginning with an understanding of dialect. The term **dialect** is used often, and it is often used with incomplete understanding. Wolfram and Christian (1989) suggest that dialect should be understood in a "technical" sense as well as the "popular" sense. Wolfram and Christian define dialect as "any given variety of a language shared by a group of speakers" (p. 1). Taylor (1990) offers a more elaborate version of the same definition: "A dialect is a variety of language that has developed through a complex interplay of historical, social, political, educational, and linguistic forces" (p. 131). All students of dialectology and sociolinguistics would agree that dialect should be understood and treated as a neutral term.

A dialect typically corresponds with other differences among groups of people who happen to be united by culture, social class, or region. That is, people who live in the same region and who share cultural, ethnic, educational, and social values tend to speak the same variety of their national language. The dialect spoken by any given group of people is neither superior nor inferior to the dialect spoken by any other group of people. It must also be understood that every speaker of a given language speaks a dialect of that language. There is no Absolute Standard English, for example, against which variations are evaluated. There are dialects of English spoken by many people and dialects spoken by fewer people, but number of speakers does not indicate superiority or correctness. Every dialect of English is linguistically correct within the rules that govern it, and every dialect of English is as valid as any other.

The popular or common lay understanding of dialect has at least two problems. First, some people use the term *dialect* as a synonym for *language*, especially when they are not adequately informed about the languages in a particular region of the world. Most people would not refer to the languages spoken by people living in Europe as dialects because they are familiar with some of the common languages of Europe, including French, Spanish, German, Russian, and so on, but they might refer to the languages spoken by people living in Africa as dialects because they do not know the languages of Africa. At the same time, these people might not realize that there are many distinct dialects of Chinese and that there are dialects of French, Spanish, German, and all major languages of the world.

A second and more troubling problem associated with the popular understanding of dialect centers on evaluating language differences as good/bad or standard/nonstandard. Such judgments are social rather than linguistic because, as we have already noted, every dialect is linguistically legitimate. A person from a northern state might judge the dialects of people from the southern states to be nonstandard or inferior, but a person from a southern state might make the same negative judgments about the speech of Yankees. In reference to English, it is best to understand that there are a number of standard dialects. A *standard dialect* is a variety of a language spoken by people of relatively high status who have economic, political, social, and educational power. Those who speak a standard dialect often maintain condescending attitudes toward other dialects and the people who speak them, but one must always keep in mind that standard is relative. The standard dialect of the rich and powerful in Texas is not the same as the standard dialect of the rich and powerful in New York, so that what is standard in one place may be nonstandard in another place.

If we accept that there are standard dialects of English, we must accept that there are nonstandard dialects as well. This is not a problem, as long as we remember that nonstandard does not mean inferior. Another term sometimes used for nonstandard dialect is **vernacular dialect.** This may be a better term because it does not connote value. *Vernacular* emphasizes what Wolfram and Christian (1989) refer to as the "indigenous community dimension of these language varieties" (p. 3).

Whether dialects are standard or vernacular, the differences that separate them occur in grammar, phonology, semantics, vocabulary, pragmatics, and all other dimensions of language. In our discussion of dialects, we consider some of these differences in several major categories of language differences: (1) regional, (2) social/cultural, and (3) gender.

What Is an Accent?

Before we continue with our discussion of dialect, we should differentiate between *dialect* and *accent*. These terms are sometimes treated as synonyms by laypersons. Is there a difference, for example, between a southern dialect and a southern accent? The two terms can be separated if one understands **accent** to indicate characteristics of speech or variations in pronunciation and **dialect** to indicate language differences as well as speech differences (Abercrombie, 1967, p. 19). Understood in this way, dialect is the broader term and subsumes accent. If a listener perceives only pronunciation differences in the speech of someone else and no language differences, he is perceiving an accent. If he hears pronunciation and language differences, he is hearing a dialect that differs from his own.

Regional Dialects

For the sake of convenience, we assume greater homogeneity within each identified regional dialect than actually exists. In fact, it is difficult to clearly separate social dialect from regional dialect. Technically, a **regional dialect** refers to a variety of language used by people living in a restricted geographic area, but within that area several social dialects may be spoken by people who are grouped by factors other than geography, including social class, ethnicity, educational level, occupation, and religion. The social dialect is influenced by the regional dialect, however, so that a group of people linked by factors such as those identified here have a different dialect in Houston than in Boston. In other words, regional and social dialects interact, producing variations within dialects of language.

As you might imagine, not all experts agree about the number of regional dialects because they do not all draw lines on dialectal maps in exactly the same places, and regional dialects are defined according to geographic boundaries. Taylor suggests that the United States has at least ten regional dialects. (1990, p. 133). According to Carver (1987), a specialist in regional U.S. dialects, there are six major regions, which can be divided into many layers and subregions. There are five places along the eastern and southern coasts of the United States from which most regional dialects have evolved: Boston, Philadelphia, tidewater Virginia, Charleston, and New Orleans (Carver, 1987, p. 7). These centers are called **cultural hearths.** In some cases, as in Boston, the original dialectal influences remain strong. In others, the original dialect has been largely lost. In all cases, American dialects constantly evolve as a result of changes in population centers. Because we tend to be increasingly mobile and increasingly connected to one another through a variety of mass media, dialects will continue to evolve, eroding many of the speech and language differences that now exist.

Our discussion of regional dialects includes samples of language differences that have been noted and explained by Carver (1987). This analysis is certainly not complete in breadth or depth but provides you with a sense of the dialectal differences that exist in the United States. Regional dialects are characterized by differences in all components of language, including phonology, grammar, and semantics, but the dimension most affected is vocabulary. Certain words that are common to the vocabularies of people living in New England may be unknown to people living in the Midwest. Some words are used and defined differently from region to region. Our discussion focuses on selected examples of these vocabulary differences in just three of the six regions identified by Carver.

The New England and Northeast Region

When many of us think about the speech of people who live in New England, especially in the Boston area, we think about what these people do with the *r*. That is, they drop the *r* when it should be present in a word, and they sometimes add it where it does not belong. The Bostonian might say *"ca"* for *car*, for example, but he might say *"tuber"* for *tuba*. As with all regional dialects, however, the most notable features of the dialects in this region are in word usage.

The past and present of New England have been powerfully influenced by the sea, and this influence is observed in the language of the people in this area. They use words such as *nor'easter* and *nor'wester* to describe the movements of winds and storms. When the wind calms, they say it is *lulling down;* when the wind increases, they say it is *breezing up*. Some words that were originally nautical terms have developed broader usage. For example, a *bulkhead* refers to a partition between compartments of a ship. The term is now used in New England to refer to the sloping doors of a cellar.

Those who came to this part of the country from England sometimes found new phenomena for which they had no vocabulary, so they adapted words to describe these things. The weather in England, for example, is fairly constant, but the weather in New England changes rapidly and often. Nautical folks in the eighteenth century referred to a sunny day as an *open* day, so that over time the expression *open-and-shut day* came to mean a day when the clouds come and go. Settlers from England were also unfamiliar with mountain passes, so, using a word known to them, they called this kind of opening between mountains a *notch*.

Many terms in the dialects of this region reflect, not influences of the sea, but experiences of rural living. *Creepers*, for example, are metal cleats fastened to boots for

The influence of the sea is apparent in New England dialects.

the purpose of providing sure footing on ice. A bobsled is called a *double runner, double ripper,* or *traverse sled.* When one hauls something, he *carts* or *teams* it. If a horse or cow is uncooperative or mean, it is described as *ugly,* but an *ugly top cow* is a bull, and not necessarily an ill-tempered bull. Cow or horse manure is called *top dressing* or *meadow dressing.* A *wheel harrow* is a farm implement used to break up clumps of plowed dirt, and a *bush scythe* is used to clear brush or weeds. When the farmer spreads his hay so that it can dry, he *tedders* it. After he tedders the hay, he *tumbles* it, which means that he stacks it for curing, and then he *mows it away,* which means that he stores it in a barn.

This region has produced many unique terms for food items. Some of these terms, such as *Boston brown bread* or simply *brown bread,* refer to recipes unique to the region, but most are terms used to name food items found throughout the country. For example, a submarine sandwich is called a *grinder,* and a soft drink is called a *tonic.* Hamburger and frankfurter are often shortened to *hamburg* and *frankfurt.* A poached egg is called a *dropped egg,* a term unique to New England dialects.

Many other terms peculiar to this region do not fit the categories already identified. For example, older residents of the region may refer to a funnel as a *tunnel,* and if liquid poured through the funnel comes out slowly, it is coming out in *dribs and drabs.* An apartment building is called a *tenement,* and a veranda or open porch is called a *piazza.* Someone who is especially rigid or fastidious is called a *fusspot* or *fussbudget.* Taking a shortcut is *cutting cross-lots.*

The Northeast region beyond New England includes New York, most of New Jersey, and Pennsylvania (Carver, 1987, p. 44), but the influences of the dialects in this region extend to the north and west. Since this portion of the region was settled by New Englanders migrating westward, many of the terms used in New England are used by other speakers in the region. Some words, however, are associated with specific areas of this region beyond New England. Although the term *cruller,* referring to a doughnut, is widely used in many areas of the country today, it was originally a word unique to speakers from the Hudson Valley. Speakers from New York refer to a freeway or expressway as a *throughway,* to curdled or sour milk as *lobbered milk,* and to a whisk broom as a *brush broom.* Speakers from the greater New York metropolitan area, including northern New Jersey, refer to a particularly large and aggressive mosquito as a *Jersey mosquito* or *Jersey bomber.* Other words are common to speakers throughout the region, including *nightwalker* for nightcrawler or large earthworm, *soda* for soft drink, *scallion* for small onion, and *grass* for asparagus. There are also slang words or phrases characteristic of the dialects in this region, including *can* in reference to buttocks, *nanna* in reference to one's grandmother, and *get a wiggle on* to mean *hurry up!*

The Northern and Midwest Region

The boundaries of this area are difficult to define with great precision, but it may be useful to think of this region as spreading from coast to coast with the Ohio River as a rough dividing line between North and South. Even though this region covers a wide geographic area, the dialects have been primarily influenced by only two cultural and linguistic hearths: New England and southeastern Pennsylvania. As these cultures moved westward across the United States, they mixed and influenced one another, eventually producing a shared dialect. There are variations within this broad dialect, of course, but our focus is primarily on the common features.

Although some dialects, including the New England dialect, still show influences of older English and include words borrowed from other European languages and American Indian languages, the dialects of this region are remarkably free of these influences. A few words such as the German word *fest,* meaning "festival" or "holiday," are retained in the dialects of the northern/midwest region, but *fest* is most often included within the words *gabfest* or *talkfest* to refer to an informal conversation or gossip session. Other self-explanatory words have been coined from the morpheme *fest,* including *beerfest, slugfest,* and *funfest.* Another word borrowed from German and used in this region is *gesundheit,* an expression used in response to a sneeze. Some speakers who use this expression may believe it means *"God bless you,"* but it is actually just a way of saying, *"I wish you good health."*

A number of slang and colloquial expressions are used throughout the country but are most common in this region. For example, when one works hard, he sweats *like a butcher.* A cigar is called a *rope,* and a cigarette is called a *coffin nail.* A common euphemism for regurgitate is *toss one's cookies.*

Speakers in this region refer to large earthworms as *nightcrawlers* and to fuzzy caterpillars as *woolly bears.* A snapping turtle is called a *snapper,* and bullfrogs are called *croakers.* Tree sap is called *pitch,* and the sugar maple tree is called a *hard maple.*

Speakers in the upper portion of the north region use *squealer* in reference to an informer, *milquetoast* in reference to someone who is shy and timid, *crusty* in reference to someone who is aggressive and nervy, and *souse* to mean a drunk. There are also phrases common to this area, as shown here. The meanings of these phrases should be clear:

I wouldn't run a marathon for *all the tea in China.*

He's always trying *to get the best of* his friends.

Jim's brother is *meaner than dirt.*

Why, I haven't seen that movie *in a dog's age.*

Our television has been *on the fritz* since the storm.

Sally is so boy-crazy. She's always *on the make.*

It's been great talking to you. *See you in church!*

Other words that are especially common in the most northern section of this region include *pollywog* for tadpole, *bloodsucker* for leech, *sticker* for a prickly weed, *sliver* for splinter, *mammoth* for large, *shuck* for removing the covering of something, and *heave* for throw.

The Southern Region

We tend to think of the speech of people who live in the southern states as representing a single dialect. In actuality, there are a variety of dialects in the South, but we treat it as one region and provide dialectal examples from throughout the region. The dividing line between North and South extends westward from central Delaware, along the traditional Mason-Dixon Line and the Ohio River to an area west of the Mississippi River, including some or all of Texas, depending on whose version of the region one accepts.

The dialects of this region are characterized by uniquely American words and phrases, including *snake doctor* for dragonfly, *calling the hogs* for snoring, *egg turner* for spatula, and *cooling board* for the slab on which a corpse is laid. Other words are adaptations of common English words, including *puny* to mean not only small and weak but also sickly, *harp* for harmonica, *rogue* for a thief or scoundrel, *spew* for gush, *slouch* for a bungler or clod, and *piddling around* for wasting time.

Because the south is primarily a rural area, a definite rural flavor is evident in the dialects of the region. Words relating to the farm experience include *hand* for farm worker, *overseer* for supervisor, *dusky dark* for twilight, *critters* for animals, *juicing* for milking cows, and *cowlot* for pasture. If a farmer works too hard, he may feel *wore out,* and if he continues to work too hard, he may *take sick* and lose weight or *fall off* a bit.

Other common words and phrases heard in the dialects of the South include *fussing* for fighting, *draw up* for shrink or squeeze, *slosh* for spill or splash, *johnny* or *commode* for toilet, *booger* for child, *sowbelly* for pork, *calaboose* for jail, *ruther* for preference, *earbob* for earring, *dead cat on the line,* meaning that something is suspicious, and *jumped the broomstick,* for getting married.

One of the more distinct subregions in the south includes Louisiana and especially the area around New Orleans. The French were among the first to settle this area, and even though settlers came from other parts of the world, including Germany, Spain, and what is now known as Nova Scotia, the French influence has remained strong through the years. It is, in fact, this French influence that gives New Orleans its unique character. The dialect of this region retains a distinct French flavor. Carver refers to this dialect as "Louisiana French" (1987, p. 141). It contains words borrowed directly from French and incorporates other words borrowed from British English, Spanish, and Indian languages. Words common to Louisiana French include *armoire* for a dresser or bureau, *gallery* for porch, *lagniappe* for modest gift or bonus, *bayou* for a marshy stream or creek, *pirogue* for canoe, *marais* for swamp, and *coulee* for dry creek bed,

Many people associate New Orleans with excellent French food. Louisiana French includes culinary terms such as *praline* (candy made with pecans and brown sugar), *gumbo* (stew containing meat or seafood and vegetables), *jambalaya* (rice with tomatoes and herbs along with chicken, ham, oysters, or shrimp), *brioche* (coffee cake), *bisque* (cream soup), and *pigeonnier* (roast pigeon).

Social/Cultural Dialects

In introducing the concept of a social/cultural dialect, it is important to reiterate that dialects are not products of biology. In this section, we consider the characteristics of three social/cultural dialects: African American English, Hispanic English, and Asian English. One must not assume, however, that all African American speakers use the same dialect. In fact, some African Americans do not speak African American English as their primary dialect and may not use African American English at all. On the other hand, many whites living in areas where the dominant dialect is African American English use the patterns of that dialect. In the same way, not all Hispanic speakers sound the same. In fact, one should not assume that speakers from a Mexican Spanish background will produce a dialect of English that is exactly the same as the dialect derived from Puerto Rican Spanish. All possible variations of English that fit within the broad African American, Hispanic English, and Asian English categories are the products of social, cultural, ethnic, educational, and occupational influences. These dialects are then influenced by regional dialects, so that African American English in Atlanta, Georgia, differs from African American English in Philadelphia, Pennsylvania, and Hispanic English in New York differs from Hispanic English in Miami.

African American English

Without question, the most studied and most controversial dialect in American English is African American English, which is also called Black Dialect, Black English Vernacular, and Ebonics (Smitherman, 1994, p. 1; Taylor, 1990, p. 140). The controversy surrounding African American English is the result of misunderstanding, ignorance, and the continuing racial prejudices that tend to divide all black/white issues into "good" and "bad." Based on what has been presented in this chapter, you should understand that good and bad have no relevance in any discussion about dialects, because no dialect is inherently superior to any other. Furthermore, it is absolutely unreasonable for any educated person to believe that all African Americans speak African American English. Although there is risk even in the following generalization, it may be relatively safe to say that African American English is the dialect spoken by most working-class African Americans living in working-class African American communities.

Each dialect of a language has its own social and cultural history. African American English has a long, diverse, complex history. According to the **creolist theory,** African American English is a complicated hybrid derived from several African languages and Portuguese, Dutch, French, and English (Taylor, 1990, p. 141). Most of the Africans brought to the United States as slaves came from the west coast of Africa. On the east coast, Swahili was the dominant language, but natives of Africa's west coast spoke hundreds of languages that, although similar in terms of phonology and syntax, had different vocabularies (Taylor, 1972). When speakers of these various languages interacted, they developed common languages so they could communicate with one another. A common language, called a **pidgin,** develops as speakers of a nondominant language accept a few key words, usually related to business or trade, from the dominant language. A pidgin begins as an informal language consisting mostly of nouns and many gestures. As it develops, the pidgin becomes more formal. The vocabulary of the dominant language is absorbed into the nondominant language, which retains revised versions of its original phonological and grammatical systems. When the pidgin becomes the primary language of a group of people, it is called a **creole** language. At this point, the original nondominant language ceases to exist. As the language evolution continues, the creole language becomes increasingly similar to the language of the dominant culture, a process called **decreolization** (Taylor, 1972, pp. 6–7; 1990, pp. 141–142). Part of the development of African American English, then, can be traced to the creolization of the west coast African languages. Elements of these creoles came with the people who were brought to America as slaves.

The influences of European languages on African American English can be traced to the trade initiatives of European countries in Africa. In the early 1500s, Portugal sent ships to West Africa for commercial purposes. Since the Portuguese traders could not learn all the African languages in this area, the Africans learned Portuguese. As one would expect, however, the Portuguese language that became the trading language of West Africa evolved into a creole, the product of Portuguese merged with various African languages. Black Portuguese came to America with the slaves who were brought to Portuguese and Spanish colonies. The Dutch took over Portuguese trading bases in the early 1600s, adding mostly Dutch vocabulary to Black Portuguese. At about this same time, England and France were becoming trading powers in Africa, and their languages were thrown into the mix. The French especially were active in the slave trade, but unlike the Dutch, they did not adopt Black Portuguese as their trade language. Their involvement in the slave markets of Africa, therefore, produced another creole, Black French. The original African American English also came to America by way of the slave trade. Unlike Black Portuguese and Black French, however, African American English became widely and firmly established in the United States because of the constant and intensive contacts between slaves and their English-speaking owners (Taylor, 1972, pp. 6–9).

African American English is a valid and valued dialect.

Although African American English has changed considerably over the years, mostly as a result of social and educational pressures, it remains a distinct dialect with its own identifiable characteristics and rules. All variations between African American English and Standard American English must be understood not as errors but as characteristics of a viable and valid dialect. According to Williams and Wolfram (1977), there are at least twenty-nine linguistic rules of African American English that vary from Standard American English rules. As should be expected, many of these twenty-nine rules overlap the rules of other dialects of Standard American English, especially the standard and nonstandard dialects of the south. Since African Americans have strong historical connections to the southern states, this overlapping of dialects should be viewed as inevitable.

A complete analysis of African American English would require an entire book. Our purposes will be met by including a summary of selected characteristics of African American English. The selections include some features most of you will readily recognize and features that may be less familiar. Unlike regional dialects that are characterized primarily by vocabulary or lexical differences, African American English differs from Standard American English in a variety of ways. There are phonological and syntactic differences as well as lexical differences.

Although the phonological system of African American English contains the same number of sounds as in Standard American English, the rules for using and combining sounds are not the same. For example, in African American English the second of two sounds in a final consonant cluster is often deleted so that *rust* is produced as *rus* and *bend* becomes *ben*. Among the most recognizable features of African

American English are the substitutions for voiced and voiceless "th." That is, "f" is commonly substituted for voiceless "th" in the word final position, as in *toof* for *tooth*, "d" is substituted for voiced "th" in the word initial position, as in *dat* for *that*, and "v" is substituted for voiced "th" when it occurs between vowels, as in *breaving* or *breavin* for *breathing*. In African American English, voiced plosives are typically devoiced in the postvocalic position so that *lid* becomes *lit* and *flag* becomes *flak*. In the word final position, "ng" is often produced as "n" as in *bringin* for *bringing* and *goin* for *going*, although this is a common feature in the speech of many people who do not use African American English. The "r" is often deleted when it occurs between two vowels so that *carrot* sounds like *cat*, and it is typically deleted when it occurs in the word final position or when it precedes another consonant, so that *car* becomes *ca* and *bark* becomes *bak*. In African American English, the "l" is often deleted in the postvocalic position and when it precedes "t," "d," "p," resulting in *te* for *tell*, *bet* for *belt*, *tod* for *told*, and *hep* for *help* (Bernthal & Bankson, 1993, p. 149; Naremore, 1980; Taylor, 1990).

Some of the grammatical differences between African American English and Standard American English center on whether a rule is obligatory or not. In Standard American English, for example, there are obligatory rules for marking plurality and possession. *Dog* is made plural by adding *s* to produce *dogs*. *Dog* is made possessive by adding *'s* to produce *dog's*. In African American English, plurality may be indicated by adding *s*, but it may also be indicated by using words that identify quantity either specifically or generally. This rule results in productions such as *I have two dog* or *I have many dog*. The rule for possession in African American English is similar. That is, possession is understood as long as the possessor is identified, resulting in sentences such as *That's Jim car* or *Mary is John mother*. In Standard American English, a marker for past tense is obligatory, but in African American English a past tense marker is not required, resulting in sentences such as *She talk to me yesterday*, or *We walk to the park last night*. In Standard American English, the copula and auxiliary forms of the verb *to be* are obligatory. In African American English, they may be deleted. For example, *He is a handsome man* might be produced as *He a handsome man*. The auxiliary verb in *They were running fast* might be deleted, resulting in *They running fast*.

Some irregular rules in Standard American English are made regular in African American English. In Standard American English, for example, the third person singular form of a verb differs from the first and second person forms, resulting in *I hit* (first person), *You hit* (second person), and *She hits* (third person singular). In African American English, the irregularity for third person singular forms is eliminated, resulting in *I hit, You hit, She hit*. The past tense copula and auxiliary forms in Standard American English change according to person and number, resulting in productions such as *I was running, You were running, He was running*, and *They were running*. The rule in African American English is regularized so that *was* is used in all cases, resulting in sentences such as *I was running, You was running, He was running*, and *They was running*. Likewise, the present tense forms that change according to person and number in Standard American English are regularized to *is* in African American English, resulting in sentences such as *I is running, You is running*, and *They is running*. In

Standard American English, the article (*a* or *an*) used depends on whether the word modified begins with a vowel or consonant, resulting in *a car* and *an automobile*. In African American English, the rule is made regular by using *a* in all cases to produce *a car* and *a automobile*. In Standard American English, *those* is used in the subject position of a sentence, and *them* is used in the object position, resulting in sentences such as **Those** cars are new, and We washed **them** yesterday. The rule in African American English is regularized so that *them* is used in both the subject and object positions, resulting in sentences such as *Them dogs are ours.*

There are at least two differences between Standard American English and African American English in the production of negation. *Ain't* is a common feature in many dialects of American English as a substitution for *am not, isn't*, and *aren't*. In African American English, *ain't* is substituted for these forms, but it is also used for *haven't, hasn't*, and *didn't* (Taylor, 1990, p. 143). For example, the sentence *She didn't go to school* becomes *She ain't go to school*. We all learned about double negatives in school, and we were all probably taught that two negatives cancel out into a positive, so that *She don't got no money* means that she does, in fact, have money. Despite the warnings, all children and many adults of all dialects use double negatives occasionally. In African American English, the rule is that the more negative terms there are, the more negative the sentence, so that *Joe ain't going to no doctor at no time no how!* conveys a fairly powerful message about what Joe intends *not* to do.

One of the most interesting characteristics of African American English is a syntactic device called *aspect* (Warren-Leubecker & Bohannon, 1989). Most readers will recognize this feature, since it is often included in imitations of African American English. When the speaker wants to convey that an action or state of being is continuing or occurs intermittently, he uses the verb *be*. For example, if the speaker is referring to someone who talks constantly and is now talking, he would say, *He be talking*. If the speaker is referring to someone who seldom talks but is now talking, he would say, *He talking*. In Standard English, both observations would be expressed in the same sentence, *He is talking*. In African American English, *been* is used to describe an action or state of being that occurred a long time ago but no longer exists. To say *Joe been sad* means that Joe was sad a while ago, but he is feeling better now. The Standard American English equivalent of this sentence is *Joe had been sad.* In African American English, the sentence *I been had this cough* means that this is not a recently developed cough but a cough I have had for a long time. What is most interesting about this feature is that there is no directly comparable version of it in Standard American English. Labov (1966) has identified aspect as a feature of several West African languages. It would be reasonable to speculate that this feature of African American English is a remnant of the creole used by the West Africans who were brought to America as part of the slave trade.

One would expect that there would be vocabulary, or lexical, differences between African American English and Standard American English, and there are. Examples abound (Smitherman, 1994). Unfortunately, the lexical characteristics of African American English change so quickly that any examples provided today could be passe by the time you read this paragraph. Some words used in African American English at the end of the twentieth century will persist in the dialect for many years.

Some will be assimilated into other dialects of American English. Many others will be faddish today and historically quaint a few tomorrows from now. Rather than focusing then on an aspect of African American English that evolves faster than our ability to record it, we will turn our attention to the forces that will drive the evolution of the dialect in the future.

Let's begin with a simple but important fact. Not all speakers of African American English will sound the same. No matter how distinctive one might believe this dialect to be, it is not a single dialect. Keep in mind that the communication system of every person who speaks African American English is also subject to the influences of the regional dialect of English spoken where he or she lives. In addition, as noted by Walker (1999, p. 41), the acquisition of African American English by each child is affected by variables such as family environment, learning strategies, the child's gender and age, the parents' occupations, and the family's socioeconomic level. As time passes, the influences of the historical factors that triggered the evolution of African American English become weakened, but a wide range of environmental factors continue to impact this dialect and all dialects.

How children in the present generation acquire language will, in the long term, affect the dialect of the language they speak. Consider the startling changes that have occurred in the written form of English from *Beowulf*, to Shakespearean English, to modern-day English. Now consider that changes in spoken language occur much more quickly than changes in written language. Among the questions that Massey (1996) suggests should direct the study and understanding of the language acquisition of African American children is this one: *What social and cultural factors account for the onset of language development and facilitate the acquisition of language?* The answers to this question will give us some clues about how African American English might change in the near future. No one can predict with any degree of certainty what will happen to any dialect of a national language in the distant future.

Certainly the interactions children have during their developing years will influence not just their language development but their cultural development as well (Taylor & Clarke, 1994). These interactions include but are not limited to the following: child/caregiver, child/family, child/peer, and child/community. If you think about all the variables subsumed within each of these interactions, you will understand that African American English is not now, nor will it ever be, a single dialect. Furthermore, if you consider the power of these interactions to influence the child's development, you will appreciate that the development of African American English will never be static. In fact, the evolution of the dialects of African American English are likely to accelerate during the twenty-first century because people are, at an ever-accelerating rate, becoming connected globally through the power of mass communication, including the Internet. No matter how much isolationists on all continents might object, we are moving toward a global society. One of the consequences of that movement is that distinctions among dialects, even distinctions among languages, will become increasingly blurred.

For the present, and in the historical short-term, dialectal differences are realities. We should understand why these differences exist, and we should appreciate the forces that push dialects to change. It might be useful to remind ourselves that we do not use language, and children do not acquire language, in a vacuum. As is true for children in every group on the planet, African American children acquire language and use language in the context of the culture into which they have been born. This means that African American children are exposed to words, the rules of syntax, semantics, morphology, phonology, and pragmatics at the same time as they are exposed to the music, literature, art, rules of interpersonal relationships, and every other component of their culture. Their language *will* be affected by these factors. Their language *will* be a product of their culture.

It must be strongly emphasized that African Americans cannot be subsumed within a single, homogeneous culture (Taylor & Clarke, 1994), so when we consider the cultural factors that might influence African American English, we must consider a very wide range of cultural factors that might impact a variety of African American English dialects. (No one ever said this was going to be easy and tidy.)

In addition to the fact that African Americans come from different places in the world's geography, we must consider that socioeconomic strata, levels of education, religious backgrounds, differences in family structure, and many other factors impact language development and language use. There is significant diversity in all these factors among African Americans. It is not surprising, therefore, that there is considerable diversity within the various dialects spoken by African Americans. Some of this diversity is within African American English, but some of the diversity can be attributed to factors that have nothing to do with African American English or even some variation of African American culture. We also need to remind ourselves, as Walker notes (1999, p. 42), that some African Americans, especially those who are well educated and members of the middle class, use Standard American English. Some of these speakers may be bidialectal, but others are not.

Table 8.1 offers a comparison of selected African American English features with those same features in what is typically regarded as Standard American English. The table provides a convenient overview of the comparisons made in this section.

Hispanic English

The history of Hispanic English is not as convoluted as the history of African American English because the historical influences in Hispanic English are connected to a single language. This is not to suggest that all forms of Spanish are the same, because that is clearly not true, but African American English is an amalgam of many distinctly different languages spoken by people from widely varying cultures. The evolution of Hispanic English followed a much more direct line from one language spoken by people whose cultures had some common denominators.

By the mid-1500s, Spain had a strong presence on the American continent. Spanish explorers moved to the west and the north across what is now Mexico and the southern portion of the United States, taking their language and their culture with them (Ramirez, 1992). Original Spanish settlements established in the 1500s that

Table 8.1 Comparison of Selected African American English Characteristics and Standard American English

Standard American English	African American English
Final consonant clusters: such as /st/ & /sk/	Tendency to delete second sound of the cluster at the end of words: *rus* for *rust* or *des* for *desk*.
Initial voiced phoneme: th /ð/ as in *that, those, them*	May substitute /d/ in the initial position in a word, as in *dat* for *that*.
Final voiceless phoneme: th /θ/ as *tooth, both*	May substitute /f/ in the final position in a word, as in *toof* for *tooth* or *bof* for *both*.
Intervocalic phoneme: /r/ as in *carrot*	May delete /r/, as in *cat* for *carrot*.
The phoneme /l/ in postvocalic position: may be a final consonant or part of a cluster (e.g., *toll* or *help*).	May delete /l/ in postvocalic position, as in *toe* for *toll*. May delete /l/ when it precedes /t/, /d/, and /p/, as in *bet* for *belt* or *hep* for *help*.
Plural -s: obligatory addition of /-s/ to the end of a word as in *I have two dogs.*	Not obliged to add /s/ if quantifier is present, as in *I have two dog.*
Possessive -s: obligatory addition of /-'s/ to the end of a word as in *That's Jim's car.*	Not obliged to add /'s/ if the possessor is identified in the sentence, as in *That's Jim car.*
Regular past tense: obligatory addition of /-ed/ to the end of a word as in *She talked to me yesterday.*	Not obliged to add /ed/, resulting in a sentence such as *She talk to me yesterday.*
Copula and auxiliary *to be* verb forms: Obligatory and contractible in certain contexts. Copula: *She is a beautiful woman* or *She's a beautiful woman.* Auxiliary: *They are running fast* or *They're running fast.*	Copula <u>may</u> be deleted, as in *She a beautiful woman.* Auxiliary <u>may</u> be deleted, as in *They running fast.* See next structure for possible exceptions.
Person and number agreement of copula and auxiliary *to be* verb forms: Copula: *They are beautiful people.* Auxiliary: *They are running.*	If not deleted, inclusion of the *to be* form may result in a lack of subject–verb agreement as in: Copula: *They is beautiful people.* Auxiliary: *They is running.*
Irregular third-person singular, present tense, as in *She kicks.*	<u>May</u> be deleted as in *She kick* instead of *She kicks.*
Articles *a* and *an:* Obligatory rule says use *a* if the word modified begins with a consonant; use *an* if the word modified begins with a vowel: *A car* versus *An automobile*	General rule is to use *a* whether or not the sound that follows is a consonant or a vowel: *A car* or *A automobile*
Pronouns *those* and *them:* The pronoun ***those*** is to be used as the subject while the pronoun ***them*** is to be used as the object. ***Those*** dogs belong to us (subject). *We washed **them** yesterday* (object).	Use ***them*** as both subject and object in sentences, as in, ***Them*** dogs belong to us.

eventually became major cities in North America include St. Augustine in Florida, Mexico City, San Juan, Santo Domingo, and Havana. In the 1600s, Spanish communities were established in what is now Texas and New Mexico, and between the mid-1700s and the early 1800s, Spanish communities were founded in California. When its territory was largest, New Spain reached from today's Panama to the southwestern boundaries of the United States (Chang-Rodriguez, 1991). New Spain, of course, eventually became Mexico. We see then that the influences of the Spanish culture and the Spanish language began when Columbus arrived in Santo Domingo in 1492 and were firmly entrenched in the Americas by the early 1800s.

A historical factor that affected the Spanish introduced to the Americas was triggered by an event in Spain. When the Moors were driven out of Spain, Queen Isabel decreed that the Castilian dialect should be spoken by all the people of Spain in order that they might become more united. This convergence of events—the defeat of the Moors, the establishment of the Castilian dialect as the national Spanish dialect, and the colonization of the Americas—meant that the Castilian dialect would also be introduced to the Spanish settlements in the Americas.

Even though the Spaniards who settled in the Americas used Spanish, it did not capture the linguistic imagination of Native Americans as Queen Isabel had hoped it would. Especially the settlers who were missionaries found that they could communicate more effectively with Native Americans in their own languages. In some cases, the Spaniards taught Spanish to a few Native Americans and encouraged them to teach the language in their own communities, but many Native Americans resisted, probably for the same reasons people resist having languages imposed on them today. That is, the substitution of a new language for one's native language is tantamount to the abdication of one's culture. It is difficult to imagine any group of people who would not resist this kind of change.

Even though Castilian Spanish was considered the most prestigious of Spanish dialects at this time, another dialect emerged as a major influence on what would become Hispanic English—Andalusian Spanish. The Spaniards who settled in the islands of the Caribbean and along the coastal areas of the Americas maintained commercial contacts with shipping companies in the southern part of Spain—Andalusia. Spanish spoken in the Caribbean and in the coastal regions of the Americas, therefore, was and continues to be heavily influenced by the Andalusian dialect (Fontanella de Weinberg, 1992).

As the first half of the nineteenth century concluded, Spanish control in the Americas was waning. Some countries, including Colombia, Peru, Bolivia, Venezuela, and Ecuador, became independent nations (Chang-Rodriguez, 1991). What is now Florida became part of the United States. Mexico, including the territory that is now Texas, gained independence from Spain. Texas then became independent from Mexico and eventually became part of the United States. Other territories that included parts or all of what are now Arizona, California, Colorado, Kansas, Nevada, New Mexico, Oklahoma, and Wyoming were added to the United States, by treaty, in 1848.

As the geography changed, the language influences changed. Changes that occurred in the Spanish spoken in Spain did not occur in the dialects of Spanish spoken

Hispanic English is a widely used dialect in the United States.

in the Americas. The people who lived in those regions that had been under Spanish control but were now under the control of the United States began to use English as their dominant language. Only those communities that were isolated—in the mountains, for example—continued to speak Spanish only. As Spanish speaking individuals have moved to states such as Texas, Arizona, and California, their Spanish has evolved to become more like the Spanish spoken in Mexico, and more changes in the twenty-first century are inevitable.

Consider that Spanish is a significantly used language in twenty-one countries in the Americas (Grimes, 1996). In some countries, it is the first language of almost all citizens. It is the first language of 90 percent or more of the citizens of Argentina, Chile, Colombia, Costa Rica, Cuba, El Salvador, Honduras, Nicaragua, Uruguay, and Venezuela. Surprisingly perhaps, Spanish is the first language of only 88 percent of Mexicans, but it may also surprise some that it is the first language of about 8 percent of the citizens of the United States (Grimes), and that percentage is likely to increase over the next several decades.

The reason these numbers are significant can be identified in one word: immigration. The influx of Spanish-speaking individuals into the United States has been strong for many years, and it will continue to be strong. There is a factor related to this immigration that cannot be ignored if we are to understand the continuing evolution of Hispanic English: Not all Spanish-speaking individuals come from the same place. They do not come from a single culture. They do not speak a homogenous brand of

Spanish. The most current United States census figures indicate that among residents of the United States who consider themselves *Hispanic,* 61 percent trace their origins to Mexico; 12 percent, to Puerto Rico; 8 percent, to Central America and the Caribbean; 5 percent, to Cuba; and another 5 percent, to South America. More than one-third of these people are first-generation immigrants (Current Population Reports, 1990; Current Population Survey, 1994). If we are to understand both the present and future of Hispanic English, we must appreciate what all of these people will bring to Hispanic English from their native dialects of Spanish and from their cultures.

Consider, for example, the powerful influence of the family among people who live in Latin America, and we are not talking here about just Mom, Dad, and siblings. In Latin American cultures, children spend considerable time with the extended family, including grandparents, aunts, uncles, and cousins. It is not unusual for a child to be a part of his extended family's activities every day. Godparents are also important players in the child's life. In the United States, being a godparent is largely ceremonial, but that is not true in Latin America. Godparents and members of the extended family are active participants in the child's life. They attend the important events in his life, of course, but they are present for mundane events as well, and they are often consulted when parents are making decisions about the child's life (Bedore, 1999, p. 161).

In Latin American cultures, language, and especially the oral expression of language, is important. A person who has extraordinary speaking talents is held in high esteem. Even when children are very young, they are strongly encouraged to participate in conversations with adults. Storytelling is also highly valued. Children are exposed to narratives early in their lives, and much of what they learn about their culture, family, even the towns and cities in which they live, is learned through narratives. They listen to these stories, and they learn how to tell them (Bedore, 1999, p. 161).

Even though we can identify factors such as these that seem to tie Latin American cultures together, we should remember that they are only loosely linked because there is considerable diversity among Latin American people, diversity in their cultures and diversity in the variations of Spanish they speak. The lessons in all this are twofold: (1) Those who speak Hispanic English are influenced in their language development and their language use, as are people who speak any language, by a multitude of factors; and (2) to appreciate the evolution of Hispanic English, we need to be aware of the range of origins from which Hispanic English is derived, including Latin America, which presents a variety of cultural, family, and religious influences and its own repertoire of Spanish dialects.

Asian English

Our focus on African American English and Hispanic English in this chapter is certainly justified by the integral role African Americans have played in the cultural history of the United States and by the demographic shifts in our nation that have made the Hispanic population an increasingly influential minority, a minority that continues to grow in numbers as well as in economic and political influence. At the same time, it is important to recognize that many of those who have immigrated to the United States over the past 40 years have come from Asia, and the projections indicate that the influx of new citizens from Asia will be strong for the foreseeable future. So what can we say about Asian English? First and foremost, we must emphasize that the cultural and linguistic diversity of those who come from Asia is staggering, so that whatever generalizations we make about Asian English must be made in the broadest possible strokes, and each generalization will be fraught with the likelihood of exceptions.

To gain more respect for the problems inherent in describing Asian English, allow yourself a brief lesson in geography and then consider the languages spoken by the people who live in the countries that comprise Asia. When most people think about Asian English, they think about a form of English spoken by people who come to the United States from Japan, China, Taiwan, Korea, and a few other countries thought of as belonging to the *Far East*. Actually, speakers of Asian English from the Far East come from, in alphabetical order, Brunei, Cambodia, China, East Timor, Indonesia, Japan, Laos, Malaysia, North Korea, Philippines, Singapore, South Korea, Taiwan, Thailand, and Vietnam.

But now, look at a map and you will see that Asia is a huge landmass that includes what we typically refer to as the *Middle East,* not just the Far East. The Middle East includes twenty-one countries: Afghanistan, Bahrain, Cyprus, Iran, Iraq, Israel, Jordan, Kuwait, Kyrgyzstan, Lebanon, Oman, Pakistan, Qatar, Saudi Arabia, Syria, Tajikistan, Turkey, Turkmenistan, United Arab Emirates, Uzbekistan, and Yemen. Very few of us would think of immigrants from these countries to the United States as speakers of Asian English. Other countries in the part of Asia that is not considered the Middle East include Bangladesh, Bhutan, Burma, India, Mongolia, and Nepal.

You should be getting a sense here that one of the problems we face in trying to describe Asian English is that we are dealing with people who come from countries that cover a very large portion of our planet. More importantly, there are not many ties, other than being in the same general geographical neighborhood, that bind all these countries together, but there is an even more significant problem. When we talk about Hispanic English, we are at least talking about the interfacing of just two languages, English and Spanish. We have already acknowledged, and we have repeatedly emphasized, that the Spanish spoken by people in Spain is not the same as the Spanish spoken by people who live in Puerto Rico, but at least it is more or less the same language.

What languages are spoken in the Far East that will interface with English when people from that part of the world move to the United States and learn our language? We can say with certainty that the most commonly spoken language is Chinese, but it is far from the only language. People who live in Japan speak Japanese. Those who live in North and South Korea speak Korean. Most people who live in Thailand speak Thai. The official language of Laos is Lao. In most of these countries, however, multiple languages are spoken. In Taiwan, for example, most people speak Chinese, but Japanese and Vietnamese are commonly spoken as well. In Thailand, in addition to Thai, people speak Chinese and Korean. Citizens of Malaysia speak Chinese,

Table 8.2 Comparison of Selected Characteristics of Asian English and Standard American English

Standard American English	Asian English
Final consonants: Obligatory rule applies.	Omissions of consonants such as /p, t, v, s, z/ are frequent.
Plural /-s/: Obligatory rule applies as in *He lost two dollars.*	May be omitted, as in *He lost two dollar.* May be added to irregular forms, as in *She saw the mans.*
Possessive /-'s/: Obligatory rule applies as in *Lane's dog is a wonderful pet.*	May be omitted, as in *Lane dog is a wonderful pet.*
Auxiliary *to be* verbs /is, are, was, were, am/ + -ing: Obligatory rule applies, in that be verbs must accompany the use of *-ing* on the end of the main verb, as in *The dog is barking loudly.*	May be either omitted or included without marking for person or number, as in *The dog barking loudly* or *They is running.*
Regular past tense /-ed/: Obligatory rule applies, as in *She kicked the ball.*	May be omitted, as in *She kick the ball.*
Articles /the, a/: Obligatory rule applies to specific types of nouns, as in *I have the keys to the car.*	May be omitted, as in *I have keys to car.*

Adapted from Cheng, L. (1987). Cross-cultural and linguistic considerations in working with Asian populations, ASHA, 29(6), 33–38.

Javanese, and Tamil. Without question, the multilanguage champion of the Far East is Singapore. Citizens of this tiny country, with a total population of about 4.2 million, speak Bengali, Chinese, East Punjabi, English, Hindi, Japanese, Java, Korean, Malay, Sindhi, Teluga, and Thai. According to the Singapore visitors' website, English is their "working language," and it is the most widely spoken of the languages used in that country, but their national anthem is sung in Malay. If you are now sufficiently exhausted by information overload, we can settle comfortably into the point that must be made and understood before you examine Table 8.2. That is, there is clearly no single Asian language that affects the production of English to create what we are calling *Asian English*. At most, there are a few common issues that arise when the languages spoken by those who immigrate to the United States from the Far East portion of Asia collide with Standard American English. We consider some of those English/Asian language characteristics, those we believe are reasonably comparable, in Table 8.2.

Cultural Diversity in the Public Schools

The controversies surrounding the legitimacies of social/cultural dialects have created problems for speakers of these dialects in all aspects of their lives, but the arenas of the most troubling and important battles have been the public schools. We have focused on the three primary social/cultural dialects in the United States, but there are many others. All of these languages and their dialects from Asia, Latin America, and Africa have mixed with all the dialects of American English to create a language confusion in many public schools that makes communication difficult at best. If the ability to communicate is diminished or lost in the educational process, all of our children suffer, but especially those who come into the schools without the advantage of speaking the same language as their teachers. In the long term, the nation suffers whenever the education of its children is compromised, and the education of those children who speak any language other than a Standard Dialect of American English is surely being compromised in many U.S. schools today. This is not a problem that is disappearing. On the contrary, it worsens as the number of children who do not speak Standard American English continues to grow. Within the next twenty years, these children will constitute the majority of our public school population (Bowman, 1989).

One solution to this problem is to insist that all children who attend public schools speak the same dialect of the same language, a solution that is as offensive as it is impractical. The United States is not now, nor has it ever been, a culturally and socially homogeneous nation. One of the great strengths of our country is its almost unlimited diversity. We are one nation of many cultures, many political points of view, many religions. We are a people of widely varying beliefs and values. The various languages of the people who come to the United States and the many dialects of those who have lived here for generations are parts of our cultural diversity. These language differences are inherent characteristics of our cultural heritages. To the extent possible in an era that absolutely requires communicative integrity, we want to preserve our language differences, and according to the principles of the American way of life, we have a right to preserve these differences.

It may be difficult for many U.S. citizens who speak versions of Standard American English to understand what all the commotion is about. After all, why should anyone object to sounding like the good people of Hometown, U.S.A.? We should all consider this issue from an empathic point of view. If you speak Standard American English, for example, how would you feel if you or your children were required to speak African American English or Hispanic English, or how would you feel if everyone were required to speak the dialect of a region other than your own? How would you feel if basic words in your vocabulary were considered slang and not worthy of inclusion in anything other than informal conversations among people like you? How would you react if the rules of your dialect were considered errors or simplifications of standard or correct rules? The problem with a single dialect, of course, is that someone must decide what is correct and proper in terms of vocabulary and all the rules that govern the way people speak. Can you think of any group of people to whom you would be willing to give this responsibility?

Perhaps you can accept the idea that dialects of a national language are inevitable. You may even accept that dialects are valuable characteristics of our cultural diversity, but what about the issue of all people speaking one language? If people choose to live in the United States, should they not speak English since English is our national language? There is no question that a single language would simplify communication, and there is no question that if all children in our public schools spoke

English with the same high degree of proficiency, the educational process would be easier and more efficient. Unfortunately, this wishful thinking just does not match the reality of our nation as it exists today. The United States cannot welcome immigrants and the cultural diversity they bring with them while insisting that they leave their heritages, including their languages, at the shore, and let us be clear about the importance of one's native language. A person's language is as much a part of her cultural heritage as her religion and feelings of nationalism. People who come here from Asia or Latin America do not come because they want to forsake their countries or their cultures. They typically come here to find a better life in a country that offers freedom of religion, freedom of political thought, and freedom from tyranny.

The problem in all this is obvious—not simple, not easily solved, not without need for accommodation, but obvious. Even though we are a multicultural, multi-political, multireligious nation, we do have a single national language. Those people who wish to take advantage of the opportunities afforded them in the United States find that understanding and speaking English are essential. Even those people who speak a dialect of American English other than what is considered a standard dialect find that many doors of social and vocational opportunity are narrowed or closed if one does not speak the language of the decision makers. There seems little question, then, that our children must be given the opportunity and encouraged to learn the national language. They must also be given the opportunity to learn those varieties of the national language that will give them the best chance of succeeding as students and as adults. We must recognize, however, that children can learn American English without surrendering the languages, cultures, and values of their native countries. Children can learn other dialects without abdicating their natural dialects and their associated cultural values. Not only is it possible to accommodate multiple languages and multiple dialects within the U.S. educational system; it is the right thing to do. The problem then needs to be addressed not by trying to make all children fit the same social/cultural mold, not even by compromise, which suggests surrender from both ends, but by accommodation. To accommodate means to adapt or reconcile. It implies that variances are allowed in a manner that promotes harmony.

In the play and film *The King and I,* one of the royal children asks Anna, the tutor, why he must learn about the cultures of other lands if the culture of Siam is so clearly superior to all others. Anna, ever the patient and wise teacher, points out that, like most people, he is viewing the world through the prism of his own experiences, shaped by the perceptions of those who have reared him. She encourages him to take a broader view, to see the larger picture of the human experience. To be a good ruler, she admonishes, one must recognize and value the contributions of all cultures. Anna could deliver the same message, with the same veracity, to those who will teach U.S. children in the twenty-first century. We live in a nation born in cultural diversity, a nation that is becoming increasingly diverse. If teachers fail to recognize and value the contributions and values of all the cultures of the people who call themselves American, they will fail to reach those who will be American in the new century.

As we begin the twenty-first century, we are seeing demographic shifts that will have profound effects on the public school system. Teachers will increasingly encounter students whose cultural backgrounds differ from their own, and classrooms will be filled by students who come from a wide range of cultural backgrounds. One of the challenges that must be met by teachers in this century is to help students accept, respect, and appreciate the cultural identities of those with whom they share the public schools (Banks, 1999).

Demographic Shifts

Since the demographic shifts that are affecting the United States are a reflection of population changes throughout the world, we should begin with the worldview. One of the driving forces behind changes in the population is people chasing resources—natural and economic. At the present time, 30 percent of the world's population lives in the Northern Hemisphere, which owns 70 percent of the Earth's resources. We see the reverse in the Southern Hemisphere. That is, 70 percent of the world's people live in that part of the earth which accounts for just 30 percent of its resources (Hodgkinson, 1998). As common sense would suggest, those who live in the Southern Hemisphere, people who are relatively poor and relatively uneducated, are moving north in search of better lives. Contrary to what might be a common perception among citizens of the United States, not all of these people are migrating to America. In fact, according to Hodgkinson, "people from Africa are moving to Europe at the same rate as people from Central and South America are moving to the U.S." (1998, p. 4).

Another factor influencing populations throughout the world is birthrate. While birthrates are declining worldwide, there are still huge disparities from continent to continent. For example, in the United States, the birthrate is 1.7 children per female. In Southeast Asia, the birthrate has declined slightly in recent years, but it is still 7.8 children per female (Hodgkinson, 1998). The big picture of birthrate provides a clearer picture of the future of the world's population. Consider that ninety-three out of one hundred children born in the world today are born in Asia, Africa, and Latin America (Banks, 1999). The long-term changes to the makeup of the world's population are profound. By the year 2010, only 9 percent of the world's population will be white compared with 17 percent in 1997, making this population the world's smallest minority (Hodgkinson, 1998).

The world's demographic shifts are mirrored in the changing U.S. population. Hodgkinson (1998) notes that "the population in the United States represents a parallel to the demographics of the Northern and Southern Hemispheres. The North is old, rich, white, well-educated and declining. The South and West are young, ethnically diverse, poorer, less educated and account for 90% of the U.S. current growth" (p. 5). Consistent with this overview, migration patterns have changed over the last one hundred years. At the beginning of the twentieth century, 97 percent of those who immigrated to the United States came from Europe. As we begin the transition to a new century, 85 percent of those immigrating to our country are coming from Asia and Latin America (Banks, 1999).

When we consider the impact that these population shifts are having and will have on the United States, we should be reminded that terms such as *Asian* and *Latin American* or *Hispanic* imply homogeneous populations that do not exist. That is, within the broad stroke *Asian* are many cultures with different languages and values.

Although there is a fairly strong language commonality shared by those who describe themselves as "Latin" or "Hispanic," there are many cultural differences, and even the language is not exactly the same from group to group. The point to be emphasized is that the influx of immigrants in these two large groups will bring wide ranges of cultural experiences and values, and they will bring substantial language differences.

The Future of the U.S. Student Population

U.S. teachers need only contemplate the basic numbers to understand the challenges that await them. By 2050, people of color will constitute 47.5 percent of the U.S. population (Banks, 1999). Within just the next decade, U.S. Caucasians will increase by 5 million; Hispanics, 9 million; African Americans, 3.8 million; Asians, 3.8 million; and Native Americans, 266,000 (Hodgkinson, 1998). Not all of this diversity and not all of these changes will be observed in every U.S. classroom, but as this century unfolds, the diversity will increase, and it will become more widespread.

By 2020, 48 percent of the students in U.S. public schools will be people of color, and what is most noteworthy is that the youngest children are, and will continue to be, the most culturally diverse (Banks, 1999). Consider that at the close of the twentieth century, 26 percent of the overall population in the United States was nonwhite, but 38 percent of the students in U.S. schools were people of color. The inescapable conclusion is that as the nation's children get older, the populations in its public schools will be increasingly diverse. Within a few decades, the Hispanic population in the country and in the schools will be larger than the African American population.

In the early decades of the twentieth century, teachers were confronted by children who spoke the languages of Europe—French, German, Italian, and so on. In today's world, teachers interact with many children who speak some version of Spanish, but there are many other languages as well, including Urdu, Hindi, Chinese, Japanese, Korean, and Arabic.

Religion is another issue that contributes to and complicates cultural diversity. A century ago, the vast majority of those who migrated to the United States were Christian or Jewish. There were Catholic Christians and many variations of Protestant Christians to be sure, and there were variations of Judaism, but the basic religion in each case was the same. Today's immigrants come from widely varying religious backgrounds. There are Hindus and Buddhists, and there are many who practice Islam. In fact, Islam is the fastest-growing religion in the United States today (Hodgkinson, 1998).

The challenges presented by trying to teach children who are so racially, culturally, ethnically, and religiously diverse are daunting. They are forcing U.S. educators to develop an instructional strategy that takes diversity into account—a comprehensive multicultural education system (Manning & Baruth, 1996). *Multicultural education* asserts, according to Banks and Banks (1997), "that all students regardless of the groups to which they belong, such as those related to gender, race, culture, social class, religion, or exceptionality should experience educational equality in the school" (p. 4). If we accept this or some similar concept of what multicultural education means, we will understand how profoundly the U.S. education system must change. To meet the needs of a culturally diverse student population, we must change curriculum. We must change the way teachers are trained. We must change the way we teach, and we must change the way we organize the educational process.

Changes in the Curriculum

Changes in curricula during the next century will be driven, in part, by attention to cultural considerations, including socioeconomic levels, family lifestyles, religions, languages, and learning styles (Manning & Baruth, 1996, pp. 40–45). Educators will be particularly careful to make their curricula *antibiased*. To create an antibiased curriculum means, according to Hohensee and Derman-Sparks (1992), that it generates "construction of a knowledgeable, confident self-identity, comfortable, empathetic interaction with people from diverse backgrounds, critical thinking about bias, and the ability to stand up for herself or himself, and for others in the face of bias" (p. 1). To create this kind of curriculum, educators must identify the cultural features in their school policies that prevent students from achieving their potentials. Once identified, these features must be eliminated or modified so that the curriculum and the school environment are culturally inclusive.

Developing a multicultural curriculum is possible only if educators operate in an intentional and systematic manner. Banks and Banks (1997, p. 233) describe four approaches educators can use to create a truly multicultural curriculum. The strategy that requires the least effort and the fewest changes to the existing curriculum is called the **contributions approach.** Teachers include information on selected heroes and holidays from a range of cultures, and they focus on a few specific characteristics of these cultures.

The second strategy is called the **additive approach.** As with the first strategy, the old curriculum is not discarded. Teachers add to the existing curriculum to take cultures other than the dominant culture into account. They expand content, of course, but they also introduce culturally related concepts, themes, and perspectives without altering the basic structure of the curriculum.

When educators use the **transformation approach,** the structure of the curriculum is fundamentally changed. It is redesigned to allow students to understand, appreciate, and value concepts, issues, events, and themes from the perspectives of a representative range of ethnic and cultural groups.

Finally, educators may choose the **social action approach,** a strategy that clearly cannot stand alone; that is, it must be used in combination with one or more of the previously identified strategies, most likely the transformation approach. As the name suggests, the social action approach leads students, through their increased understanding about cultural diversity, to make decisions about how best to address social issues affected by cultural differences. Going further, students actually take action to solve problems that are created by cultural differences. They assume responsibility for the problems shared by people who come from widely diverse backgrounds but who are committed to living together as people whose common bonds are stronger than their differences.

Ideally, of course, all four of these strategies will be used to develop a curriculum that is relevant to all students, a curriculum that facilitates understanding and respect for all people and all cultures.

Although schools in the twenty-first century will rely far less on books than schools in the twentieth century, textbooks and other printed instructional materials will still be used. Teachers in the new century who will be teaching an increasingly diverse student population must take care to use materials that are as bias-free as possible. Gollnick and Chin (1991, p. 2) suggest that teachers should be aware of at least six forms of bias that can be found in textbooks and other printed instructional materials: (1) invisibility, (2) stereotyping, (3) selectivity and imbalance, (4) unreality, (5) fragmentation and isolation, and (6) language bias.

Escamilla (1993) suggests that textbooks should not use sidebars to include information about multicultural issues because sidebars suggest that this information is less important than the information in the body of the text. Textbooks should also avoid a "superhero" approach that suggests that only a few selected individuals from a particular ethnic group have made contributions. Instead, the overall contributions of an ethnic group should be emphasized with reference to some of the major players in these contributions. Finally, Escamilla asserts that textbooks should not be written in a "one size fits all" manner. That is, authors should not write about Hispanic contributions as though they come from a single source. There is not a single African culture or a single Asian culture. Native Americans and African Americans can trace their cultural backgrounds to many different groups of people. The contributions of each group must be recognized and valued, no matter how convenient it might be to envision that all Africans come from the same place, that all Asians hold the same values, and that all Hispanic people maintain the same beliefs.

The Training of Teachers in the Twenty-First Century

The majority of teachers in the United States are now, and have been throughout the history of the republic, white females. Except for the female part of the description, the personal and cultural backgrounds of teachers have been wholly consistent with the young people sitting in their classrooms. We begin this century with white female teachers addressing student bodies that are more and more divergent from them in their personal and cultural experiences. It seems inevitable that as the cultural chasm between teachers and students widens, problems in the instructional process will develop. One solution to this problem is to integrate teaching staffs, making them more representative of the cultural differences that mark America's present and future. Another solution, which must occur no matter how diverse teaching staffs become, is to make sure that teachers—all teachers—are sensitive to the cultural differences among their students. This means, of course, that white female teachers must understand and appreciate the cultural experiences of African American, Hispanic, Asian, and Native American students, but it also means that African American teachers must understand and appreciate the cultural experiences of those students whose backgrounds differ from their own.

Any program designed to help twenty-first-century teachers prepare for culturally diverse student bodies must include three components: awareness, knowledge, and skills (Sue, Arredono, & McDavis, 1992). Teachers must become **aware** of their own beliefs, values, and biases, and they must understand how they view their own students. A teacher who lacks appropriate awareness and sensitivity is likely to bring her personal biases into the classroom, biases that will be recognized by her students and will influence how they respond to the teacher and to the learning process. If a teacher acquires **knowledge** about other cultures, she will be able to integrate that knowledge into class material. Her awareness and knowledge will lead to enhanced teaching **skills.** She will shape her teaching style to take into account the cultural differences in her classroom. Her interpersonal skills will be improved to the extent that she learns that one communicative style will not be effective with all students, that how people talk to one another is influenced by their cultural experiences.

Some experts provide fairly specific guidelines about what should be included in a teacher education program to ensure that issues of cultural diversity are adequately addressed in teacher training. Carmen Coballes-Vega (1992, p. 1) identifies five specific inclusions. First, there should be at least one course in multicultural education that stresses the importance of taking the needs of all students into consideration in the instructional process. Second, the teacher education curriculum should provide information about the history and culture of students from a representative range of ethnic, racial, linguistic, and cultural backgrounds. Third, future teachers should be informed about the contributions of people from various cultures to literature, art, music, science, technology, medicine, law, and so on. Fourth, information about first- and second-language acquisition should be provided, and future teachers should learn instructional strategies designed to help students who have limited competence with American English. Finally, this preparation should not be limited to the classroom. Those who will teach culturally diverse students must have field experiences, including student teaching experiences, with children from varying backgrounds.

The Changing Classroom

Carger (1997) asserts that efforts to create an educational experience that is truly multicultural must include more than just cosmetic adjustments to our current system. Even if we make the kinds of curricular changes the experts recommend to address cultural diversity, and even if teacher training programs include courses and experiences designed to make teachers more sensitive to their culturally diverse students, more needs to be accomplished if we are to assure that all students achieve the degree of academic, social, and vocational success we believe they deserve. Carger suggests that educating multicultural students does not happen through a *recipe* approach. Teachers must help students experience "an individualized, lifelong process of learning, discovery, accepting and trying—a little like developing gourmet cuisine versus ordering fast food" (p. 39). This means that a teacher who is serious about being an effective multicultural teacher will immerse students in multicultural literature, art, and music. She will invite guests from widely varying cultural backgrounds into her classroom to share their life stories. She will find ways to give students learning experiences that will expose them to cultural perspectives that differ from their own, perhaps through field trips. Most important, the teacher will lead students to think about, reflect on, and embrace the cultural differences among people rather than allowing them to reject reflexively what they do not understand or what does not fit neatly into their own life experiences.

Within the context of the history of the United States, it might seem a little strange that dealing with cultural diversity is a *problem.* After all, the United States is a nation built by people from widely varying backgrounds. We describe our nation as a *melting pot.* Unfortunately, it has always been true in the United States that differences matter more than they should. We have managed to survive our differences for the duration of our history because even if people have not been voluntarily tolerant of the differences, our laws have mandated tolerance; and when the laws have been found wanting, they have been amended to guarantee tolerance, or new laws have been drafted to protect those who have been, for one reason or another, unprotected. As we face a new century, the situation is changing because the population is changing. Groups we describe as *minorities* are becoming larger. They are gaining political and economic strength. They will no longer be content with legal tolerance. All people in the United States, no matter their racial, ethnic, religious, or cultural backgrounds, are demanding equal rights and equal access to the opportunities that are, in aggregate, the American Dream. Teachers, whether they want the responsibility or not, are on the front lines of the changes that will make this a truly multicultural nation in the sense that differences are not just recognized, not just tolerated, but *celebrated.*

Houston (1999) repeats the common mantra that people gain strength from their differences. He observes that the population of the United States is like a building found in an ancient city, a building formed by rocks of varying shapes and sizes that have been carved and fitted together perfectly. This kind of building, because it was so powerfully constructed, has stood for centuries—impervious to the ravages of war, violent weather, and the passing of time. If we manage to put the diverse pieces of our population together in a manner that optimizes the strengths of all our people and recognizes their unique values, our nation will long endure. This process begins in the classrooms of the twenty-first-century.

Gender Differences in Language

In Chapter 6, we briefly discussed the emergence of gender differences in language. We noted that many of the language differences between men and women begin to show up in the communicative efforts of children as young as four and five years, and children recognize gender differences in the messages of others at a very young age. As we consider gender differences in language, we must always keep in mind that some differences between the sexes may be explained on the basis of biology, but very often they reflect variations in the way males and females are socialized. It is highly likely that many of the gender differences we observe in language are socialized differences and are not biologically based. We should take care, therefore, to understand these as differences without drawing unwarranted conclusions about how they have developed or what they mean.

Assuming Gender Roles

Consider the following riddle that has made its rounds for several generations. A young man was in a serious automobile accident and suffered injuries that required immediate surgery. He was rushed to the emergency room of the nearest hospital. It was obvious that the young man needed surgery, but the surgeon on duty, although not the patient's father, declined to perform the operation, saying, "I can't operate on this patient because he's my son." Why did the surgeon refuse to operate? Some people speculate that the surgeon was the patient's stepfather. Others assume that the surgeon was confused because the patient resembled his son. Some people, who are not myopic about gender roles, correctly conclude that the surgeon could not operate because she was the patient's mother.

When my youngest daughter was about eight years old, she came home from school one day in an especially excited mood. She could not wait to announce that she had decided what she wanted to be when she grew up: a nurse. When I asked why she did not want to be a doctor, she laughed, saying boys are doctors and girls are nurses. This was certainly not a perception consciously or deliberately taught at home, and when I asked her where she got the idea that girls could not be doctors, she could not say. Gender roles are so powerfully socialized, even though sometimes in subtle ways, that we may grow up and accept our roles without ever giving any thought to their origins or their validity.

Even though linguists argue about how much language affects the way we perceive things, most would agree that language does shape the way we think just as surely as the way we think shapes our language. Are perceptions of gender roles shaped by language? Are perceptions of gender roles reflected in the language we use? Both questions must be answered in the affirmative. Men refer to their boats and cars as *she*. Draw your own conclusions about what these references suggest. When men refer to women as *babes* and *chicks*, what do we learn about their perceptions of women? When boys and girls grow up hearing the sexist labels we attach to both men and women, why are we surprised that they accept the stereotypical perceptions reflected in the labels?

Some gender differences in language are almost imperceptible but just as meaningful as the slang terms we use to identify men and women. Richmond and Gorham (1988) studied the use of gender referents in the written language of children in grades 3 through 12. The task was to write a story about a hypothetical classmate of unspecified gender. After reading a brief description of this student, the subjects were instructed to write a story about "how the hypothetical classmate would do in school." The investigators found that the male subjects of all ages used significantly more masculine referents (e.g., *he, his, him, the boy*) and fewer neutral referents (e.g.,

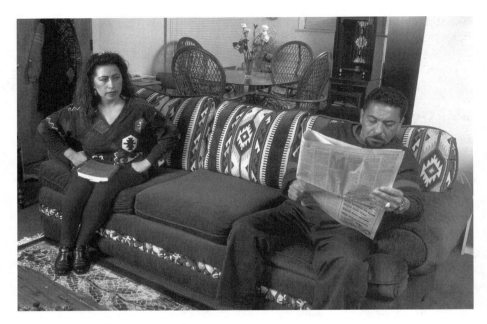

The gender gap in communication.

they, their, the student) than did the female subjects. Their female subjects, especially those in the lowest and highest grades, used nearly as many masculine referents as neutral referents. The males at all grade levels used almost no feminine referents (e.g., *she, her, the girl*). Among the female subjects, the number of feminine referents declined dramatically as age increased. Richmond and Gorham concluded that the trends in their research tend to support an earlier assertion (Nilsen, 1977) that young boys tend to perceive a neutral person as being male, and young girls tend to perceive a neutral person as being female, but the female perception does not endure. As females learn the language rule that when gender is not identified, assume male, they are less likely to perceive neutral persons as female. Boys, on the other hand, continue to perceive neutral persons as male, a perception reinforced by common language usage. In such subtle but powerful ways are language differences between the sexes created.

He Said . . . She Said

We have already identified some gender differences in Chapter 6. Let's review the highlights. Even though men and women include the same words in their vocabularies, they tend to select different words when they talk (Thorne, Kramerae, & Henley, 1983). Men tend to use profane and crude words more often than women, and women are more likely than men to use polite words such as *please, thank you,* and *you're welcome* (Greif & Berko-Gleason, 1980). Women also use words such as *darling, lovely,* and *adorable* more often than men and are more likely to name shades of colors. Men talk more than women (Swacher, 1975). Men are more likely to interrupt during conversations than women and are more likely to interrupt women than men (Parlee, 1979). Only about one-third of the new topics introduced into conversation by women are retained, but almost all of the new topics introduced into conversation by men are retained (Ehrenreich, 1981). Mothers talk to their preschool daughters more than they talk to their preschool sons (Cherry & Lewis, 1976), and fathers use more endearing nicknames for their daughters than for their sons (Berko-Gleason & Greif, 1983).

Even though some writers caution that there is little solid empirical evidence of gender differences in American English (Warren-Leubecker & Bohannon, 1989), many writers and readers find the possibilities of sex-related language differences interesting and potentially enlightening. Are some differences clearly biological? Do language differences by gender tell us anything about what it means to be a man or woman? Is sexism reinforced by the way men and women use language, especially in reference to one another? Can we change the way people think about gender roles by changing the way they use language? We cannot satisfactorily answer all of these questions, but we can add some additional grist for your thoughts about these matters.

At least one aspect of oral communication is, to some extent at least, biologically determined. The voice of the average man is lower in pitch than the voice of the average woman because adult males tend to have longer, thicker vocal folds than women. What is interesting, however, is that some of the vocal differences between men and women may be environmentally or socially determined. For example, women adjust their voices so that they sound like women, and men adjust their voices to sound like men (Sachs, Lieberman, & Erickson, 1973, p. 78). This means that a man may force his habitual pitch lower than it naturally should be, and a woman may force her habitual pitch higher than it should be to match some unspecified social standards for male and female voices.

Another aspect of speech that may be socially determined is vocal variation. Women tend to use a wide range of pitches in all speaking situations, and they use their voices more expressively than men. Men tend to use their voices in a somewhat subdued and monotonous manner when they talk to adults, but they use much greater vocal variation when they talk to young children (Warren-Leubecker & Bohannon, 1984). In other words, although both genders have the capability of vocal variation, men are much more selective about when and with whom they vary their voices.

What We Have Here Is a Failure to Communicate

Gender differences in communication are no more apparent than when men and women try to talk to one another. Sometimes even the most innocent topics create tension, frustration, and anger because men and women seem to be on different pages of the communication manual. Why do we have so much trouble talking to one another? When and why did the trouble begin? Deborah Tannen, a linguist and author of the best-selling *You Just Don't Understand: Women and Men in Conversation*, believes she has some answers to these questions.

According to Tannen (1990), the failure of men and women to communicate can be traced to the way boys and girls grow up. Although brothers and sisters may grow up in the same house with the same parents, they grow up in different worlds. Boys tend to play in large groups, and their play is activity oriented. Their games have winners and losers, and there are elaborate rules about which the participants frequently argue. Boys brag about their own skills and argue about who is best. Speech is used in the context of play to achieve status and establish a hierarchy of superiority. They tell stories and jokes, and they interrupt and challenge one another to determine who is the quickest or wittiest. Boys with high status give orders to those with lower status. Speech is used as a tool of aggression, not only to establish one's status, but to defend one's position when verbally attacked.

Girls, according to Tannen (1990), play and communicate in very different ways. They tend to play in small groups or in pairs. Many of their activities, such as jump rope or playing house, do not have winners and losers. In fact, taking turns and sharing in the experience are emphasized, not winning. They do not boast about their skills but are often self-deprecating because they want to be accepted and not be offensive. Rather than giving orders, girls are more inclined to try to manipulate the behaviors of others by offering suggestions or indicating their preferences. They do not maneuver for status because they are concerned that such maneuvering will cause others not to like them. Speech is used as a means for interacting with other people and for sharing feelings and thoughts.

Given their early life experiences, it is not surprising that adult men and women communicate differently, and that these differences often make communication between the sexes difficult. Tannen (1990) argues that while all people need intimacy and independence, women are more concerned with intimacy and men are more concerned with independence. The relative importance each gender gives to these needs is clearly reflected in the ways they talk to members of their own sex and to members of the opposite sex. Men use talking to convey information, to solve problems, to establish their positions within hierarchies of status. They often perceive the words of others as threats to their independence or challenges to their status. Many men who feel a strong need to be self-reliant are comfortable in giving information or advice to others but are not at all comfortable about accepting advice or information. Women, on the other hand, use talking to connect and interact with other people. They are very comfortable in using language to express their feelings. They talk to share, to demonstrate that they understand how the other person feels, and to be supportive. Many women are just as comfortable receiving information and advice as they are in giving it.

Of course, all of these observations are generalizations. Some women, in some circumstances if not all, communicate as men do and with the same apparent motivations. Likewise, some men have many of the communicative traits identified here with women. Furthermore, it is probably safe to assume that all speakers, regardless of gender, share some of the communicative needs and characteristics of the opposite sex some of the time. Nevertheless, the generalized differences are interesting.

Have you ever wondered, for example, why someone who is talkative in one situation may be silent in others? There are many explanations, of course, but Tannen (1990) suggests that there are gender reasons in many cases. Men tend to engage in what she calls "report talking"; that is, they use talking to inform, impress, or persuade. This is the kind of talking one does in public settings such as at work, in meetings, or at parties. A man who is very talkative in these settings may be relatively silent at home because at home he does not have to prove himself. At home he is free to be quiet. Women, on the other hand, engage in what Tannen calls "rapport talking." They talk to establish, maintain, and cultivate relationships. They engage in very personal forms of communication. A woman who is talkative at home, a setting that allows for personal communication, may be relatively quiet in public settings because she is less comfortable in the role of information conveyor and more fearful of the negative and personal reactions her words might prompt. This gender difference creates a real and common problem. A wife cannot understand why her husband does not want to talk at home even though he cannot shut up at parties, and a husband cannot understand why his wife insists on talking at home when she says little or nothing in public meetings. The wife interprets her husband's silence at home to mean that he does not care about what she thinks or feels. The husband interprets his wife's insistence on conversation at home about what he perceives as trivial matters as nagging. What we have here is a classic case of a failure to communicate about communicative needs and expectations.

In *Talking from 9 to 5—Women and Men in the Workplace: Language, Sex and Power*, Tannen (1994) suggests that the gender differences in communication can be observed in the way men and women try to get things done at work, the way they interact with their bosses and those they supervise, the way they develop relationships with their co-workers, and the way they try to position themselves to move up the corporate ladder. Even though some of these differences may cause you to smile or giggle knowingly, few of them will surprise you.

Tannen (1994, pp. 27–28) notes, for example, that while men at work are very willing to give information, they are reluctant to seek information. It may be that they are concerned about what others will think about them if they admit they do not know everything, and they may believe that asking for information puts the person who asks in a one-down relationship with the person from whom information is being solicited. Women, on the other hand, are quite willing to seek information. They apparently place far more importance on getting information they need than on how others will perceive them if they ask.

The communicative aggressiveness we observe in young boys continues to be part of the male style at work (Tannen, 1994, pp. 29–30). When men negotiate for the division of duties, for example, they will often try to grab what they want as early in the negotiating process as possible. A woman is more likely to open negotiations by asking the other person what he or she would like to do. If the other person is a man, he will likely interpret the question to be an invitation to seize what he wants, but the woman is probably extending an invitation to discuss the division of responsibilities before any decisions are made. The woman, just as she did as a child, attempts to be conciliatory in negotiations. She tries to create a win–win situation in that each party has a chance to identify what he or she would like to do and to explain why. After the discussion, the responsibilities will be divided according to ability and interest to the satisfaction of everyone. It does not always work out this way, of course, but that's the plan.

In reference to boys and girls, Tannen (1990) notes that boys play and interact in a manner that places a premium on being right, being the best, and being confident. Girls often react negatively to other girls who are too sure of themselves, too sure they are always right, or who are too confident for any reason. These same tendencies show up in adults at work (Tannen, 1994, pp. 35–36). Men are "more likely to downplay their doubts," whereas women are "more likely to downplay their certainty." It is interesting and revealing that adults of both sexes react to girls the same way that girls react to overly confident girls. While boys are often praised for being aggressive, girls are expected to keep their confidence and their aggressiveness in check. It does not require much of a stretch to see how these perceptions and expectations spill over into the adult world of work. A man who is assertive and confident is viewed positively. A woman with the same traits is often viewed negatively, by both men and women.

Conversation, including casual conversation, is a necessary part of the work experience. The fact that men and women talk differently can lead directly to communication breakdowns. A common communicative habit on the part of women is saying, "I'm sorry," when an apology is not called for and when an apology is not intended (Tannen, 1994, pp. 43–46). For example, a woman might give instructions to a subordinate. The subordinate, because of inattention or incompetence, fails to carry out the instructions. When the woman and the subordinate discuss what happened, the woman might begin by saying, "I'm sorry. . . ." She is not apologizing in this case; she is trying to restore communicative balance. It's her way of saying, "We obviously had a breakdown in communication. Let's try again." Unfortunately, a man listening to or taking part in this exchange might perceive that the woman is putting herself down. Men, you see, are far less likely than women to apologize, even when apologies are appropriate.

Tannen (1994, p. 56) notes that the communicative rituals of apologizing, softening criticism, and thanking are more common in women than in men. All of these rituals depend on mutuality or balance. If a woman apologizes, for example, in a situation that clearly does not call for an apology and the other person accepts the apology, balance has been lost and the woman may be frustrated. If the other person dismisses the apology by saying something like, "There's no need to apologize. I'm the one who forgot what time we were supposed to meet," mutuality or balance has been maintained.

There are also communicative rituals involved in confrontational situations, and men and women tend to react differently to confrontation. Tannen (1994, p. 61) implies that men enjoy confrontation and women do not. Whereas men seem to thrive in situations in which there are winners and losers, women would rather work things out so that all parties save face and remain friends.

The gender differences related to conversational topics follow through from childhood to adulthood. When men talk to men at work, their conversations are laced with comments about sports and politics. When women talk to women at work, they include comments about their personal lives, and women who are reluctant to share in these personal exchanges are viewed as cold or aloof. The topic differences are important because when people share a workplace, they establish personal and professional relationships by talking to one another, and the line between personal and professional is always a little fuzzy. It should be easy to understand why a man working in an office staffed by mostly women, if closed out of the personal conversations, would feel somewhat ostracized at a professional level. It is also easy to understand that a woman who does not feel welcome to join men when they talk about the NFL, the assets and liabilities of the 3-4 defense, and who will go high in next year's draft will also feel left out as a co-worker.

Can the Gender Gap Be Bridged?

Is it possible for men and women to change the ways they talk and listen to one another? It is possible, of course, but as Tannen (1990, 1994) notes, most people expect the other person to change. We tend to view the way we communicate as not being in need of repair and probably as being superior to the way the other person communicates. A more reasonable expectation for both men and women is that we learn to understand and appreciate the communication needs, expectations, and strategies of both sexes. Two personal examples may illustrate common problems and reasonable solutions.

> For many years, my wife and I have repeated the following scenario more times than I care to admit. She comes home from work after a troubling day during which she has felt overwhelmed by the volume of her work and frustrated by confrontations with one or more people with whom she must interact in the course of fulfilling her duties. I have always listened, but not always patiently, and certainly not with understanding, because as I listen, I am identifying the problems and conflicts that I believe are contributing to her vocational unhappiness. My responses to her are suggestions about how to solve her problems. She reacts with irritation to my suggestions. I am hurt because I believe I am trying to be helpful. In the context of Tannen's (1990) explanations of gender differences in communication, I now understand that my wife's recounting of the events of the day has nothing to do with identifying problems that beg for solutions. She wants to share with me, to be intimate about her feelings of frustration and anger. She does not want my advice. She just wants me to listen and express support and understanding. Knowing her needs, I am trying to become a better listener, and if necessary, I will bite my lip until I draw blood to prevent myself from offering advice when advice is not requested.
>
>   The second example is really the flip side of the first. When I have a particularly trying day, I want to retreat into the silence my home offers. For at least a few hours, I do not want to talk to anyone. Over the years, my wife has often interpreted this silence to mean that I am not happy to be home or that I am angry or upset about

something. Because she is a rapport talker, she wants to connect with me. As my silence continues, she presses me for reasons, and if I say that nothing is wrong and I just do not want to talk, she perceives rejection. Now that she recognizes and understands the gender differences that account for my silence, she is more tolerant of my reticence. She leaves me alone for a time to revel in my quiet retreat. I, in turn, recognize that she has a powerful need to connect during our first few hours at home, so I compromise my silence after what seems an appropriate interval and give her an opportunity for the rapport talking she needs.

The conversational style differences between the sexes become problems only to the extent that we allow them to be problems. Understanding and compromise will not eliminate the differences, but they will do much to eliminate the gender friction that can be caused by the differences.

In closing this section, we must emphasize that just as there is no language or dialect that is superior to any other language or dialect, there is no right or wrong about the way men and women talk. The conversational style of each gender has validity and value. Some of the disagreements that occur between men and women are exacerbated by differences in conversational style. When men and women argue, for example, men often use logical and reasonable arguments and accuse women of being too emotional. If we understand that because men use language to convey information and to impress and persuade, they tend to argue in a manner that emphasizes logic and reason, and that because women use language to connect and establish rapport, they tend to argue in a manner that emphasizes feelings and attitudes, the argument can focus on the issue of the conflict and not on the manner in which the argument is being waged. In the final analysis, we should consider that we may communicate best as we develop an integrated style of communication which includes elements of the male and female styles. Perhaps that is the most important lesson to be learned from gender differences in language and communication.

Review Questions

1. Identify language differences you associate with each of the seven variables that influence the acquisition of language and language behaviors according to Taylor (1990).
2. Differentiate the following terms: *language, dialect,* and *accent.*
3. What are the issues surrounding the use and understanding of labels such as standard dialect and non-standard dialect?
4. What are some of the factors that account for the development of regional dialects in the United States?
5. Identify some of the lexical features of the dialects spoken in each of the following regions and offer an explanation for how these dialectal features have developed: New England Region, Northern and Midwest Region, and the Southern Region.
6. Trace the origins of African American English, incorporating explanations of the terms *pidgin, creole,* and *decreolization.*
7. How does the production of negation in African American English

compare to the production of negation in Standard American English?

8. What is the syntactic device *aspect?* Provide examples of aspect expressed in African American English.

9. Discuss the social and cultural factors that are likely to contribute to the continuing evolution of African American English in the twenty-first century.

10. Trace the origins of Hispanic English, and account for the influences that have resulted in the varying dialects within Hispanic English.

11. Why is it impractical and, in the opinions of many experts, wrong-minded to insist that U.S. students speak a uniform dialect of American English?

12. What are the demographic shifts in the world and in the United States that are affecting the present and future cultural diversity of U.S. schools?

13. What are the goals of a *comprehensive multicultural education system?*

14. What are the advantages and disadvantages of the four strategies suggested for developing a multicultural curriculum in U.S. schools?

15. How will the increasingly diverse nature of the student body in U.S. schools affect the way teachers are recruited and trained?

16. What are the possible ramifications of not addressing multicultural issues in U.S. public education?

17. What do gender differences in communication seem to suggest about differences between women and men, girls and boys?

18. How do gender differences interfere with communication between women and men?

19. How might gender communication differences affect how work is conducted when a woman is the boss and many of her subordinates are men? When a man is the boss and many of his subordinates are women?

20. How might a woman's communicative strategies affect her ability to negotiate for a raise or for a promotion?

21. Can the gender gap be bridged? If so, how? If not, why not?

References and Suggested Readings

Abercrombie, D. (1967). *Elements of general phonetics.* Edinburgh: University Press.

Allen, H., & Linn, M. (Eds.). (1986). *Dialect and language variation.* Orlando, FL: Academic Press.

Bailey, G., & Maynor, N. (1989). The divergence controversy. *American Speech, 64,* 12–13.

Banks, J., & Banks, C. (1997). *Multicultural education: Issues and perspectives* (3rd ed.). Boston: Allyn & Bacon.

Banks, J. (1999). Multicultural education in the new century. *School Administrator, 56,* 4–7.

Battles, D. (1983). Social dialects. *ASHA, 25,* 23–24.

Bebout, L., & Arthur, B. (1992). Cross-cultural attitudes toward speech disorders. *Journal of Speech and Hearing Research, 35,* 45–52.

Bedore, L. (1999). The acquisition of Spanish. In O. Taylor & L. Leonard (Eds.), *Language acquisition across North*

America: Cross-cultural and cross-linguistic perspectives. San Diego, CA: Singular.

Berko-Gleason, J., and Greif, E. (1983). Men's speech to young children. In B. Thorne, C. Kramerae, & N. Henley (Eds.), Language, gender, and society. Rowley, MA: Newbury House.

Bernthal, J., and Bankson, N. (1993). Articulation and phonological disorders. Upper Saddle River, NJ: Prentice Hall.

Bowman, B. (1989). Educating language-minority children: Challenges and opportunities. Phi Delta Kappan, 71, 118–120.

Bryen, D. (1978). Variant English: An introduction to language variation. Upper Saddle River, NJ: Merrill/ Prentice Hall.

Campbell, L. (1993). Maintaining the integrity of home linguistic varieties: Black English vernacular. American Journal of Speech–Language Pathology, 2, 11–12.

Campbell, L. (1994). Discourse diversity and Black English vernacular. In D. Ripich & N. Creaghead (Eds.), School discourse problems (2nd ed.). San Diego, CA: Singular.

Carger, C. (1997). Attending to new voices. Educational Leadership, 54, 39–43.

Carver, C. (1987). American regional dialects: A word geography. Ann Arbor: University of Michigan Press.

Chang-Rodriguez, E. (1991). Latin America, her civilization and culture. New York: HarperCollins.

Cheng, L. (1987, June). Cross-cultural and linguistic considerations in working with Asian populations. ASHA, 29(6), 33–38.

Cherry, L., & Lewis, M. (1976). Mothers and two-year-olds: A study of sex differentiated aspects of verbal interaction. Developmental Psychology, 12, 278–282.

Coballes-Vega, C. (1992). Considerations in teaching culturally diverse children. [On-line]. Retrieved from ERIC Digest (ED 341648).

Cole, P., & Taylor, O. (1990). Performance of working class African-American children on three tests of articulation. Language, Speech, Hearing Services in Schools, 21, 171–176.

Crago, M., Eriks-Brophy, A., Pesco, D., & McAlpine, L. (1997). Culturally based miscommunication in classroom interaction. Language, Speech, and Hearing Services in Schools, 28, 245–254.

Craig, H., & Washington, J. (2002). Oral language expectations for African American preschoolers and kindergartners. American Journal of Speech–Language Pathology, 11, 59–70.

Craig, H., Washington, J., & Thompson-Porter, C. (1998). Average c-unit lengths in the discourse of African American children from low-income, urban homes. Journal of Speech, Language, and Hearing Research, 41, 433–444.

Craig, H., Connor, C., & Washington, J. (2003). Early positive predictors of later reading comprehension for African American students: A preliminary investigation. Language, Speech, and Hearing Services in Schools, 34, 31–43.

Cummins, J. (1989). A theoretical framework for bilingual special education. Exceptional Children, 56, 111–119.

Current Population Reports. (1990). 1990 census of population and housing. Washington, D.C.: U.S. Census Bureau. [On-line]. Available URL: http://www.census.gov/cdrom/lookup

Current Population Survey (March, 1994). *Hispanic origin.* Washington, D.C.: U.S. Census Bureau. [On-line]. Available URL: http://www.census.gov/population

Dillard, J. (1973). *Black English: Its history and usage in the United States.* New York: Vintage.

Edwards, W., and Winford, D. (1991). *Verb phrase patterns in Black English and Creole.* Detroit, MI: Wayne State University Press.

Ehrenreich, B. (1981). The politics of talking in couples. *Ms, 5,* 43–45, 86–89.

Escamilla, K. (1993). Integrating Mexican-American history and culture into the social studies classroom. In L. Gronlund (Ed.) *Striving for excellence: The national education goals* (Vol. 2, pp. 53–54). Washington, D.C.: Educational Resources Information Center.

Fasold, R. (1984). *The sociolinguistics of society.* London: Basil Blackwell.

Figueroa, R. (1989). Psychological testing of linguistic-minority students: Knowledge gaps and regulations. *Exceptional Children, 56,* 145–152.

Fontanella de Weinberg, M. (1992). *Spanish in America.* Madrid: Mapfre.

Francis, W. (1987). *Dialectology: An introduction.* New York: Longman.

Gollnick, D., & Chin, P. (1991). Multicultural education for exceptional children. [On-line]. Retrieved from ERIC Digest (ED 333620).

Greif, E., & Berko-Gleason, J. (1980). Hi, thanks, and goodbye: More routine information. *Language in Society, 9,* 159–166.

Grimes, B. (Ed.) (1996). *Ethnologue: Languages of the world* (13th ed.). Dallas, TX: Summer Institute of Linguistics.

Hakuta, K., & Garcia, E. (1989). Bilingualism and education. *American Psychologist, 44,* 374–379.

Hammer, C., & Weiss, A. (1999). Guiding language development: How African American mothers and their infants structure play interactions. *Journal of Speech, Language, and Hearing Research, 42,* 1219–1233.

Hammer, C., & Weiss, A. (2000). African American mothers' views on their infants' language-development and language-learning environment. *American Journal of Speech-Language Pathology, 9,* 1226–140.

Harbaugh, M. (1990). Celebrating diversity. *Instructor, 100,* 45–48.

Haskins, J., & Butts, H. (1973). *The psychology of black language.* New York: Harper & Row.

Hodgkinson, H. (1998). Demographics of diversity for the 21st century. *Education Digest, 64,* 4–7.

Hohensee, J., & Derman-Sparks, L. (1992). Implementing anti-bias curriculum in early childhood programs. [On-line]. Retrieved from ERIC Digest (ED 35114692).

Houston, P. (1999). The accelerating change of American diversity. *School Administrator, 56,* 6–7.

Labov, W. (1966). *The social stratification of English in New York City.* Washington, D.C.: Center for Applied Linguistics.

Manning, M., & Baruth, L. (1996). *Multicultural education of children and adolescents* (2nd ed.). Boston: Allyn & Bacon.

Massey, A. (1996). Cultural influences on language assessment and intervention. In A. Kamhi, K. Pollock, & J. Harris (Eds.), *Communication development and disorders in African American children: Research, assessment, and intervention.* Baltimore: Brookes.

Naremore, R. (1980). Language variation in a multicultural society. In T. Hixon, L. Shriberg, & J. Saxman,

(Eds.), *Introduction to communication disorders*. Upper Saddle River, NJ: Prentice Hall.

Naremore, R., & Hopper, R. (1990). *Children learning language* (3rd ed.). New York: Harper & Row.

Nilsen, A. (1977). Sexism in children's books and elementary teaching materials. In A. Nilsen et al. (Eds.), *Sexism and language*. Urbana, IL: National Council of Teachers of English.

Parlee, M. (1979). Conversational politics. *Psychology Today, 5,* 48–56.

Ramirez, A. (1992). *The Spanish of the United States: The language of the Hispanics*. Madrid: Mapfre.

Richmond, V., & Gorham, J. (1988). Language patterns and gender role orientation among students in grades 3–12. *Communication Education, 37,* 142–149.

Ripich, D., and Creaghead, N. (Eds.). (1994). *School discourse problems* (2nd ed.). San Diego, CA: Singular.

Robbins, J. (1988). Employers' language expectations and nonstandard dialect speakers. *English Journal, 77,* 22–24.

Sachs, J., Lieberman, P., & Erickson, D. (1973). Anatomical and cultural determinants of male and female speech. In R. Schuy & R. Fasold (Eds.), *Language attitudes: Current trends and prospects*. Washington, D.C.: Georgetown University Press.

Schneider, E. (1989). *American earlier Black English*. Tuscaloosa: University of Alabama Press.

Smitherman, G. (1994). *Black talk, words and phrases from the hood to the amen corner*. New York: Houghton Mifflin.

Sue, D., Arredona, P., & McDavis, R. (1992). Multicultural counseling competencies and standards: A call to the profession. *Journal of Counseling and Development, 70,* 477–486.

Suhor, C. (1988). "English only" movement emerging as a major controversy. *Educational Leadership, 46,* 80–81.

Swacher, M. (1975). The sex of the speaker as a sociolinguistic variable. In B. Thorne & N. Henley (Eds.), *Language and sex: Difference and dominance*. Rowley, MA: Newbury House.

Tannen, D. (1990). *You just don't understand: Women and men in conversation*. New York: Morrow.

Tannen, D. (1994). *Talking from 9 to 5—Women and men in the workplace: Language, sex and power*. New York: Avon.

Taylor, O. (1972). An introduction to the historical development of Black English: Some implications for American education. *Language, Speech, and Hearing Services in the Schools, 3,* 5–15.

Taylor, O. (Ed.). (1986). *Nature of communication disorders in culturally and linguistically diverse populations*. San Diego, CA: College-Hill.

Taylor, O. (1990). Language and language differences. In G. Shames & E. Wiig (Eds.), *Human communication disorders* (3rd ed.). Upper Saddle River, NJ: Merrill/Prentice Hall.

Taylor, O., & Clarke, M. (1994). Communication disorders and cultural diversity: A theoretical framework. *Seminars in Speech and Language, 15,* 103–113.

Terrell, S. (1983). Effects of speaking Black English upon employment opportunities. *ASHA, 25,* 27–29.

Terrell, S., & Terrell, F. (1993). African-American cultures. In D. E. Battles (Ed.), *Communication disorders in multicultural populations.* Stoneham, MA: Butterworth-Heinemann.

Thorne, B., Kramerae, C., & Henley, N. (Eds.) (1983). *Language, gender, and society.* Rowley, MA: Newbury House.

Van Keulen, J., Weddington, G., & De-Bose, C., (1998). *Speech, language, learning, and the African American child.* Boston: Allyn & Bacon.

Walker, M. (1999). The acquisition of African American English: Social-cognitive and cultural factors. In O. Taylor & L. Leonard (Eds.), *Language acquisition across North America: Cross-cultural and cross-linguistic perspectives.* San Diego, CA: Singular.

Warren-Leubecker, A., & Bohannon, J. (1984). Intonation patterns in child-directed speech: Mother–father differences. *Child Development, 55,* 1379–1385.

Warren-Leubecker, A., & Bohannon, J. (1989). Pragmatics: Language in social contexts. In J. Berko-Gleason (Ed.), *The development of language* (2nd ed.). Upper Saddle River, NJ: Merrill/Prentice Hall.

Washington, J., & Craig, H. (1994). Dialectal forms during discourse of poor, urban, African American preschoolers. *Journal of Speech, Language, and Hearing Research, 41,* 618–626.

Washington, J., & Craig, H. (2002). Morphosyntactic forms of African American English used by young children and their caregivers. *Applied Psycholinguistics, 23,* 209–231.

West, C., & Garcia, A. (1988). Conversational shift work: A study of topical transitions between women and men. *Social Problems, 35,* 551–571.

Wiener, F., Lewnau, L., & Erway, E. (1983). Measuring language competency in speakers of Black American English. *Journal of Speech and Hearing Disorders, 48,* 76–84.

Williams, R., & Wolfram, W. (1977). *Social dialects: Difference versus disorder.* Rockville, MD: American Speech–Language–Hearing Association.

Winsboro, B., & Solomon, I. (1990). Standard English vs. the American dream. *Educational Digest, 56,* 51–52.

Wolfram, W., & Christian, D. (1989). *Dialects and education: Issues and answers.* Upper Saddle River, NJ: Prentice Hall.

9

One Tongue—Two or More Languages

The previous chapter addressed diversity in American English, a phenomenon born, in part, by the influences of immigration on the English language. From the founding of the United States through the middle decades of the twentieth century, there was a general consensus that when people moved to the United States, they should *melt* into the culture, and that included learning to speak English. As the twentieth century blurred into the twenty-first century, the nation was faced with a new reality. That is, many people moving to the United States were eager to embrace the "American dream," but they were not al-

ways eager to abandon their native cultures and their native languages in the process.

There are those who continue to argue that if you want to be an American, you must speak the national language, but another view is being expressed, and the voices expressing that view are growing in number. That is, being an American is not the product of the language one speaks. To be true to the principles on which this nation was founded, these voices assert, we must be tolerant of people who choose to keep one foot firmly planted in their native cultures while determinedly placing the other foot in the mainstream culture of the United

States of America. The pluralism these people advocate includes *bilingualism*—the maintenance of one's native language and the mastery of English. In this chapter, we will consider a range of issues associated with bilingualism, including the following:

- The language implications of our changing demographics
- Defining *bilingualism*
- Differentiating *simultaneous* and *successive* bilingualism

- The influence of dual language use on cognitive development and function
- *Subtractive* and *additive* bilingual environments
- The optimal age for learning a second language
- *Code mixing, transfer,* and *interlanguage*—products of dual language development
- Stages of language development in *simultaneous bilingualism* and in *successive bilingualism*

A s I type these words, the more than 6 billion people on this planet speak about 4,000 languages, and that does not include Sarkhanese, a language my high school friend, Mike, and I invented while we attended the Schutz School in Alexandria, Egypt. Actually, there is considerable debate about how many languages there are, because the experts do not agree on whether we should include a major dialect of a language as a separate language. This argument seems somewhat moot when you consider that, in some cases, dialects of a given language are so disparate that two people speaking two different dialects cannot understand one another. If we include major dialects as separate languages, the total number of languages used in the world today might be in the range of 6,000.

You might try this question in a trivia battle: What are the ten most commonly spoken languages in the world today? Mandarin Chinese is at the top of the list, followed, in order, by English, Hindustani, Spanish, Russian, Arabic, Bengali, Portuguese, Malay-Indonesian, and French. Did you get them all in your first attempt? By the way, Sarkhan is a fictional country that serves as the backdrop for *The Ugly American,* written by William J. Lederer and Eugene Burdick in 1958. The national language of Sarkhan would be Sarkhanese. Since Sarkhan did not really exist, Mike and I took the liberty of developing a fictitious language for the fictitious country. It was, as you might guess, an adolescent product that accurately reflected the shallow end of our collective intellectual pool.

When you consider the number of languages spoken by the world's population and when you consider the rapidly changing demographics of the Unites States of America, the debate that continues to rage in our country about *one language* versus *bilingualism* might seem quaint and clearly out of touch with reality. The reality is that trying to limit our rapidly increasing and increasingly diverse population to one language is something akin to piling thousands of tons of sand on our coastal beaches in an effort to thwart rising ocean levels caused by global warming. That is a climate battle we will lose, and given the changes occurring in our population, we will not be limited to one language in the United States, no matter how hard we hug English to our chests as our national language. Bilingualism was a subject of interest two generations ago. Today bilingualism is a fact of life for many. Tomorrow it will be a fact of life for many more.

The Changing Face of America

In the preceding chapter, we presented some of the demographic evidence of a changing nation, in the context of public education. We want to expand on that evidence in this chapter to paint a more complete and detailed picture of the United States in the early years of the twenty-first century and to give the reader a clearer idea about the changes that await us over the next forty to fifty years, changes that will impact every aspect of our society, including the language or languages that will bind us together, or, if we are not adequately prepared and accepting, drive segments of our society apart.

According to the United States Census Bureau, there were 281.4 million people in the United States in 2000, an increase of 13.2 percent from 1990. This was the largest growth over a single decade in the history of our country. To the surprise of no one who pays attention to the national news, the greatest growth occurred in the West and in the South. The smallest increases were in the Midwest and the Northeast. Every state experienced some growth. Only the District of Columbia saw its population decrease (U.S. Census Bureau, 2000).

Overall growth of the population, and even differentiated increases by geographic segments, do not tell the whole story about what is happening in the United States. Consider, for example, that among people who are five years and older, 18 percent report that English is not the language they speak at home. Placed in some meaningful context, while the number of people older than five years grew by 25 percent from 1980 to 2000, the number of people who speak a language other than English at home increased more than twofold over that same time frame (U.S. Census Bureau, 2000). Put another way, 10.2 million Hispanics spoke Spanish at home in 1980. By 2000, that number rose to 24.7 million (Pew Hispanic Center Survey Brief, 2002).

The most commonly spoken language in the United States, other than English, is Spanish. Of the 47 million who reported in 2000 that they speak a language other than English at home, nearly 60 percent speak Spanish. Interestingly, only about half of those who speak Spanish report that they speak English well (U.S. Census Bureau, 2000). The third most common language spoken in the United States is Chinese, followed by French and then German (U.S. Census Bureau, 2000).

Because Spanish is the most common non-English language used in the United States, the focus of this chapter will be on people who speak English and Spanish, with one or the other as the dominant language. Note that many of the issues raised in this particular form of bilingualism would affect people whose bilingualism includes a language other than Spanish. One needs only look at recent trends to appreciate that in the foreseeable future, the focus of people who are concerned about bilingual issues must be on Hispanics. The number of people living in the United States who consider themselves *Hispanic* or *Latino* increased by 142 percent from 1980 to 2000. Hispanics and Latinos now account for 13 percent of the total population in our country, and that number is projected to grow during the coming decades (Pew Hispanic Center Survey Brief, 2002).

What Does It Mean to Be Bilingual?

As you have surely discovered by this point in our journey together, nothing in the area of language is ever easy. Terms that seem self-explanatory somehow defy simple definitions. The term *bilingual*, on the surface, seems to mean *two* (bi) *languages* (lingual). The fundamental obstacle to a simple definition can be summed up in a single word, *proficiency*. That is, how competent must a person be in two languages to be considered bilingual? Most of us know snippets of other languages, and many of us routinely use words from other languages. If, as an English-speaking person, I know a few French words, that does not make me bilingual. How much French do I need to know before I would be considered bilingual? Good question. Tough answer.

Deciding whether or not a person is bilingual is further complicated when the person is a child who is in the language acquisition period of development. Such a child is only partially competent in the language that will be her dominant language. How skilled in a second language must she be before she is considered bilingual? Good question. Tough answer.

In the ideal model of bilingualism, the speaker—adult or child—functions well in both languages. The speaker is comfortable and competent speaking English with his English-speaking friends, for example, but when his Spanish-speaking grandmother comes into the room, he transitions easily and smoothly into Spanish. In the *ideal* model of bilingualism, there is no dominant language. The speaker owns both languages equally. In the vast majority of cases, however, there is a dominant language. A child, for example, might speak Spanish exclusively at home. He speaks English at school and to his English-speaking friends, but even at school, he speaks Spanish to his Hispanic friends, so even though he is competent in English, he is a more accomplished speaker of Spanish.

Dopke (1992) suggests that we should distinguish between individuals who are *productive* bilinguals and those who are *receptive* bilinguals. The productive bilingual is truly competent in both languages even if one is more dominant than the other. The receptive bilingual clearly has a dominant language and can understand a second language, perhaps even read a second language, but is not a proficient speaker in that language.

The question remains, "How proficient must a person be in two languages before she is considered bilingual?" We must begin by acknowledging that objectifying proficiency or competence for a person who speaks one language is problematic. There are instruments designed to measure a child's receptive vocabulary, her syntactic knowledge, her morphological inventory, her pragmatic skills and then compare the results against norms established by employing these instruments with large groups of children who are judged to be "normal" within specified age groups, but ultimately these judgments are not as objective as they seem. If we are honest about this kind of assessment, we will confess that we judge a monolingual child to be proficient if she can engage in conversation, make her wants, needs, and opinions known, and if she does a reasonably good job of constructing utterances according to the rules of her language, recognizing that even the most competent adult speaker violates some of the rules some of the time.

If a child's proficiency is essentially equal in two languages, and if he meets whatever standards are established for *language competence* in those languages, he is bilingual, and his bilingualism is considered *balanced*. In most cases, he will be more proficient in one language than in the other, but even in the nondominant language, he is minimally competent. A child meeting this standard is also bilingual, but the stronger of the two languages is *dominant* (Kohnert, 2004). According to Hakuta (1990), "The range (of bilingualism) can be from native-like control of two or more languages to possessing minimal communicative skills in a second or foreign language."

Bilingual Development—Different Views, Different Terminology

As we have seen in other areas of the study of language, the problem of defining bilingualism is obfuscated by varying terminologies and by the varying interpretations of the phenomenon, i.e., bilingualism, which drives the terminologies. Two versions of bilingualism in the context of development will make this point nicely even if their differences tell us more about what we do not know than what we do know.

Simultaneous and Successive (Sequential) Bilingualism

Simply stated, if a child learns two languages at the same time, that is **simultaneous acquisition.** If she acquires one language, and having mastered that language, learns a second language, that is **successive acquisition,** also called **sequential acquisition.**

Unfortunately, what can be simply stated is not so simple. Experts argue, for example, about the age factor in determining if acquisition is truly simultaneous. Some writers have argued that the term *simultaneous acquisition* should only be used if the child acquires both languages before her third birthday (McLaughlin, 1978). Some writers apply an even stricter standard. That is, bilingual acquisition is simultaneous only if the child learns two or more languages from birth (Padilla & Lindholm, 1984). De Houwer (1995) also asserts that the cutoff age for determining simultaneous bilingualism must be set before three years, and she uses different terminology to make the acquisition difference clearer. She says that the child who acquires two languages from birth experiences **bilingual first language acquisition,** a term that does make sense. That is, during the language acquisition period, the child becomes competent in both languages, presumably at an equal rate. De Houwer uses the term **bilingual second language acquisition** to describe the child who begins the process of acquiring one language before exposure to the second language. Exposure to the second language, in order to fit De Houwer's understanding of the term, comes at least one month after birth but before the child's second birthday.

Whatever the exact age we use to distinguish between a bilingual child who has been exposed to two languages from the beginning of his life and the bilingual child who learns one language and then another, there is general agreement among those who have studied the development of children who learn two languages very early in their lives that they encounter special challenges. We will examine some of these issues in more detail later in this chapter, but at this point, we need to establish that in the beginning, there are confusions between the two languages, some mixing of the vocabularies and rules. Over time, the child separates the two languages as he becomes increasingly aware of the differences between them. If, however, one language is dominant, as is usually the case, its vocabulary and grammatical rules may continue to have undue influence on the nondominant language. This would mean, for example, that if a person's dominant language were Spanish, and the nondominant language were English, his English would always sound like English spoken by a Spanish-speaking person, even if he were quite facile in English.

How dominant a language is for a bilingual speaker depends, in large part, on the nature of inputs he receives while he is learning two or more languages and on how thoroughly he is immersed in the communities in his environment that use each language. If, for example, a child lives in a household in which Spanish is the only language spoken, and especially if he lives in a neighborhood in which Spanish is the overwhelmingly dominant language, Spanish will be his dominant language even if he is exposed to English six hours a day in school. At the same time, the degree to which Spanish dominates depends on how much exposure he receives from English media, including radio, television, and films. Even these few variables—home, community, mass media, school—should give you the idea that bilingualism exists on a continuum ranging from two languages used equally to one language as clearly dominant. All of this serves as a logical segue to an understanding of successive or sequential bilingualism.

To appreciate *successive bilingualism* in its most usual form, consider the Hispanic child who lives with parents and members of her extended family who speak only Spanish. She is immersed in this environment for the first three or four years of her life, with few excursions into English-speaking segments of the culture. By the time she is ready for preschool, she is clearly monolingual. She speaks Spanish, even though she might know a few words of English. Beginning in preschool, she is systematically exposed to English. If she is not exposed to English until she is five years old, she will understand English before she is able to speak it, and is not likely to achieve significant strength in her bilingual language system until she is in the sixth or seventh grade (Kohnert & Bates, 2002). If the child is thoroughly acculturated in her school community and in her peer community, English will become her dominant language, but if she maintains stronger ties to her Hispanic community and culture than to the mainstream English-speaking culture, Spanish will remain her dominant language.

Dual Language Learner—A Different Perspective

Another term used to describe the child who uses two languages is **dual language learner** (Genesee, Paradis, & Crago, 2004, p. 3). This term subsumes simultaneous and successive (sequential) acquisition. That is, all children who acquire two languages, no matter when they acquire them, are dual language learners. The distinction made is between **simultaneous bilingual** children and **second language** children. A simultaneous bilingual child learns two or more languages from the beginning of his life, or is exposed to a second language within the first year. If two languages are acquired, neither is dominant. Each is considered the child's *first* or *dominant* language.

A second language child acquires one language through the age of three years. She acquires a second language only after the first language has been established. You may recognize that this description perfectly matches the more traditional successive (sequential) acquisition explanation.

Genesee and his colleagues agree with others that timing of exposure to the second language is important in understanding the experiences of dual language learners, but they suggest we also need to consider the role of the *ethnolinguistic communities* of these children (Genesee et al., 2004, p. 6). In a **majority** ethnolinguistic community, the language is used by a strong majority of the citizens. It has value and status because it is associated with socioeconomic power. It is the language of the government and of the community's most influential institutions. In the United States, members of the majority ethnolinguistic community speak English. The language of a **minority** ethnolinguistic community is used by far fewer people, has less social value, and is not associated with political or economic power. In Tokyo, Japanese is the language of the major ethnolinguistic community, but in the United States, Japanese is the language of a minority ethnolinguistic community.

With this terminology in mind, consider some of the possibilities for dual language learners: (1) A child is a member of a major ethnolinguistic group who is learning two languages from the beginning of his life. A child in the United States, for example, might be born to two English-speaking parents, but they ask his Spanish-speaking nanny to immerse him in Spanish. (2) A child is a member of a major ethnolinguistic group who, after learning his first language, is exposed to a second language. An English-speaking child, for example, might attend a Spanish-immersion preschool beginning at three years. (3) A child is a member of a minority ethnolinguistic group who is exposed to two languages from the beginning of her life. A child born in the United States to Hispanic parents might be enrolled in an English-only day care program shortly after her birth. She remains in English-only educational settings even though her parents speak to her in Spanish. (4) A child who is a member of a minority enthnolinguistic group is exposed to a second language only after her first language is established. For example, a child is born in an Hispanic family in which only Spanish is spoken and is not exposed to English until she begins preschool at the age of three years (Genessee et al., 2004, pp. 7–8).

At this point you should appreciate that children who speak two languages are not homogenous. There are differences tied to language community, socioeconomic status, parents' educational backgrounds, how intentional the family is about facilitating bilingualism, the age at which the child is exposed to a second language, and too many other variables to list.

Cognition and Language Development in Bilingualism

As we established early in this book, cognition and language are closely related, and there are connections between cognitive development and language development. If a child is acquiring two languages rather than one, does the relationship between cognition and language change in any fundamental way? Is the child's innate intellectual capacity for language overloaded when he attempts to learn two languages at the same time? Given that children have for centuries demonstrated that they can master two, three, four, or more languages at the same time, the obvious answer to that question is *no*. The more troubling question centers on the possible cognitive damage that might be done when a child learns two languages. In the early 1900s, there were claims that teaching a child a second language could suppress intellectual function and cause emotional problems (Hakuta, 1986). In a review of research on bilingualism and possible links to personality problems, Diebold (1968) concluded that bilingualism could cause schizophrenia in the most severe cases and lesser adjustment problems in many cases. Other research suggested that bilingual children, because they appeared to have limited linguistic abilities, were retarded in verbal intelligence, if not in overall intelligence. By all accounts, however, this research was either biased to support the views of those who were trying to discourage immigration of Europeans to the United States in the early 1900s, or the research designs were simply flawed. In many of these studies, the bilingual subjects were children from socioeconomic backgrounds that were lower than those of the monolingual children with whom they were being compared. In addition, the bilingual children were often tested in their nondominant language, giving the impression that their language skills and their cognitive abilities were lower than they actually were. We certainly recognize today that these factors—socioeconomic class and dominant versus nondominant language—are critically important variables in research that compares groups of children.

In carefully controlled studies, the results have been starkly different. This body of research suggests that bilingualism does not adversely affect cognitive development but, in fact, strengthens it. Bilingual children perform better than monolingual children on a number of cognitive tasks, including selective attention, forming concepts, and reasoning analytically. In addition, children who speak two or more languages are more cognitively agile or flexible than children who speak just one language (Bialystok, 1999; Hakuta, Ferdman, & Diaz, 1989).

It is also noteworthy, especially to people who are specifically interested in the language aspects of cognition, that bilingual children are superior to monolingual children in their metalinguistic skills; that is, in their ability to use language to think about, analyze, and describe language (Bialystok, 2001; Ricciardelli, 1992). Bilingual children are more aware of the arbitrariness of words as symbols than monolingual children. They are more adept at identifying grammatical and semantic errors, and they have greater phonological awareness.

Questions remain about exactly why and under what conditions bilingualism enhances cognitive function, and we do not know precisely how, or even if, the brain is organized differently when a person is fluent in two languages, but research over the past several decades has effectively dispelled the notion that the effects of bilingualism on cognition and on cognitive development are deleterious.

Cognition and a Second Language: Two Views

Even among those who accept the obvious fact that the child can acquire two languages simultaneously without a significant or long-term negative impact on cognitive function, there is disagreement about what might happen in the earliest phases of development if the child is exposed to two or more languages. According to the **limited capacity hypothesis** (Genesee et al., 2004, p. 43), the child has the innate ability to acquire one language completely, but she does not have the ability to acquire two or more languages simultaneously without suffering some reduction in competence in one or both languages.

An opposing, and decidedly more positive, view is that the child does, in fact, have the cognitive capacity to acquire two languages at the same with no ill effects. Genesee and his colleagues (2004, p. 43) use a computer analogy to explain this view. The child's brain is like the hardware in a computer that gives the computer a tremendous capacity for processing information. Computer software is added to the computer to allow for complex and sophisticated multitasking. Inserting a second language into the child's brain is like adding more software. If the hardware is sophisticated enough and powerful enough, we can add many elements of software, and the computer continues to function smoothly and flawlessly. Assuming the child's brain has the vast capacity for processing information that we believe it does, adding a second language will not slow down or diminish the effectiveness of cognitive or linguistic processing.

A Footnote to the Cognitive Debate in Bilingualism

All experts in bilingualism would agree, as we have already established in this chapter, that not all children who speak two languages are the same. They acquire their languages under different circumstances, in different social and language environments, with different expectations from their caregivers, some with formal educational assistance and some without, and at different ages. Genesee and his colleagues (2004, pp. 54–55) note another difference that might affect the impact of acquiring two languages on cognition. Even if this difference does not affect cognition, it is a difference worth noting.

Many of the children included in the studies in the early years of the twentieth century lived in what have been identified as **subtractive bilingual environments.** In this environment, a child who speaks a minority language gives up his minority language when he acquires the majority language. In the process of giving up his first language, this child gives up his heritage, his culture. The child who lives in an **additive bilingual environment** has a much different life experience. This child is encouraged to retain his first language and to embrace his native culture while he learns the majority language and embraces a second culture. What is interesting about this contrast, from a cognitive point of view, is that the research that showed negative effects of bilingualism on cognitive function was conducted primarily on children from subtractive bilingual environments. The more recent research, showing cognitive advantages derived from bilingualism, involved children from predominantly additive bilingual environments. Common sense, together with the research data, would suggest that a child's cognitive abilities, including concept formation, selective attention, reasoning, and metalinguistic abilities would be enhanced by increasing competence in two languages, both of which are valued, both of which are used frequently, as is true in an additive bilingual environment. In this circumstance, the child simply has more language information available to him, and he can directly compare one language to the other in terms of vocabulary, grammar, phonology, and so on. Not only would this presumably enhance his overall understanding of language, all the language data would be grist for cognitive exercise. If one language is being systematically erased while another is being acquired, as in the subtractive bilingual environment, it is difficult to imagine that any cognitive advantage would accrue because language data would be lost, not gained.

Learning a Second Language—The Optimal Age

Is there an optimal age for learning a second language? Is there a kind of "acquisition window," an age span during which a second language can be mastered, and once that window closes, it's difficult or impossible to learn a second language? The answer to both of those questions can be found in the lyrics to the theme song of FOX Network's situation comedy *Malcolm in the Middle*. The song, *Boss of Me,* is performed by They Might Be Giants. The opening lyrics follow: "Yes, no, maybe. I don't know. Can you repeat the question?" Now, wasn't that helpful?

Let's begin with something we know for sure. We know that adults, even adults who are considered *senior citizens* or *elderly* can, and do, master second languages, some with relative ease. We also know that some people seem to have a facility for mastering languages, and others seem to struggle in the process. My father was in the former category. As a soldier during World War II, while he was in his late 20s, my father attended intensive language training at Georgetown University and, in a matter of months, learned to speak French well enough that he was scheduled to be dropped into German-occupied France to serve as a spy for military intelligence. The war ended just months before his scheduled drop, so he never had the chance to put his French to the test, but years later, when he was in his 40s, he learned to speak Korean—actually two different dialects of Korean—in about six months. The people in South Korea with whom he worked as a vocational education advisor for the Agency for International Development were stunned by his facility with the language. Several years later, he was assigned to a new position in Libya, and learned Arabic, a task he completed well enough in just three months that he was understood easily by the people with whom he worked in Benghazi. Meanwhile, my father's oldest son and my brother's only brother invested four years in high school and college classes learning French. While I was a student in Munich, Germany, I spoke French—the international language at the time—well enough that I could find a restaurant and a restroom, and that was about it. My French always evoked laughter because, as is true of other linguistically inept people who acquire a second language, I always sounded like an American tourist *trying* to speak French.

The question then is not, *can* someone learn a second language later in life, because that is a simple question with a simple answer—*yes*, although some clearly do better than others in becoming bilingual. The more important question is whether there is a period of time in a person's life that is optimal for acquiring a second language. The answer to that question is not so simple. See the lyrics to *Boss of Me*.

Research does not point to a clear age demarcation, an age before which acquiring a second language is easy and after which acquiring a second language is difficult. Some experts believe that adolescents and adults might actually have an advantage over very young children in learning a second language, in the early stages at least, because older learners bring stronger cognitive abilities and well-developed metalinguistic skills to the process. Collier (1988) asserted that children between eight and twelve years are the most proficient second language learners. Adults who learn a second language are not as adept as younger learners in acquiring the grammar and the phonology of a second language, and the difficulties in these areas tend to increase as adults age. Furthermore, as one would guess, when a person learns a second language as an adult, she tends to rely heavily on the rules of her first language to understand and formulate in the second language (Sanders, Neville, & Woldorff, 2002). There is, however, no evidence that age, in itself, is an impediment to acquiring a second language.

If a second language is forced upon a person, as is the case when someone immigrates to the United States and must learn English in order to function in the mainstream society and the public schools, age does seem to be a factor, especially when the person's first language is quite dissimilar to English. When Chinese-speaking children immigrate to the United States before they are nine years old, they tend to acquire English easily and are so proficient in English within a year that it has become their dominant language (Jia & Aaronson, 2003). Those who come to the United States after the age of nine years tend to retain Chinese as their dominant language and never become as competent in English as younger immigrants. As one would expect, age is less a factor in acquiring English for immigrants from European countries, because their native languages have the same historical roots as English and share considerable common ground with English.

As with all aspects of bilingualism, we must be cautious when we focus on a single factor, such as age, because no factor operates in a vacuum. For example, Chinese children, in addition to learning a new language when they come to America, are also being immersed into a culture that differs radically from what they experienced in their native country. European immigrants, especially those from the most industrialized countries, experience far less culture shock than immigrants from what are called third world countries. Consider too, that a child who speaks Chinese will, all other factors being equal, acquire English more easily and proficiently if his parents place him in an environment that offers exposure to English under circumstances that are supportive and encouraging. The Chinese-speaking child is more likely to retain Chinese as his preferred language while learning English if Chinese continues to be spoken at home and if his native language and culture are valued. Even something as basic as childcare can be a factor. If a Chinese-speaking preschool child is in the care of his grandmother who speaks only Chinese, and if he is in her care eight to ten hours every day, we should not be surprised that he acquires English more slowly than a Chinese-speaking preschool child who is in the care of a nanny who speaks only English.

There is also danger in trying to understand the developmental experiences of the bilingual child only in the context of what we know about the monolingual child. Why would we assume that the experiences of these two populations would be the same, especially when we compare monolingual children who have been born and reared in the United States with bilingual children who were born in one country and then moved to the United States? The cultural and social experiences of these two groups of children are dramatically different. Their language experiences are different, and there is every reason to believe that there are aspects of their cognitive experiences that differ. What is remarkable is that in spite of these differences, monolingual and bilingual children acquire language in very much the same way and according to the same general schedule (Bialystok, 2001, p. 88).

In returning to the never-ending argument about nature versus nurture, we reasonably conclude that the innate capacity for acquiring language does not die when one reaches thirteen or sixteen or seventy. We retain the biological ability to learn language as long as we live with healthy brains, intact sensory mechanisms, and functional speech mechanisms. We must also recognize that learning is a factor in language acquisition, whether it's one language or two or three, and no matter the age of the learner. We may assume that, for adults, the experience of acquiring a second language is extremely learning-intensive, and it may be for some adults, but for others, including my father, learning a second, third, or fourth language is more a process of exposure and social practice than study and drill. We should also not ignore the fact that learning is important in linguistic development for the very young child if the child is learning one language or two. The capacity for language may be innate, but the conventions of the child's language or languages are learned (Bialystok, 2001, p. 88).

In thinking about an optimal or critical age for learning a second language, we should keep in mind the possibility, nay the likelihood, that in the process of learning a second language, the learner is assisted by her competence in her first language. Schiff-Myers (1992) suggests that when a child learns a second language during the school years, she is able to use the metalinguistic skills she acquired in mastering her first language to facilitate acquisition of the second language.

We began this section with a statement of fact, that people *can* learn a second language, no matter how young or old they might be. We will end with another statement of fact. Although children might be slower in acquiring a second language than adults, in the early stages of acquisition, and even if they might experience some *language confusion* in the early months and years of development, over the long term—all other factors being equal—younger learners will outperform older learners in the second language. That's not a revelation unique to language. It's true for nearly everything human beings learn. If two people with equal innate talent begin piano lessons or tennis lessons at the same time, and one of those people is three years old, and the other person is sixty years old, the three-year-old person will eventually reach a greater level of proficiency in those activities than the adult. It is not true that "You can't teach an old dog new tricks," but it is true that the challenge in learning becomes more difficult as we tack years onto the old dog.

A Closer Look at Simultaneous Bilingualism

No matter how you slice the debates about bilingualism, one dimension consistently looms large—possible differences between simultaneous bilingualism and successive, or sequential, bilingualism. For that reason, we are going to take a closer look at what we know about each of these categories of bilingualism and what has been speculated about the experiences of children who fit into each category.

Two Languages or a Single Hybrid Language?

Since, in simultaneous bilingualism, the child is presumably acquiring two languages at the same time, there is debate about whether the child, in the beginning, is actually acquiring two separate languages or a rather convoluted single language hybrid that includes elements of both languages.

The **unitary language system hypothesis,** postulated by Virginia Volterra and Traute Taescher (1978), suggests that the child who is exposed, more or less equally, to two languages from birth, in the first stage of language development, actually functions with a single language that is a hybrid of two distinctly different languages, a hybrid that includes vocabulary and grammatical rules from both languages. As development continues into a second stage, the child differentiates the vocabularies of the two languages, but continues to rely on the hybrid grammatical system she developed in the first stage. In the third and final stage, the child differentiates the grammatical systems of the two languages, resulting in a kind of surgical separation of the two languages. The evolution from "unitary" to "separate" is not unlike what happens with conjoined twins who, prior to surgery, share organ systems and, after successful separation surgery, function independently.

Fred Genesee (1989) offers an opposing view in what he calls the **dual language system hypothesis.** In this case, the name accurately describes the argument. That is, the child who is exposed to two languages from birth uses two separate language system from the very beginning. The child, according to this hypothesis, does not go through stages in which a conjoined language system is gradually differentiated into two language systems.

Research provides more support for the dual language system hypothesis than the unitary language system hypothesis. While simultaneous bilingual children will occasionally mix vocabulary, and while they might occasionally use rules from one language with vocabulary from the other, they do not produce these confusions frequently or in a consistent manner that would suggest they are *rule-governed*. Even more telling, there is no evidence that these children produce truly hybrid, or amalgamated, rules of grammar, something we would expect in the first stage of development if the unitary language system were valid.

The Impact of Community on Simultaneous Bilingualism

As we have already noted several times, if we are to understand bilingualism in any form, we cannot overlook the context in which the two languages are learned. In the case of simultaneous bilingualism, we have to consider which language is most highly *preferred* in the child's home and which language is most highly *valued* in the larger community. We must consider if the child's family encourages him to retain his native language in the face of pressures outside the home to extinguish that language in favor of the language of the majority population.

When children grow up in countries that have traditions of bilingualism, many of the *community issues* are not operative, but these issues certainly are operative in the United States. Hispanics who migrate to the United States, for example, must confront these issues and decide if they will retain Spanish only, if they will teach their children to speak English only, or if they will encourage their children born in the United States to be bilingual by exposing them to both languages from birth. Even if they choose bilingual, there is still the question about which language will be favored, or if equal value will be ascribed to each. These are not easy decisions because they are embedded in larger questions about culture and heritage.

Even if parents decide that their child is best served by remaining truly bilingual, there are forces beyond the home that might shape the child's ultimate linguistic destiny. When it becomes clear to an Hispanic child, for example, that the educational system strongly values English over Spanish, she might decide that little is to be gained by maintaining Spanish. Portes and Rumbaut (2001) found that adolescent immigrants from Asian and Latin countries quickly developed a preference for English. When they were in junior high school, almost three-fourths of the children they surveyed preferred English to their first language. By the time they graduated from high school, nearly nine of ten preferred English. While some people might look at these numbers and conclude that the death of bilingualism is simply one of the costs of becoming an "American," we feel compelled to point out that there are clear downsides to the death of bilingualism in a child. We have already noted that there are cognitive advantages to bilingualism, and there are metalinguistic advantages as well. Furthermore, since language is so inextricably connected to culture and heritage, it's difficult to imagine what cogent argument could be made to support the idea that a child is best served by disassociating himself from his origins, especially in a country like the United States of America that characterizes itself, with considerable pride, as a nation of immigrants.

Monolinguism vs. Simultaneous Bilingualism—Developmental Differences?

Does simultaneous bilingualism cause developmental differences? The easy answer to this question is *no*. Children who are exposed to two languages from birth follow the same overall developmental patterns and hit developmental milestones at the same ages as children who are exposed to just one language (Genesee et al., 2004, p. 85). Bilingual children experience the same challenges in language development as monolingual children and make the same kinds of "mistakes" in grammar and phonology. If a bilingual child does make a unique mistake, it is most likely the product of the unique influences one of his languages exerts on the other. We should also note that we see the same variability in rate of language development among simultaneous bilingual children as we see in monolingual children (Genesee, p. 78).

Into this simple depiction of developmental harmony, we must inject an important qualification. That is, even though in simultaneous bilingualism the child is exposed to two languages from birth, it is highly unlikely that the exposure will be exactly equal, which means that one language is *dominant* and the other is *nondominant*. If, during the developmental period, the child is exposed more often and more deliberately to one language than the other, there is no reason to believe that the development of both languages will be exactly equal. The dominant language will, of course, be accelerated in development in comparison to the nondominant language, but over time, if exposure to both languages remains reasonably strong and consistent, the developmental differences will diminish. Even when the differences are most pronounced, however, one should not conclude that the child is proficient in the dominant language and incompetent or semi-competent in the nondominant language (Genesee et al., 2004, p. 80). Competence or proficiency is always relative, and there is something else to consider. The dominant language at three or four years might be the child's nondominant language by the time he is eighteen.

In a less enlightened time, researchers believed that exposure to two languages retarded development. The evidence they often cited was smaller vocabulary size in the bilingual child. While that may appear to be true, especially if it's the vocabulary of the nondominant language that is measured, when the vocabularies of both languages are combined and when we account for the conceptual bases of the words included in both languages, the size of the vocabularies of simultaneous bilingual children are the same as those of monolingual children during the developmental period (Pearson, 1998; Pearson, Fernandez, & Oller, 1993).

Code Mixing—Serious Problem or Bump in the Road?

To argue that the child exposed to two languages from birth *never* confuses the two languages would be silly and not conformant to facts or common observations. My youngest sister, Jinny, was exposed to Korean and to English at birth, and the exposures were fairly equal during the earliest stages of her language development. She often used Korean words in otherwise English sentences, and she used English words in Korean constructions. She also confused grammatical rules. Code mixing is the norm for bilingual children and adults (Genesee et al., 2004, p. 111). Is this a serious problem? On the contrary, the fact that most of the bilingual child's code-mixing issues are grammatical means that she is mastering the syntactic systems of the two languages. She could not mix elements of the two grammars unless she was mastering both of them and unless she was able to draw from one grammar to insert one of its rules into the other grammar. A fact of linguistic life for the bilingual code mixer is that she mixes less and less as language development proceeds.

Genesee and his colleagues (2004, p. 111) make the argument that code mixing is a *communicative resource*. That is, the child draws upon her greatest competencies in each language to create a communicative effort that is more complete than it would be if either language were used alone. We should also consider that code mixing, like every other dimension of bilingualism, is a product of the child's familial, community, and cultural experiences. In other words, code mixing is not just a language phenomenon. What is mixed and how it is mixed may well be influenced by factors in the child's life that go beyond the boundaries of language.

A Closer Look at Successive or Sequential Bilingualism

Recall that dual language usage is considered *successive* or *sequential* bilingualism if one language is established before the speaker—child or adult—is exposed to a second language. The second exposure could occur when the child is three years old and moving into the latter stages of language development, or it could occur when he is taking language classes in high school or college, or it could occur when he is taking a *Berlitz-Brighton* language course as an older adult.

Depending on when the exposure occurs, the challenges involved in acquiring the second language will differ. If the exposure comes in the child's third year of life, there may be more initial confusions than if the exposure comes in his thirtieth year of life, but if exposures to both languages remain consistent and rich, and if both languages are highly valued in his life, proficiency in both languages will usually be greater if the exposure is early.

Transfer—Keeping One Foot in the First Language

Assuming the dual language learner is a child, we would expect that in the early stages of exposure to the second language, the child's productions in that language would be influenced by his first language expertise. When the child applies something from his first language to the second language, we call that *transfer*, a process that may be reflected in grammar, vocabulary, and phonology. The casual observer might notice transfer most easily in the bilingual individual's pronunciations. If, for example, the speaker's second language contains sounds that do not occur in his first language, he might adjust his production of words containing those unfamiliar sounds to conform to the phonology he knows best, resulting in quaint pronunciations. At one time, transfer was viewed negatively, as an impediment to effectively learning the second language. We now understand that transfer is a healthy phenomenon, that when the child transfers something he knows from his first language to his productions in the second language, he is using his first language as a kind of linguistic resource to advance his acquisition of the second language (Genesee et al.,

2004, p. 131). Some transfers, like pronunciations shaped by his greater comfort level with the phonology of his first language, might remain, especially if the second language exposure comes later in life, but most transfers will fade away as the process of separating the two languages moves to completion.

How Quickly Is the Second Language Learned?

Most adults are impressed by how quickly very young children learn everything they learn. When I watch my elementary school-age grandchildren sit at a computer, I am amazed by how quickly they become computer geeks. I am equally impressed when I watch youngsters learn to play the piano, or learn the basic skills in baseball, soccer, or basketball. Because most of us are awed by the capacities of young minds and young bodies to learn at breakneck speed, we assume that young children will learn a second language quickly and easily. In fact, the process is not as rapid as we might imagine (Genesee et al., 2004, p. 133).

We must, of course, keep in mind that acquiring a second language will not be the same experience or occur at the same rate for all children, any more than learning the piano or learning soccer will be the same experience for all children, even if the amount of exposure to the language, the piano, or soccer is exactly the same. Every child is unique. Each child's unique circumstances determine the rate at which a new skill or a second language will be mastered. Some Spanish-speaking children, after just one year of English immersion, will be able to use English conversationally. Others will be functional in English after one year, but will not reach conversational competence in that time span. Why do some children advance more rapidly than others? Aside from the obvious possible differences in the quantity and quality of exposure, some children are simply more motivated than others. Children who are more gregarious and social advance more quickly in the second language than children who are shy and withdrawn (Wong Fillmore, 1983), and although it's difficult to quantify, some people simply have a greater aptitude for language learning than others (Carroll, 1981, p. 93). So, how quickly do these children master their second language? The answer, of course, is that it depends on many factors, but what can be said with absolute certainly is that rate of acquisition is highly variable, and what can be said with a reasonable degree of confidence is that some children are proficient in the second language within one year and most are proficient within two, three, or four years (Genesee et al., 2004, p. 137).

Attrition—Influence of the Second Language on the First

The child probably uses proficiency in his first language to help him learn a second language, as evidenced by transfer. In many cases, the once dominant first language fades, and the second language becomes dominant. This process is called **attrition** (Genesee et al., 2004, p. 143). In attrition, the first language might simply become the child's nondominant language, or it might fade away entirely so that the formerly bilingual child becomes essentially monolingual.

Under what conditions does attrition occur? Your educated guesses will almost certainly match the facts. If, for example, an Hispanic child moves to the United States and speaks Spanish as his first language and then enters school in a district in which only English is spoken in its classrooms, and if all of the child's friends speak only English, and if the child's parents are eager to become completely assimilated into the dominant culture, it is easy to imagine what will happen. The child first becomes bilingual, using his proficiency in Spanish to help him master his new language, English. Over time, as Spanish becomes devalued and as he finds fewer and fewer opportunities to use it, his proficiency in Spanish declines, and his proficiency in English improves. Attrition has occurred.

The journey from dual language to single language by means of attrition is not inexorable, and most experts with interests in language or child development would argue that it is not desirable. No matter what a child brings to life from the genetic pools that merge into his conception, he is also a product of his environment. That environment includes his culture, his immediate and extended family, and his social community. The connections between language and the most critical components of the child's environment are powerful. Although it might seem an overstatement to some, others would agree that when the child's first language is allowed to die, the child's cultural background is wounded, and some important part of the child's identity dies as well. Unless there are extenuating circumstances that would seem to require extinguishing one of a bilingual child's two languages—and it's difficult to imagine what those circumstances would be—the child is a more enriched human being when he is encouraged to retain his first language, and by extension, embrace his native culture. There are, as we have already noted several times, metalinguistic and cognitive advantages that are derived from proficiency in two or more languages. One could argue that even these advantages are not as important to the *wholeness* of the life experience as the cultural, social, and psychological advantages that thrive in the context of dual language proficiency.

Stages of Language Development in Bilingual Children

We conclude this chapter by examining two attempts to describe stages of language development in children who are exposed to two languages. You should appreciate at this point that, as difficult as it is to describe stages of language development in monolingual children, it is considerably more difficult to identify stages of development in children who are bilingual. Whatever conclusions we draw about the nature of these stages and the ages at which they are reached, we must remember that they are, at best, generic and necessarily vague because there are simply too many factors beyond the acquisition of language that will impact how a given bilingual child will progress through language development. Consider just some of the variables: (1) Bilingual children are exposed to different languages, (2) They grow up in different familial, social, and cultural environments, (3) In some homes, the minority language is highly valued, and in other homes it is deliberately extinguished, (4) The frequency and quality of exposure in each language is sometimes radically different from child to child, and (5) Some, but not all, bilingual children attend preschool, and the preschool experience can either reinforce the use of two languages or discourage it. The influence of these and other variables make the experience of acquisition for these children anything but homogeneous. We can all agree that describing stages of development that will accurately fit all dual language children is impossible. In spite of the obstacles, it is important to at least consider the progression of development for these children, especially in comparison to monolingual children, so that we might appreciate the unique challenges they face. Even if the stages fail to capture all, or even most, bilingual children, they will give us at least a general idea about how the language experiences of these children evolve as they move through the developmental process.

We will consider two, often overlapping, views of language development in bilingual children. Robert Owens (2005, pp. 418–422) describes three stages of language development in simultaneous bilingualism and three stages in successive bilingualism. Patton Tabors (1997) describes four stages in successive bilingualism, or *second language learning.*

Owens' Stages of Development in Simultaneous Bilingualism

In Stage 1, the child has two different language systems and chooses one system over the other depending on the communicative context or the communicative purpose in any given circumstance. She might, for example and logically, use one system with adults who speak one language and the other system with adults who speak the other language. In the beginning, the child combines the phonologies of the two languages into a single system, but she begins to ascribe the correct phonology to the correct language by twenty-four to thirty months, and she has them well separated by the time she is three years old, at least well enough that she knows the phonology of her native language.

By the time the child enters Stage 2, she has two separate vocabularies for her two languages, but she uses one grammatical system in both languages. The words she adds to her vocabularies are drawn from specific contexts, and if she acquires a word in one language, she typically does not learn its equivalent in the other language right away. In terms of syntax, she tends to learn constructions that are applicable in both languages before she learns the constructions that are unique to each language, and as common sense would suggest, she learns simple constructions earlier than more complex constructions. If the construction for a given syntactic rule is easier in one language than the other, she will learn the simpler version first.

In Stage 3, the child is fairly consistent in keeping the vocabularies and syntactic systems of the two languages separate. The interference that remains occurs primarily in syntax, when the child applies a rule from one language in producing a construction in the other language. There are very few instances of code mixing in the child's productions by the time she is three or four years old, and some of those mixes seem to occur when the child attends to code mixing in the speech of adults with whom she interacts. In other words, the child seems to be learning what her caregivers model for her, mixes and all.

Owens' Stages of Development in Successive Bilingualism

In considering the stages of successive or sequential bilingualism, remember that exposure to the second language can occur at any age. Although many factors can influence the ultimate degree of proficiency in the second language, it is generally true that it is more difficult to become highly proficient in a second language if the exposure occurs in the late teens or later—not impossible, but more difficult. Again, generally speaking, if the person acquiring a second language has a strong need for that language, if she is highly motivated, if her attitude about acquiring the language is positive, and if she identifies with the community in which that language is dominant, she is likely to become proficient in that language. To these generalizations, one more needs to be added. Since this group is exponentially heterogeneous, any stage concept applied to this group must be vague enough to be sufficiently ubiquitous to include the developmental experiences of most, if not all, of its members.

In describing the stages of development for successive bilingualism, Owens excludes the acquisition of a second language as the result of formal classes. With that in mind, in Stage 1, the child develops personal and social relationships with people in the community who use the second language. At this point, the relationships and communicative exchanges between the child and users of the second language are more important than any specific linguistic advances that might be made. In fact, the child's productions in the second language during the first stage are usually limited to the most basic of vocabulary words and to standard phrases, including common social gesture expressions. The child's primary language commitment is to listen to what is being said, to find repeating linguistic patterns that might provide clues about topics of conversation, and to act as though he knows what is being said as a way of establishing relationships. The child might be an *other-directed* communicator in this stage, using whatever means he can to get his message across, using the few words and phrases from the second language he knows, along with a full range of nonverbal communications. He might be *inner-directed,* which means that he stays on the periphery of communicative exchanges and might seem to be introverted. In fact, he is very much engaged in the communicative process, but rather than focusing on expressing his own messages, he is trying to figure out what is being said, and he is analyzing the language forms contained in the productions of others. He uses private speech to practice constructions he hears and uses the fragments he does understand to covertly form expanded productions.

In Stage 2, the child makes a concerted effort to communicate in the second language, using whatever he does understand without worrying about the grammatical or morphological nuances. That part of mastery will come later. For now, he is a *messenger,* and he uses all resources available to him in the second language, no matter how unrefined the linguistic pieces are, to say what he wants to say. In this second stage, we might hear the child use what is called **interlanguage,** a kind of language hybrid that combines rules from his dominant language, rules from the second language, and rules the child invents to bridge any gaps between the two. Interlanguage should not be understood as a deficient form of either language. It is the child's unique, but clearly rule-governed, language system. Over time, the child's interlanguage evolves to reflect his growing proficiency in the second language and his overall developing linguistic competence.

When the child enters Stage 3, his focus is on correctly applying the rules of the second language. Note that the child developing successive bilingualism begins the process of acquiring the second language having already established some degree of proficiency in his first language, so he is able to use the metalinguistic awareness nurtured in his first language to help him analyze, understand, and master the second language. Using the knowledge he has gained in his first language and insights he has developed about his second language, he understands the importance of sequential ordering in language. As he monitors the speech of those who speak the second language, he discovers the rules for sequencing in that language, and he applies those rules in his own productions. His first language experiences have taught him that specific contexts affix meanings to words, and that a single word, depending on varying contextual associations, can have several meanings. He applies that knowledge as he sorts out and organizes the words of his second language. In the beginning, he keeps his productions as simple as they need to be so he can correctly preserve the rules he is learning, but as his confidence in the second language grows, his utterances become more elaborate. You should recognize this progression, because this is exactly what we observe in the monolingual child. The monolingual child uses single words before he uses phrases. He uses simple phrases before he uses complex phrases. He uses simple sentence forms before he embeds and conjoins. The successive bilingual child goes through the same process . . . twice, the first time in his first language and then again in his second language.

Tabors's Stages of Second Language Acquisition

Patton Tabors (1997) concluded that there are four stages in second language acquisition, based on a study she conducted with preschool children who were acquiring English as their second language. Tabors noted, as we have repeatedly emphasized, that there was a great deal of variation among these children. The variation in development was so great, in fact, that some children seemed to skip a stage while others seemed to remain in that stage much longer than one would expect. Tabors's stages, therefore, should be viewed as she intended them to be viewed—as general descriptions of what a mythical, prototypical child is likely to experience in the step-by-step process of acquiring a second language. There is no suggestion in her conclusions that all second language children will progress through these stages in the same way or according to the same timetable.

In Stage 1, called the *home language use* period, the child uses her first, or native, language in settings where only English is spoken. This stage typically does not last long, often just a few days, because the child figures out that her native language is not working in this environment.

Stage 2 is called the *nonverbal period.* As the name suggests, the child depends heavily on nonverbal communication to convey her messages. The assumption is that the child is acquiring English receptively at this point, but there is very little expressive language in English, and in some cases, none at all. It is important to reinforce, however, that the child is communicating nonverbally, and through those communications, she is interacting with the people around her who are speaking English. This stage might last a few weeks or a few months. Younger children tend to remain in the nonverbal period longer than older children. Perhaps the key element in this stage is the development of relationships and social interactions, which presumably will help motivate the child to make stronger attempts to use English.

When the child begins to produce English utterances, she has moved into Stage 3, also called the period of *telegraphic and formulaic use.* Early in Stage 3, she is not producing complete sentences and there is very little that is original in what she says. Most of her productions are direct replications of constructions formulated by others. Tabors noted that most of the earliest English utterances she heard produced by the preschool children she observed were single-word productions used to label, count, or identify color. The first multiple-word productions Tabors heard were imitations of phrases such as, "Excuse me," and "I don't know," and she believed these productions were imitations of whole phrases with little or no understanding of the individual words that made up each phrase. This is probably a safe assumption, since adults do the same thing when they learn bits and pieces of a second language in preparation for a trip to a foreign country. An American, for example, who visits Japan might memorize the phrase that means, "Can you direct me to the nearest restroom?" without knowing where one word ends and the next begins. It's not hard to imagine that a child faced with the daunting task of learning a second language would do the same thing. As the child nears the end of Stage 3, she begins to utter sentences that are productive. A sentence is considered *productive* if at least portions of the construction are original and if the child draws from her English vocabulary and from some rudimentary version of an English grammar in order to formulate it. In terms of abiding by all aspects of the rules system for English, these sentences are not perfect. They may be far from perfect, but the child is showing the first signs of genuine proficiency in her second language.

The shift from Stage 3 to Stage 4 is not dramatic, but when the child's productions in English are truly productive, she has moved into Stage 4. The child's English constructions are original, not imitated fragments taped together into something that sounds like English. She has apparently mastered the basics of English language rules and is rapidly filling in remaining gaps in her English competence. This does not mean that she sounds like an American speaking English. She does not. Even if she is young, she will retain remnants of the accent identifiable with her first language. She will mispronounce words. She will make incorrect vocabulary choices. She will make grammatical and morphological errors, but we should all be quick to recognize that, except for lingering accent, monolingual English-speaking children make these errors as well. We should accept that some aspects of less than perfect English productions are the result of the child's learning a second language, but others are the result of simply learning language.

Bilingualism—Good, Bad, or Inevitable?

Especially in light of evidence suggesting that cognitive and metalinguistic advantages accrue from dual language exposure, it would be difficult for any reasonable person to conclude that bilingualism is a bad thing. Most language people, including the authors of this book, would argue vehemently that bilingualism is an entirely positive phenomenon, and not just because of the cognitive and metalinguistic advantages. Language is so thoroughly embedded into a child's culture, his social consciousness, and his personal identity that efforts to subtract a first language when the child moves to the United States and is exposed to English could be viewed as insensitive. At the very least, subtracting the first language is entirely unnecessary. Whatever minor difficulties might occur as a result of code mixing, interlanguage, or transfer errors fade quickly as the child's proficiency in the second language increases. The time frame for mastering the second language, even if the child is in the middle elementary school years before he is exposed to English, is typically three to five years. Although there are likely to be social and academic problems during the transition from monolingualism to bilingualism, those problems need to be weighed against the long-term advantages of being able to communicate with proficiency in two languages. As we look at the unfolding of the twenty-first century, we might also consider that dual language use may be inevitable for a majority of people who live in the United States. Bilingualism is already a fact of life for many. If the demographics of the United States continue to change as they have changed over the past forty years, we will be a more pluralistic nation than ever, and that might mean pluralism in language. Stay tuned.

Review Questions

1. What do the changing demographics in the United States suggest about the future of our country? How will these changes affect you personally?

2. How does the concept of *proficiency* affect our understanding of *bilingualism?*

3. What do the terms *simultaneous bilingualism* and *successive (sequential) bilingualism* mean, and what is the significance of the difference between the two?

4. What does *dual language learner* mean, and how does that term relate to *simultaneous* and *successive* forms of bilingualism?

5. What is an *ethnolinguistic community*? What is the difference between a *majority* and a *minority* ethnolinguistic community?

6. What do we know about the connection between bilingualism and cognition? How do we explain the apparent contradiction in findings between the older studies (i.e., early twentieth century) and current studies?

7. What is the *limited capacity hypothesis*?

8. What do the terms *subtractive bilingual environment* and *additive bilingual environment* mean? What are the advantages and disadvantages

of each environment for developing children?

9. What is the *optimal* age for acquiring a second language?

10. Explain the *unitary language system hypothesis* and the *dual language system hypothesis*.

11. What is *code mixing*? Is this a serious problem for the bilingual child? Why or why not?

12. What is meant by *transfer* in the language development of the bilingual child? Is transfer a liability or an asset in development?

13. What is *attrition* in bilingualism? How does it occur? How can it be prevented?

14. Identify and briefly describe the three stages of development in si-

multaneous bilingualism, according to Robert Owens.

15. Identify and briefly describe the three stages of development in successive bilingualism, according to Robert Owens.

16. Identify and briefly describe the four stages of development in second language acquisition, according to Patton Tabors.

17. What is *interlanguage*? Is interlanguage an asset or a liability for the child who is acquiring a second language?

18. Is bilingualism in the twenty-first century United States good, bad, or inevitable?

References and Suggested Readings

Bedore, L. (2004). Morphosyntactic development. In B. Goldstein (Ed.), *Bilingual language development & disorders in Spanish-English speakers.* Baltimore: Paul H. Brookes.

Bhatia, T., & Ritchie, W. (1999). The bilingual child: Some issues and perspectives. In W. C. Ritchie & T. Bhatia (Eds.), *Handbook of child language acquisition* (pp. 569–646). San Diego: Academic Press.

Bialystok, E. (1992). Attentional control in children's metalinguistic performance and measures of field independence. *Developmental Psychology, 28,* 654–664.

Bialystok, E. (1997). Effects of bilingualism and biliteracy on children's emerging concepts of print. *Developmental Psychology, 33,* 429–440.

Bialystok, E. (1986). Factors in the growth of linguistic awareness. *Child Development, 57,* 498–510.

Bialystok, E. (1988). Levels of bilingualism and levels of linguistic awareness. *Developmental Psychology, 24,* 560–567.

Bialystok, E. (1999). Cognitive complexity and attentional control in the bilingual mind. *Child Development, 70,* 636–644.

Bialystok, E. (2001). *Bilingualism in development: Language, literacy, & cognition.* Cambridge, United Kingdom: Cambridge University Press.

Bosch, L., & Sebastian-Galles, N. (2001). Early language differentiation in bilingual infants. In J. Cenoz & F. Genesee (Eds.), *Trends in bilingual acquisition* (pp. 71–94). Amsterdam: John Benjamins.

Carroll, J. (1981). Twenty-five years of research on foreign language aptitude. In K. C. Diller (Ed.), *Individual differences and universals in language learning aptitude.* Rowley, MA: Newbury House.

Carroll, S. (1999). Putting 'input' in its proper place. *Second Language Research, 15,* 337–388.

Carroll, S. (2001). *Input and evidence.* Amsterdam: John Benjamins.

Collier, V. (1987). Age and rate of acquisition of second language for academic purposes. *TESOL Quarterly, 21,* 617–641.

Collier, V. (1988). The effect of age on acquisition of a second language for school. *Forum, 2,* Winter 1987/1988.

Cummins, J. (2000). *Language, power and pedagogy: Bilingual children in the crossfire.* Clevedon, England: Multilingual Matters.

de Houwer, A. (1990). *The acquisition of two languages from birth: A case study.* Cambridge, MA: Cambridge University Press.

de Houwer, A. (1995). Bilingual language acquisition. In P. Fletcher & B. MacWhinney (Eds.), *Handbook of child language* (pp. 219–250). Oxford: Basil Blackwell Ltd.

de Houwer, A. (1998). Environmental factors in early bilingual development: The role of parental beliefs and attitudes. In G. Extra & L. Verhoeven (Eds.), *Bilingualism and migration* (pp. 75–95). Berlin: Mouton de Gruyter.

Delgado-Gaitan, C. (2001). *The power of community: Mobilizing for family and schooling.* Lanham, MD: Rowman & Littlefield.

Diebold, A. (1968). The consequences of early bilingualism in cognitive and personality formation. In E. Norbeck, D. Price-Williams, & W. M. McCord (Eds.), *The study of personality: An interdisciplinary appraisal* (pp. 218–245). New York: Holt, Rinehart & Winston.

Dopke, S. (1992). *One parent one language: An interactional approach.* Amsterdam: John Benjamins.

Dopke, S. (2000). The interplay between language-specific development and cross-linguistic influence. In S. Dopke (Ed.), *Crosslinguistic structures in simultaneous bilingualism* (pp. 79–103). Amsterdam: John Benjamins.

Genesee, F. (1976). The role of intelligence in second language learning. *Language Learning, 26,* 267–280.

Genesee, F. (1989). Early bilingual development: One language or two? *Journal of Child Language, 16,* 161–179.

Genesee, F. (2003). Rethinking bilingual acquisition. In J. M. de Waele (Ed.), *Bilingualism: Challenges and directions for future research* (pp. 158–182). Clevedon, England: Multilingual Matters.

Genesee, F., Nicoladis, E., & Paradis, J. (1995). Language differentiation in early bilingual development. *Journal of Child Language, 22,* 611–631.

Genesee, F., Paradis, J., & Crago, M. (2004). *Dual language development & disorders: A handbook on bilingualism & second language learning.* Baltimore: Paul H. Brookes.

Goldstein, B. A. (Ed.). (2004). *Bilingual development & disorders in Spanish-English speakers.* Baltimore: Paul H. Brookes.

Grosjean, F. (1998). Studying bilinguals: Methodological and conceptual issues. *Language and Cognition, 1,* 131–149.

Gutierrez, V. (2004). Narrative development and disorders in bilingual children. In B. Goldstein (Ed.), *Bilingual language development & disorders in Spanish-English speakers.* Baltimore: Paul H. Brookes.

Gutierrez-Clellen, V., & Dreiter, J. (2003). Understanding child bilingual acquisition using parent and teacher reports. *Applied Psycholinguistics, 24,* 267–288.

Hakuta, K. (1986). *Mirror of language: The debate on bilingualism.* New York: Basic Books.

Hakuta, K. (1990). *Bilingualism and bilingual education: A research perspective.* Washington, D.C.: National Clearinghouse on Bilingual Education.

Hakuta, K. (1994). Distinguishing among proficiency, choice, and attitudes in questions about language for bilinguals. In G. Lamberty, & C. Garcia Coll (Eds.), *Puerto Rican women and children: Issues in health, growth and development* (pp. 191–209). New York: Plenum Press.

Hakuta, K., & D'Andrea, D. (1992). Some properties of bilingual maintenance and loss in Mexican background high-school students. *Applied Linguistics, 13* (1), 72–99.

Hakuta, K., & Diaz, R. (1985). The relationship between degree of bilingualism and cognitive ability. In K. Nelson (Ed.), *Children's language* (Vol. 5, pp. 319–344). Mahwah, NJ: Erlbaum.

Hakuta, K., Ferdman, B., & Diaz, R. (1989). *Bilingualism and cognitive development: Three perspectives and methodological implications.* Los Angeles: University of California.

Hakuta, K., Goto Butler, Y., & Witt, D. (2000). *How long does it take English learners to attain proficiency?* (Policy Report 2000-1) Davis, CA: University of California Linguistic Minority Research Institute. On-line. Available at www.stanford.edu/hakuta/Docs/HowLong.pdf

Hakuta, K., & McLaughlin, B. (1996). Bilingualism and second language learning: Seven tensions that define the research. In D. Berliner & R. Calfee (Eds.), *Handbook of educational psychology* (pp. 603–621). New York: MacMillan.

Hammer, C., Miccio, A., & Rodriquez, B. (2004). Bilingual language acquisition and the child socialization process. In B. Goldstein (Ed.), *Bilingual language development & disorders in Spanish-English speakers.* Baltimore: Paul H. Brookes.

Hammer, C., Miccio, A., & Wagstaff, D. (2003). Home literacy experiences and their relationship to bilingual preschoolers' developing English literacy abilities: An initial investigation. *Language, Speech, and Hearing Services in Schools, 34,* 20–30.

Jackson-Maldonado, D. (2004). Verbal morphology and vocabulary in monolinguals and emergent bilinguals. In B. Goldstein (Ed.), *Bilingual language development & disorders in Spanish-English speakers.* Baltimore: Paul H. Brookes.

Jia, G., & Aaronson, D. (2003). A longitudinal study of Chinese children and adolescents learning English in the United States. *Applied Psycholinguistics, 24,* 131–161.

Jia, G., Aaronson, D., & Wu, Y. (2002). Long-term language attainment of bilingual immigrants: Predictive variables and language group differences. *Applied Psycholinguistics, 23,* 599–621.

Kohnert, K. (2004). Processing skills in early sequential bilinguals. In B. Goldstein (Ed.), *Bilingual language development & disorders in Spanish-English speakers.* Baltimore: Paul H. Brookes.

Kohnert, K., & Bates, E. (2002). Balancing bilinguals, II: Lexical comprehension and cognitive processing in children learning Spanish and English. *Journal of Speech, Language, and Hearing Research, 45,* 347–359.

Kohnert, K., Bates, E., & Hernandez, A. (1999). Balancing bilinguals: Lexical-semantic production and cognitive processing in children learning Spanish and English. *Journal of Speech, Language, and Hearing Research, 42,* 1400–1413.

Maneva, B., & Genesee, F. (2002). Bilingual babbling: Evidence for language differentiation in dual language acquisition. In B. Skarabela et al. (Eds.), The *Proceedings of the 26th Boston University Conference on Language Development* (pp. 383–392). Somerville, MA: Cascadilla Press.

McLaughlin, B. (1978). *Second-language acquisition in childhood.* Mahwah, NJ: Erlbaum.

Miccio, A., Hammer, C., & Toribio, A. (2002). Linguistics and speech-language pathology: Combining research efforts toward improved interventions for bilingual children. In J. Alatis, H. Hamilton, & A-H. Tan (Eds.), *Georgetown University Round Table on Languages and Linguistics 2000: Linguistics, language and the professions* (pp. 234–250). Washington, D.C.: Georgetown University Press.

Nicoladis, E., & Genesee, F. (1996a). A longitudinal study of pragmatic differentiation in young bilingual children. *Language Learning, 46(3),* 439–464.

Nicoladis, E., & Genesee, F. (1996b). Word awareness in second language learners and bilingual children. *Language Awareness, 5(2),* 80–89.

Nicoladis, E., & Secco, G. (2000). Productive vocabulary and language choice. *First Language, 20(58),* 3–28.

Owens, R. (2005). *Language development: An introduction* (6th ed.). Boston: Allyn & Bacon.

Padilla, A., & Liebman, E. (1975). Language acquisition in the bilingual child. *Bilingual Review, 2(1, 2),* 34–55.

Padilla, A., & Lindholm, K. (1984). Child bilingualism: The same old issues revisited. In J. Martinez, & R. Mendoza (Eds.), *Chicano psychology* (pp. 369–408). Orlando, FL: Academic Press.

Paradis, J., Nicoladis, E., & Genesee, F. (2000). Early emergence of structural constraints on code-mixing: Evidence from French-English bilingual children. In F. Genesee (Ed.), *Bilingualism: Language and cognition* (pp. 245–261). Cambridge, MA: Cambridge University Press.

Pearson, B. (1998). Assessing lexical development in bilingual babies and toddlers. *International Journal of Bilingualism, 2(3),* 347–372.

Pearson, B., Fernandez, S., Lewedag, V., & Oller, D. (1997). Input factors in lexical learning of bilingual infants (ages 10 to 30 months). *Applied Psycholinguistics, 18,* 41–58.

Pearson, B., Fernandez, S., & Oller, D. (1993). Lexical development in bilingual infants and toddlers: Comparison to monolingual norms. *Language Learning, 43,* 93–120.

Pearson B., Fernandez, S., & Oller, D. (1995). Cross-language synonyms in the lexicons of bilingual infants: One language or two? *Journal of Child Language, 22,* 345–368.

Petitto, L., Katerelos, M., Levy, B., Gauna, K., Tetreault, K., & Ferraro, V. (2001). Bilingual signed and spoken language acquisition from birth: Implications for the mechanism underlying early bilingual language acquisition. *Journal of Child Language, 28,* 453–496.

Pew Hispanic Center/Kaiser Family Foundation (2002). Update: March 2004. *2002 National Survey of Latinos:*

Summary of Findings. Washington, D.C. Online at: www.kff.org or www.pewhispanic.org

Polka, L., & Sundara, M. (2003). Word segmentation in monolingual and bilingual infant learners of English and French. In M. J. Sole, D. Recasens, & J. Romero (Eds.), *Proceedings of the International Congress of Phonetic Sciences, 15,* 1021–1024.

Portes, A., and Rumbaut, R. (2001). *Legacies: The story of the immigrant second generation.* Berkeley and Los Angeles, CA: University of California Press.

Ricciardelli, L. (1992). Bilingualism and cognitive development in relation to threshold theory. *Journal of Psycholinguistic Research, 21,* 301–316.

Ricciardelli, L. (1993). Two components of metalinguistic awareness: Control of linguistic processing and analysis of linguistic knowledge. *Applied Psycholinguistics, 14,* 349–367.

Romaine, S. (1995). *Bilingualism* (2nd ed.). Oxford: Blackwell Publishers.

Sanders, L., Neville, H., & Woldorff, M. (2002). Speech segmentation by native and nonnative speakers: The use of lexical, syntactic, and stress-pattern cues. *Journal of Speech, Language, and Hearing Research, 45,* 519–530.

Schiff-Myers, N. (1992). Considering arrested language development and language loss in the assessment of second language learners. *Language, Speech, and Hearing Services in Schools, 23,* 28–33.

Tabors, P. (1997). *One child, two languages: A guide for preschool educators of children learning English as a second language.* Baltimore: Paul H. Brookes.

U.S. Bureau of the Census. (2000). Update April, 2001. *Languages spoken at home.* Retrieved October 25, 2004, from www.census.gov

U.S. Bureau of the Census. (2000). Update March, 2004. *U.S. Interim Projections by Age, Sex, Race and Hispanic Origin.* Online at www.census.gov/ipc/www/usinterimproj/

Volterra, V., & Taeschner, T. (1978). The acquisition and development of language by bilingual children. *Journal of Child Language, 5,* 311–326.

Wong Fillmore, L. (1979). Individual differences in second language acquisition. In C. Fillmore, D. Kempler, & W. S.-Y. Wang (Eds.), *Individual differences in language ability and language behavior* (pp. 203–227). San Diego: Academic Press.

Wong Fillmore, L. (1983). The language learner as an individual: Implications of research on individual differences for the ESL teacher. In M. Clarke & J. Handscombe (Eds.), On TESOL '82: *Pacific perspectives on language learning and teaching* (pp. 157–173). Washington, D.C.: Teachers of English to Speakers of Other Languages.

Zentella, A. (2002). Latina languages and identities. In M. Suarez-Orozco & M. A. Paez (Eds.), *Latinos: Remaking America* (pp. 321–338). Berkeley: University of California Press.

Zuniga, M. (2004). Families with Latino roots. In E. Lynch & M. Hanson (Eds.), *Developing cross-cultural competence* (3rd ed., pp. 179–198). Baltimore: Paul H. Brookes.

10

Speech and Language Disorders

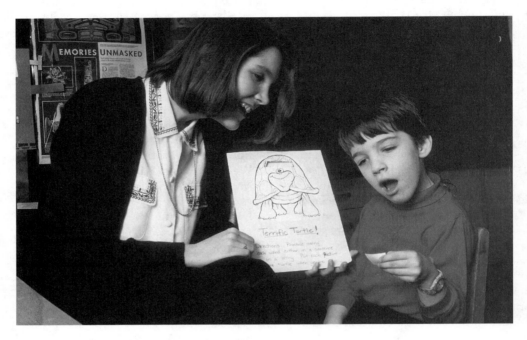

CHAPTER OBJECTIVES

The overwhelming majority of humans acquire speech and language without difficulty, but occasionally problems arise, either during the acquisition period or later in life after speech and language have been normal for a time. Communication disorders develop for many reasons, including environmental deprivation, faulty learning, emotional conflicts, disease, and physical trauma. In this chapter, we consider some common speech and language disorders, with special attention to those disorders most likely to affect children. Specifically, this chapter is designed to facilitate understanding of the following topics:

- Differentiating between normal and abnormal speech and language
- The classification of communication disorders
- The use of the terms *organic* and *functional* when categorizing disorders according to etiology
- Phonological disorders
- Language impairments
- Voice disorders
- Fluency disorders, with an emphasis on stuttering

The acquisition of speech and language is so natural that we may not truly appreciate the complexities and power of human oral communication unless or until something goes wrong. In the United States, about 10 percent of the population have speech, language, or hearing problems (Larkins, 1985; Leske, 1981a, 1981b), and this number is likely to increase as people live longer. Some may be surprised that this many people have communication disorders. When we consider how much language knowledge the child must acquire, how quickly he acquires it, and the incredible neuromuscular mechanisms that must be coordinated to make speech work, we must be amazed that more people do not have communication problems. In fact, it's a wonder how any of us master the mysterious and magical processes of speech and language.

Falling Short of Normal Communication

Before we proceed, it is important to note that the 10 percent prevalence figure we have cited tells only part of the story about how many people have communication problems. If we exclude hearing disorders, for example, the prevalence figure drops considerably. Fein (1983) suggests that the prevalence of speech and language disorders in the United States is about 4 percent. Shewan (1988), using numbers from several sources, suggests it may be about 6 percent. More important, Shewan and Malm (1990) emphasize that a single prevalence figure for speech and language disorders is misleading, because communication disorders are not evenly distributed throughout the population. Prevalence figures vary depending on age, gender, racial/ethnic background, and even geographic region.

Defining Communication Defects

In this chapter, we will examine the major communication disorders affecting children. We must begin by addressing the issue of **abnormality.** What constitutes a communication defect? This may seem a simple question, but it is, in fact, such a difficult question that experts in speech–language pathology have failed to come to any uniform definition. The problem in defining communication defects becomes immediately obvious when we try to define **normal** speech and language.

How many words are included in a normal vocabulary? How fast is normal speech? What is a normal voice? How hesitant or nonfluent must speech be before we call it stuttering? How precisely must one produce speech sounds to be considered normal? We trust you are beginning to see a trend here. The range of normal along every dimension of speech is tremendous. We have no exact standards for how much language a normal speaker has or even for how well he uses the language he has. We have vague ideas about acceptable male and female voices, but most of us have a tolerance for voices that go beyond even our own standards. We may notice that well-known television journalists such as Tom Brokaw and Barbara Walters have some problems with "r" and "l," but few of us would consider these individuals speech-defective. There are people we would all agree are normal speakers who are more nonfluent than other people we would all agree are stutterers. So how do we determine what a communication defect is?

One of the most widely used definitions of defective speech is offered by Van Riper and Erickson (1996): "Speech is impaired when it deviates so far from the speech of other people that it (1) calls attention to itself, (2) interferes with communication, or (3) provokes distress in the speaker or the listener" (p. 110). The advantage of this kind of definition is that it focuses our attention on what might be called the keys of communication abnormality. Van Riper and Erickson suggest, in fact, that their definition can be reduced to three key adjectives: *conspicuous, unintelligible,* and *unpleasant* (p. 111). The disadvantage of this definition, in either the long or short form, is that it is very subjective. Nevertheless, it provides an appropriate foundation for understanding what is meant by disordered or defective communication.

Most communication disorders, in their most severe forms, are **conspicuous.** You have perhaps observed a severe stutterer whose face becomes distorted as he struggles to get out a single word. Maybe you have listened to a person with a cleft palate who is so excessively nasal that you pay more attention to the quality of his voice than to the content of his words. Whenever speech is so far removed from normal that listeners' attentions are more drawn to the manner of speech than to the message being conveyed, it may be considered defective. Keep in mind, however, that a manner of speech conspicuous to one person might be ignored or considered perfectly normal by someone else. The nasal quality of a Texas dialect might be very conspicuous in Iowa but would be unnoticed in Dallas.

When speech differences reduce **intelligibility**—that is, when they interfere with the ability of listeners to understand what is being said—there is probably a communication disorder. We have all listened to youngsters who do not have complete sound systems. They leave out so many sounds, or substitute for them, that we can understand little of what they are trying to say. A speaker's voice might be so hoarse, or nasal, or breathy that we literally cannot understand the words he is trying to speak. Fluency problems can sometimes occur with such frequency and severity that intelligibility is reduced. One might conclude that reduced intelligibility is a fairly exact parameter of defective speech, but such a conclusion would not be entirely justified. When a child is twenty-four months old, we would not expect her speech to be completely intelligible, and if we could understand only half of what she was trying to say, we would probably not consider her speech defective; but if the same child, at the age of six years, was still only 50 percent intelligible, we would undoubtedly agree that her speech was defective. In addition, reduced intelligibility might be the consequence of regional or cultural dialects, and, as we established in Chapter 8, dialectal differences are not considered defects.

Deciding what is **unpleasant** to the speaker or his listeners might be the most troubling aspect of understanding disordered speech. We have grown up hearing the expression "Beauty is in the eye of the beholder." "Unpleasant" is also the product of individual perception. The range of tolerance for speech differences is as wide as the range of tolerance for all other human differences. In the speech–language pathology business, we sometimes talk about colleagues with "long ears," which means these people hear problems most of us would ignore. They have little tolerance for speech differences. Other people can and do accept almost all kinds of speech differences as normal unless the differences reduce intelligibility. It would probably be fair to say that we would not call speech defective, on the basis of listeners' perceptions, unless *many* people find the difference unpleasant.

The only single perception that really matters is that of the speaker. If she considers her speech difference to be unpleasant, it really does not matter whether anyone else agrees, especially if the rest of us cannot persuade her that nothing is wrong with her speech.

The Classification of Communication Disorders

Communication disorders are usually classified according to their symptoms or their causes. When we classify by **symptoms,** we identify four disorder categories: (1) **phonological** disorders, which are problems with the production of speech sounds; (2) **language** impairments, which include difficulties in understanding or using the symbols of speech; (3) **voice** disorders, including a wide range of abnormalities in the laryngeal tone from the vocal folds to the resonating cavities that modify that tone into what we recognize as the voice; and (4) **fluency** disorders, which are problems affecting the rhythm, rate, or forward flow of speech.

When we classify communication disorders by **causes** or **etiologies,** we must first differentiate between organic disorders and functional disorders, and this differentiation is not as simple as it may first appear. One might assume that these terms represent opposite ends of a continuum, that functional means nonorganic. It is not accurate to use these terms as though they represent a dichotomy.

An **organic** disorder is caused by a demonstrable pathology of an organ system. If, for example, a child with a cleft palate cannot produce a "p" sound because every time she puts her lips together to build up pressure for the production of "p," the air escapes through the opening in the roof of her mouth and out of her nose, this is clearly an organic articulation problem. Or, if a child's voice has been normal until his vocal folds become infected and swollen, and his voice becomes hoarse, this is an organic voice problem.

Now consider what *functional* means. A disorder is considered **functional** if, after using the best diagnostic procedures and technologies available, we fail to identify a pathology of an organ system. This does not necessarily mean that there is not a pathology. It simply means that if there is an organic etiology, we have not been able to identify it. We generally use the term functional to describe disorders that we believe are the result of learning, psychological, or environmental factors, but we need to be careful that we do not think of functional and nonorganic as synonyms.

Not many years ago, depression was widely understood as a psychological problem. We now understand that depression can be the result of biochemical imbalances that can be treated with medications. Until recently, alcoholism was viewed as strictly an environmental problem. We now understand that some people are genetically predisposed to alcoholism. These and similar conditions afflicting human beings cannot be easily dismissed as nonorganic, although there are undoubtedly cases of depression and alcoholism that are psychological and environmental.

Many children have problems with phonology or language that are identified as functional communication disorders. In some cases, there may be organic etiologies we are not able to identify. In many other cases, children have speech and language problems for reasons that have nothing to do with the integrities of their organ systems. If, for example, a child is reared in an environment that provides little or no speech and language simulation, or if she is reared by parents who are physically or emotionally abusive, we will not be surprised if there are communication disorders; and if the child's speech and language patterns are consistent with environmental or psychological causative factors, we will feel comfortable referring to these patterns as functional communication disorders.

Against this broad introductory background, we now examine some of the common communication disorders we see in children. The main headings refer to symptomatic categories, but we also consider etiologies within each category.

Phonological Disorders

For the past twenty years, speech–language pathologists have been in something of a quandary about the terminology used to describe speech sound disorders. Prior to the quandary, we referred to these problems as *articulation* disorders, but over the past two decades we have come to understand that the production of speech sounds is not limited to the speech apparatus; that it is more directly connected to language than we once thought; and that it is a rule-governed process, not just a mechanical process. We needed another, more comprehensive, term. The term that has been widely adopted is *phonology. Articulation* has been retained, but it is more narrowly defined today than it was twenty years ago. Some people might regard this fussing about terms to be much ado about little, but the difference between *articulation* and *phonology* is important in reference to understanding the etiologies of speech sound production problems and treating these problems.

Fey (1992) notes that "the notion of phonology and its role in Speech Pathology is a source not just of debate, but of bewilderment" (p. 225). The problem, it seems, is that many people are convinced that if we adopt the term *phonology,* we are obligated to discontinue using the term *articulation.* The fact is, the two terms, when used properly, coexist without difficulty. What we are obligated to do is to understand how these two terms are related to one another conceptually. Fey offers an excellent beginning point by defining articulation as "the processes involved in the planning and execution of smooth sequences of highly overlapping gestures of the speech organs" (p. 225). In short, articulation is concerned with the motor aspects of speech production.

Conceptually, *phonology* is a much broader term. It subsumes articulation but goes far beyond the physical production of speech sounds to include the perceptual and cognitive aspects of speech sound production and understanding, as well as the rule system that governs how sounds are combined. In acquiring his speech sound system, for example, the child must learn that some consonants can be sequenced and others cannot. He must learn that some consonants can be used to open and close syllables, whereas others can only be used to open syllables or only to close syllables.

Clarifying the terms *articulation* and *phonology* leads us to a better understanding about how speech sound problems are categorized. To say that a child has an **articulation** problem means that she cannot physically produce a given sound. It is not in her inventory of sounds. For example, the child who cannot produce an "s" because her cleft palate will not allow her to trap air in her mouth so that she can force air through the narrow constriction between her tongue and alveolar ridge has an articulation problem. Another child might be able to produce "s" in isolation and correctly in some contexts, but she does not produce it correctly in all contexts. Perhaps she deletes "s" in the postvocalic position because she deletes all sounds that, given a place and manner of articulation, can be either voiced or voiceless. Perhaps she produces "s" when it is a single sound but deletes "s" when it occurs in sequences. If the child has the physical ability to produce "s" and produces it correctly in some contexts but not in all contexts, she has a **phonological** disorder in the sense that she is having a problem with some aspect of her speech sound system, but she does not have an articulation disorder because she is physically capable of producing the target sound.

Because it is not always possible to isolate articulation from the other processes involved in speech production, it is best to categorize all speech sound production problems as *phonological disorders.* Those phonological disorders associated with structural defects in the speech mechanism or with neuropathologies that affect the function of the mechanism are properly called *articulation disorders.* Structural problems that might cause articulation disorders include cleft lips and cleft palates, tongues that are too large or too small, tongues that are not capable of full range of movement because their connective tissues insert too close to their tips, and dental malocclusions. Any abnormality that interferes with the natural movements of the structures in the mouth or that makes normal contact points difficult or impossible has the potential to create an articulation disorder. If the structures are normal, but they are not properly innervated by the central nervous system because of damage or disease, the net result might also be articulation disorders. Neurological damage can cause movements to be slow, weak, labored, or imprecise. Since normal speech is ballistic, and since it requires precise synchronization of movements, any neurological problem that slows it down, interferes with coordination, or reduces accuracy, can result in articulatory products that fall short of normal.

The majority of phonological disorders are *functional.* That means, as noted earlier, that these disorders are caused by factors that are not organic, or if they are caused by organic factors, we cannot prove those origins because our diagnostic procedures and technologies are not sensitive or sophisticated enough. Common causes of functional phonological disorders include habit strength and a range of environmental influences that cause a child's speech and language experiences to be less than ideal for normal development. We also know that there are connections between phonological disorders and reduced intelligence, hearing problems, and perceptual deficits. Basically, anything that interferes with the reception of speech and language during the acquisition period or anything that reduces the accurate processing of the speech and language information the child is receiving can negatively impact his communication output, and that might include phonological disorders. It should be noted that while some of these causal factors are clearly organic, the resulting phonological disorders are considered functional because the organic problems are not in the speech mechanism itself.

Language Impairments

Terminology is a problem without end in all behavioral sciences, and that certainly includes the related disciplines of speech–language pathology and audiology. We had to deal with a terminology issue in the previous section on phonological disorders, and we revisit the tangled issue in this section.

The word *language* did not appear in the name of the national professional association until 1979. Prior to that time, the national organization was called the American Speech and Hearing Association (ASHA). The association decided to add *language* to make it clear to all other disciplines that speech–language pathologists assess, diagnose, and treat language disorders. The national organization changed its name to the American Speech–Language–Hearing Association, but it retained the ASHA acronym because it was the well-established short-form name of the professional organization and because there was concern that people might hurt themselves trying to say *ASLHA.*

There is a point to this little story. For many years, the term *language disorders* seemed adequate to describe the broad category of problems people of all ages might have with language, but as is fashionable in the perception of some and necessary in the perception of others, some experts concluded that *disorders* in reference to language had outlived its semantic usefulness.

The argument about this particular term centers on the use of a single term to describe problems that are truly differentiated, or should be differentiated. Over the years, terms such as *language delay, language disorder,* and *language impairment* have been used to describe problems in language understanding and production grounded in limited skills, but the surface interpretation of these terms is not the same. Most people, whether or not they are expert in language matters, would understand *language delay* to mean that the language of a given child is immature for her age, that it fails to meet normative standards. A child with a language delay is acquiring language, but she is acquiring it more slowly than we expect she should. *Language disorder,* according to ASHA, is "impaired comprehension and/or use of spoken, written, and/or other symbol systems. This disorder may involve (1) the form of language (phonology, morphology, syntax), (2) the content of language (semantics), and/or (3) the function of language in communication (pragmatics) in any combination" (Ad Hoc Committee on Service Delivery in the Schools, 1993, p. 40). Clearly, *language disorder,* as defined by ASHA, goes well beyond *delay,* so how do we extricate ourselves from this little semantic quagmire?

Owens (1999) advocates use of the term *language impairment*. It is his view that *impairment* is a broader, more inclusive term that accommodates both *delay* and *disorder*, and reason seems to be on his side. Not only does the term nicely accommodate delay and disorder, but it allows us to avoid the arguments that invariably occur about the kinds of language problems exhibited by certain communicative populations. Do individuals who are mentally retarded, for example, produce delayed language or disordered language? We can deftly avoid the potential discomfort of the question by describing the language as *impaired*. Reread the ASHA definition of *language disorder* and compare it to Owens's (1999) definition of *language impairment* as "a heterogeneous group of developmental and/or acquired disorders and/or delays principally characterized by deficits and/or immaturities in the use of spoken or written language for comprehension and/or production purposes that may involve the form, content, and/or function of language in any combination" (p. 4). This definition is certainly broad enough and inclusive enough to cover everything that could possible go wrong with language. We can only hope that someday in a galaxy not too far away, automobile bumper-to-bumper warranties will be as comprehensive. In any case, for all the reasons we have identified here and for all the reasons implied in the plethora of *and/or*'s, we shall use the term *language impairment*.

What follows is an introductory overview of the major diagnostic categories associated with various language impairments common to children. The reader must approach this information on the tiptoes of an important caution, however. We use categories in this discussion as an organizational convenience. In doing so, we will be making generalizations about mythical typical children. Real children are rarely considerate enough to behave exactly as they are described in any category of any set of behaviors, and that includes language. We tried to make that point in reference to stages early and often in this book, and we are now making that same point about language impairment categories. It is highly unlikely that any child, even correctly deposited into a given category, will exhibit all of the characteristics associated with that category. It is quite likely that a given child will exhibit characteristics associated with two or more categories, as well as a few characteristics of her own idiosyncratic category. Human beings, even when they walk and talk in small packages, are very complex creatures who defy all attempts to place them into tidy, clearly differentiated, categorical boxes. Just as present-day physicians are taught in medical school to treat people and not just organs or diseases, speech–language pathologists are taught from day 1, or late in day 2, that we treat individual people. Even when several individual people appear to have the same communication problem with the same etiology, we should expect differences because differences are the rule, not the exception. It is easy to fall into the trap of describing the speech of a client as "cleft palate speech," for example, as though all people with cleft palates produce speech in exactly the same way. It may also seem appropriate to talk about "autistic language" or "mentally retarded language," but although such terms may have a certain face validity, they are worthless descriptions. In fact, they are worse than worthless because they perpetuate stereotypes that can be harmful to the people to whom they are attached. Within the following discussion, therefore, you are strongly encouraged to keep in mind that significant variability exists within categories and across categories.

Specific Language Impairment

It should come as little surprise, after considering the problems we have experienced trying to define the broader category of language impairment, that there would be disagreements about how to describe and understand specific subcategories of language impairment. Though we can perhaps come to agreement about etiological subcategories such as mental retardation or autism, there has been considerable debate about the descriptive and causal boundaries for what is called **specific language impairment,** or **SLI.** Perhaps the most widely applied description has been offered by Leonard (1987), who observes that children with SLI "exhibit significant limitations in language functioning that cannot be attributed to deficits in hearing, oral structure and function, or general intelligence" (p. 1). Consider what Leonard is suggesting in this description. The etiologies of specific language impairments are essentially unknown. As one might imagine without working up an intellectual sweat, this a pretty heterogeneous group of language-impaired children. In fact, research by Aram (1991), Stark and Tallal (1988), and others have led language experts to conclude that several identifiable subgroups are evident within the larger SLI population.

Even though few common denominators seem to connect the language impairments of SLI children, some generalizations about their language behaviors seem warranted. Craig (1993) notes, for example, that there are qualitative and quantitative differences between SLI children and children who have normal language when they are matched for mental age. SLI children seem to experience failure in the classroom more often than their peers. These failures are typically blamed on pragmatic problems. That is, SLI children have trouble initiating interactions with other children, and they have problems with conversational turn taking. In general, SLI children use pragmatic functions we would expect of younger children. They have trouble adjusting their language to fit particular speaker–listener interactions, and they do not effectively repair conversations when failures occur.

SLI children do not acquire their first words as early as other children, and their vocabulary growth is slower than normal. They sometimes have difficulty naming things, probably not because they have word retrieval problems but because they do not possess adequate mental dictionaries. SLI children, in comparison with younger children with comparable MLUs, have fewer grammatical morphemes, including auxiliary verbs, tense and number markers for verbs, and function words such as conjunctions, articles, and prepositions. Whereas younger children with comparable MLUs tend to make random pronoun errors, SLI children tend to use the same pronoun repeatedly, whether or not it is applicable.

Mental Retardation

In the case of mental retardation, we should begin with the common ground. There is no dispute about the fact that a connection exists between mental retardation and language impairment, and there is no dispute about the fact that the severity of language impairment is correlated with the degree of mental retardation. Please keep in mind, however, that "mentally retarded language" is a meaningless description. It is meaningless, in part, because the mentally retarded continuum stretches a considerable distance. Some individuals at the mild end of the continuum use language quite well. Individuals at the severe end are often noncommunicative, and we find a wide range of language abilities between the extremes.

Before we consider the generalizations we can make about the language abilities of mentally retarded individuals, we need to establish some form of definition of **mentally retarded.** The definition most often used today was established by the American Association on Mental Retardation (AAMR). Mental retardation, according to an AAMR committee, is "significantly subaverage general intellectual functioning existing concurrently with deficits in adaptive behavior and manifested during the developmental period" (Grossman, 1983, p. 1). We can almost hear some readers groaning that this sounds like a statement a committee would generate. This complaint duly noted, the definition has significant value if we consider its constituent parts. What does it mean, for example, to function at a "significantly subaverage intellectual" level? A person meets this criterion if he has an IQ of 68 or lower, an IQ cutoff determined by appropriate statistical manipulations. What is meant by "deficits in adaptive behavior"? A person demonstrates *adaptive behavior* by functioning in an independent and socially responsible manner. Conversely, a person exhibits *deficits* in adaptive behavior when she demonstrates an inability to function independently or behaves irresponsibly in common social situations. What is meant by the "developmental period"? As presently understood, the developmental period extends from the moment of conception to adulthood (Nelson, 1993, p. 98). Most important, how many of these three criteria must be met before a person is classified as mentally retarded? The answer is simple and quite clear. A person must meet all three criteria to meet the AAMR definition of mental retardation.

Keeping in mind that wide individual variations exist among mentally retarded individuals in terms of their speech and language abilities, Kamhi (1981) observes that children with mental retardation experience more language difficulties than normally developing children even when they are matched for mental age. That is, a typical child with mental retardation who is six years old but who has a mental age of three years will have more trouble with language than a normally developing child whose chronological and mental ages are three years. It is also noteworthy that even when children with mental retardation have other developmental problems, including neuromuscular difficulties or social skill deficits, language impairment is usually the most critical problem they face. Language impairment may, in fact, be the single most defining characteristic of this population.

Owens (2004, p. 24), after thoroughly reviewing the literature, provides an excellent summary of the language behaviors of mentally retarded children. Even though these children exhibit gestures and intentions that are similar to those used by normally developing children, they tend to be submissive conversational partners and are not as effective as their mental age–matched peers in clarifying their messages when misunderstandings occur. Children who are mentally retarded acquire morphemes in the same order as other children, and the sequence in which they produce varying types of sentences is similar to that of normal children, but they tend to use shorter and less complex sentences than their mental age–matched peers. Whereas all children begin with word meanings that are concrete, children with mental retardation do not make the change from concrete to abstract meanings as quickly and easily as other children, and their word meanings remain restrictive. They experience a slower vocabulary growth, and they have more trouble with figurative forms of language than their mental age–matched peers. Children with mental retardation tend to use phonological processes that are typical of younger children, and they are slower to suppress these processes than their peers who have normal intellectual abilities. Finally, these children produce more articulation, or motor production, errors than other children.

If we put all these pieces together, we understand that children with mental retardation acquire language forms more slowly but in the same order as normally developing children. In some cases, when we match children with mental retardation and normally developing children for mental age, they perform about the same. In other cases, even when we account for mental age, children with mental retardation are less effective in their use of language and more restricted in their use of the language forms they do have than their mental age–matched peers.

Autism

The term **autism** typically conjures up images of children who are withdrawn into their own egocentric worlds, children who appear to have rejected reality in favor of a fantasy place that other people cannot reach, children who engage in a wide range of abnormal and socially unacceptable behaviors, children whose language is severely impaired. Autism was first named as a syndrome, or aggregate of symptoms that in combination describe a condition, by Leo Kanner, a child psychologist, in 1943. The American Psychiatric Association, in 1987, categorized autism as a *pervasive developmental disorder* and described autism as an impairment involving a stringent repertoire of activity, a limited range of behaviors, a severely reduced interest level, and little or no social interaction.

According to the National Society of Autistic Children, autism develops in 4 out of 10,000 children, and it is more common in males than females by a ratio of 4:1. The onset of autism usually occurs before thirty months. Physical appearance is normal, but motor, social, and cognitive development tends to be erratic. Children with autism do not react to sensory stimuli the same way other children do. That is, they tend to be either hypoactive or hyperactive in response to visual and/or auditory stimuli. Sometimes their responses are ritualistic, and they are intolerant of any environmental changes. These children may appear to be preoccupied with mechanical devices at the same time that they seem uninterested in establishing contacts with people. Their speech and language problems include echolalia, mutism, and failure to use abstract terms. They also experience cognitive difficulties, even when, on occasion, they seem to be gifted in one particular area, such as math. They not only have trouble relating to people, but sometimes even to objects, and to events. Children with autism tend not to show affection. Their play behaviors are often unusual, ritualistic, and perseverative, and when they are interrupted while they are playing or manipulating objects, they often become agitated (Ritvo & Freeman, 1978).

The cause of autism has not been established, but there is speculation that it may be a genetic disorder, that it may result from a degenerative neurological disease, or that it may be an autoimmune disease. Prognosis is uncertain in all cases but is considered poor for children with autism who are not talking by the time they are five years old. At this time, there is no single established treatment, but most treatments stress educational and behavior modification principles, with emphases on teaching small segments of information and strictly controlling inappropriate and maladaptive behaviors.

The primary focus of concern for children with autism, as it is for children with mental retardation, is severe language impairment. According to Tager-Flusberg (1985), all individuals with autism have impairments that affect their ability both to understand language and to produce language. Paul (1987) notes that half of the population with autism fails to develop functional language and more than a few communication skills of any kind. Beyond this general and not very positive view, we can make a number of generalizations about the language abilities of children with autism.

These children have difficulty establishing the kind of mutual attention that is necessary for communicative exchanges. They have trouble initiating conversation and using language to inform, skills that are basic to social interactions (Wetherby, 1986). These children lack conversational turn-taking skills, and they utilize a very limited range of communication functions (Donnellan & Kilman, 1986; Mirenda & Donnellan, 1986). Considering our general description of individuals with autism, it is not surprising that these children have difficulty with abstract words. They struggle to retrieve words, and they have trouble expressing their emotions. Children with autism often refer to themselves with second-person *(you)* and third-person pronouns *(he, she)*. They often construct sentences without regard to underlying meaning (Bartolucci, Pierce, Streiner, & Eppel, 1976). The least affected component of language is phonology, although phonological problems are common in this population. The sequence of phonological development is the same as for normal children, and development is not distinctly delayed (Fay & Schuler, 1980).

In summary, the language problems of children with autism are diverse because they are members of a diverse population. Some of these children eventually use functional language, but just as many never do. Some of the language problems associated with autism seem to be the result of developmental delay, but other problems seem to go beyond delay. When children with autism are matched for mental age with mentally retarded, SLI, and normally developing children, the syntactic abilities of the children with autism are equal to the syntactic abilities of children with mental retardation and SLI children. What does this mean? According to Swisher and Demetras (1985), it may mean that children with autism construct sentences differently than normally developing children, that they derive surface structures from incompletely understood deep structures. Taking into account research on the development of all components of language, Swisher and Demetras conclude that there is evidence of delay, but in some cases, there is also evidence that these children follow developmental patterns that are unique. And we will reiterate one more time that, given what we know about the characteristics of autism, it is not surprising that there would be evidence of unusual developmental patterns.

Brain Injury

The general category of brain injury includes **traumatic brain injury (TBI),** resulting from a blow to the head that might occur in a fall or automobile accident, as well as the kind of brain injury that occurs in a **cerebrovascular accident (CVA),** commonly called a *stroke.* In this section, however, brain injury will be limited to traumatic brain injuries affecting children. In the United States, there are about one million victims of TBI who are children and adolescents. Some of these young people will experience complete, or nearly complete, recoveries from their brain injuries. Sadly, others will remain in essentially vegetative states for the remainder of their lives.

This next sentence should be annoyingly familiar: Children with traumatic brain injury are members of an extraordinarily heterogeneous group. This means, as we should now be able to chant in unison, that they will exhibit widely varying behaviors over a wide range of severity, and in the case of TBI, for varying periods of time. In addition, we must note that the language impairments associated with TBI differ in some respects from the language impairments that have developmental etiologies.

In their review of studies focusing on the effects of traumatic brain injury on children, Ewing-Cobbs, Fletcher, and Leven (1985) found that these injuries affect general intellectual functioning, memory, psychosocial skills, academic performance, and, of course, language. Depending on the severity of the injury and on the site and extent of the damage, problems in these areas might persist for weeks or months, or they might be permanent. Compounding the problems identified by Ewing-Cobbs et al., these children tend to be highly distractible. They tend to perseverate, and to have low thresholds for frustration. Imagine for a moment the combination of these behavioral characteristics and language impairment, academic problems, and the social challenges inherent in interpersonal relationships. To say that traumatic brain injuries, even those in the mild and moderate categories, can be life altering is something of an understatement.

As with the other categories of language impairment we have already discussed, we must be careful to acknowledge that whatever generalizations we make about the language impairments of TBI children are just that, generalizations. Here, then, are a few generalizations. These children often make statements during conversations that are not topic focused. They have problems organizing their thoughts into language forms, and they have difficulty expressing complex ideas. Language that is automatic, including the language we use when we greet one another, tends to be unaffected by TBI; but when language is intentional or purposive, and when it is important, communication becomes more difficult. Individuals with traumatic brain injuries often struggle to name things, and they have problems with word retrieval even if their vocabularies are relatively intact. The sentences they produce tend to be long, aimless, fragmented, and inappropriate. TBI children typically do not have phonological problems as a result of their brain injuries, but they might have some articulation difficulties associated with injury-induced dysarthria and/or apraxia. It is not unusual for children with traumatic brain injuries to experience some problems with language comprehension. They might, for example, have problems affixing meanings to the syntactic structures of sentences, but most of these children will be able to interpret the sentences included in ordinary conversational exchanges.

A Few Words about Other Categories

Learning disabilities may hinder language development. Many people believe that mental retardation and learning disability mean the same thing. They do not. A child with a learning disability may have a normal or superior intellectual capacity. You will best understand learning disability by taking the term literally. This is a child with a deficit that renders traditional learning strategies ineffective, perhaps useless. If, for example, a child sees visual stimuli backward or scrambled, she will have problems learning to read. If she is unable to group auditory sounds into appropriate segments, she will have problems organizing and interpreting spoken language, because she may have difficulty grouping sounds into words and words into sentences. Children with learning disabilities often have difficulty attending to, sorting, or organizing stimuli, and they may have deficits in memory. Try to imagine learning language with these problems. The normal child learning language attends, even if unconsciously, to thousands of language samples each day. She is eventually able to sort through all those samples to figure out how verbs and nouns differ, how to organize words into subjects and predicates, and everything she learns about language is stored in memory. A deficit in any of these or related areas can have a significant impact on language acquisition and may result in language impairment. Treatment focuses on helping the child compensate for her learning disability by teaching her to rely more heavily on learning skills not affected or by helping her discover alternative learning strategies.

It will surprise no one that **hearing loss** and **deafness** are related to language impairments, and it should be obvious that, all other factors being equal, the greater the hearing loss, the greater the language impairment is likely to be. The deaf child lives in a speech-impoverished environment, no matter how much speech is generated by his parents and siblings and no matter the quality of those models. If the deafness is congenital, it is unrealistic to hope for normal speech. If the child has had normal hearing during the speech and language learning period and then becomes deaf, the outlook for oral communication is much more promising, but it will still fall short of the language quality we expect from normally hearing children. Consider the fact that adults who have had normal speech and normal hearing throughout their lives and who become deaf in adulthood experience some deterioration in the quality of speech (Goehl & Kaufman, 1984). It should be emphasized that hearing losses, even deafness, do not preclude language. The congenitally deaf child has the same natural language abilities as the hearing child, but he will best receive and express language visually. For this reason, most experts today recommend that the deaf child be provided opportunities for acquiring a visual language communication system as early as possible.

Some Summarizing Thoughts So Far

This section has presented some of the factors that might be responsible for language impairment, but certainly not all of them. A comprehensive analysis of the possible etiologies of language impairment goes beyond the scope of this book. The important message is that anything that affects the way language develops and anything that affects the way language is received, processed, understood, or produced can result in language impairment.

No matter how narrowly experts might define a category of language impairment, there will always be a great diversity of language behaviors produced by the people who "fit" into that category. No matter how hard experts try to arbitrarily limit the possibilities by establishing strict categorical criteria, that diversity proves that language is an extraordinarily complex phenomenon produced by incredibly complex human creatures. When language is acquired normally and used routinely, people take this uniquely human gift for granted. Only when there is failure do we begin to appreciate how awesome, complicated, and impossible language really is.

Voice Disorders

Most people are impressed by the ability of some birds, such as the mynah or parrot, to imitate human speech. Even more impressive is the ability of humans to imitate the sounds produced by birds, other animals, musical instruments, machines—almost any kind of sound imaginable. This virtually unlimited imitative ability is made possible because of the extraordinary range and versatility of the human voice mechanism, including the larynx and the resonating cavities. Within this range, determining what is a so-called "normal" voice is an exceedingly difficult task. Although many voices can be identified as unusual, surveys conducted by experts in this disorder indicate that about 1 percent of adults and perhaps as many as 6 percent of children have voices that can be considered abnormal or disordered (Miller & Madison, 1984; Silverman & Zimmer, 1975). When a voice is disordered, there is a problem with pitch, loudness, and/or quality.

Pitch can be atypical in three ways. It can be too high, too low, or it can be monotonous. There are three common loudness problems. A voice can be too loud or too weak, of course, and if there is no voice at all, we have a condition known as **aphonia.** Over the years, the terminology in the area of voice quality disorders has been cacophonous, and there has been no agreement among the experts about how to define or explain these disorders. If we allow the chaff of disagreement to blow away, however, we can say that there are disorders of *resonance* and there are disorders of *laryngeal tone*. In terms of resonance, a voice can be too nasal, or it can lack nasality when nasality is required. In terms of laryngeal tone, a voice can be harsh or breathy, or it can be hoarse, if harsh and breathy are combined. It is very important to stress that on a practical level, we cannot separate pitch, loudness, and quality. Each affects and is affected by the others. For example, when people describe a voice as *breathy*, that is a quality judgment, but a breathy voice is also weaker in volume and usually lower in pitch than a normal voice.

Fluency Disorders

When most people, even many speech–language pathologists, talk about fluency disorders, they limit their consideration to **stuttering.** In fact, stuttering is just one of the fluency disorders therapists are called on to treat. Obviously, there are common denominators among fluency disorders, but it is important to differentiate among them because they are not just shades of the same disorder. They have different etiologies and different symptomatologies.

Any disorder characterized by hesitations, repetitions of speech segments, or prolongations of sounds that impedes the forward flow of speech is a fluency disorder. Beyond this commonality are many differences. Fluency problems often accompany neuropathologies. People with epilepsy or cerebral palsy or people who have suffered strokes or head injuries often have fluency problems along with other communication disorders. Whether all of these conditions should be called *stuttering* is the subject of considerable debate (Hulit, 2004).

Developmental Stuttering

For purposes of this discussion, *developmental stutterers,* or simply *stutterers* with no qualifying adjectives, are individuals who are normal neurologically and who do not have serious psychological problems. Consider, however, that even if we limit ourselves to this population, we encounter another problem. All speakers occasionally experience fluency failures. All speakers repeat syllables, words, even phrases. They all stumble, hesitate, revise, add superfluous interjections, and produce all the other behaviors associated with stuttering. It is not as easy to differentiate between stuttering and normal fluency failures as you might imagine. You might be tempted to conclude that the difference is frequency of fluency failure. That is, people who stutter fail more often than people who do not stutter. While frequency of fluency failure is one factor in the difference, it is not the only difference, and it may not even be the most important difference. As noted in the opening of this chapter, some people we would all agree are stutterers have fewer fluency breakdowns than some people we would all agree are normal speakers. Stutterers and nonstutterers actually have more similarities as communicators than they have differences (Hulit, 2004). They are separated as much by their **perceptions** of speech, speaking situations, sounds, words, and listeners as by the struggle associated with stuttering.

One of the most difficult problems we face in discussing stuttering, as indicated in the preceding paragraph, is defining it (Bloodstein, 1995; Guitar, 1998; Silverman, 1996; Wingate, 1997). Experts over the centuries have argued about what stuttering is, what causes it, why it seems to run in families, why it is more common in males than in females, why some children spontaneously recover from it and others do not, and how to treat it. Suffice it to say that even though much has been written about stuttering, and even though it is among the most investigated of all communication disorders, there is still far more we do not know about stuttering than we know.

We need only sample definitions and/or descriptions of stuttering to appreciate the nature and extent of the mystery and debate that surround it:

> Stuttering is a psychoneurosis caused by the persistence into later life of early pregenital oral nursing, oral sadistic, and anal sadistic components. (Coriat, 1933, p. 167)

> Stuttering is an evaluational disorder. It is what results when normal nonfluency is evaluated as something to be feared and avoided; it is, outwardly, what the stutterer does in an attempt to avoid nonfluency. (Johnson, 1946, p. 452)

> Stuttering is that class of fluency failure which is the consequence of classically conditioned negative emotion. (Brutten & Shoemaker, 1967, p. 35)

> "I will, however, for the purpose of this text describe or define *stuttering* or *stuttered* speech as *typically* involving: (1) sound or syllable repetitions; (2) sound prolongations, (3) monosyllabic whole-word repetition; or (4) within-word pause." (Conture, 2001, p. 5)

> Stuttering occurs when the forward flow of speech in interrupted by a motorically disrupted sound, syllable, or word, or by the speaker's reactions thereto. (Van Riper, 1992, p. 15)

> All of the surface features of stuttering are reducible to two underlying tendencies, that of producing utterances with abnormal muscular tension and that of fragmenting them. Stuttering, in short, is speech transformed by tension and fragmentation. (Bloodstein, 1993, p. 137)

> Traditionally, stuttering has been viewed as a disorder in which the "rhythm" or fluency of speech is impaired by interruptions, or blockages. For many ordinary purposes such a definition is adequate. . . . Yet it cannot be denied that what we identify as stuttering is sometimes evident not only in the intermittent impairment of fluency, but also in the rate, pitch, loudness, inflectional patterns, articulation, facial expression, and postural adjustments of the speaker and that there are stutterers for whom its features are not always confined in an easily identifiable manner to discrete "moments." (Bloodstein, 1995, p. 1)

Defining stuttering is so fraught with difficulty that many authors avoid defining it. They might share with their readers definitions crafted by others, and they might offer their insights about the limitations of these definitions, but they do not enter the fray. We have shared examples of definitions but will not criticize them. With or without any encouragement to do so, you will draw your own conclusions about what each definition might contribute to our understanding of this disorder.

One might suggest that if experts cannot agree on a definition of stuttering, anything else they might say on the subject lacks credibility. It certainly would be easier if we had a universally accepted definition, but the fact is countless conditions afflict human beings that are not fully understood, do not have irrefutable and universally accepted definitions, and defy exacting diagnoses. Knowledge tends to advance by inches, not miles. We understand these problems to the extent we can at any point in time. We design the best diagnostic strategies, the best intervention programs, and the best preventive measures we can, based on what we know or what we think we know. Do we make mistakes in the process? Of course we do, but we continue to advance our knowledge, and based on that knowledge, we systematically reduce the mistakes engendered by ignorance. With this perspective in mind, let's consider some of what we do know about stuttering.

Developmental stuttering is a disorder that begins in childhood, usually between the ages of two and six years. Many children who begin to stutter spontaneously recover by the time they are about six years old. Some experts, based on empirical research, believe that about 40 percent of young stutterers spontaneously recover; a few place the recovery rate as high as 80 percent. Stuttering is much more common in males than in females. When children are young, the ratio is about 2:1. By adulthood, the ratio is 4:1 or 5:1.

When stuttering begins, it is relatively simple and uninvolved. The child who stutters repeats single-syllable words or the first syllable of multisyllabic words, and he stutters without struggle, awareness, or concern.

Early stuttering is usually episodic. That is, weeks or months go by when speech is relatively nonfluent, followed by weeks or months when speech is relatively fluent. The episodes of fluent speech and nonfluent speech might continue for several years until the child enters a fluent period and never has another episode of excessive nonfluency. Such a child has *spontaneously recovered.* If stuttering continues, the behaviors increase in number and become more complicated. The stutterer becomes more aware that he is producing fluency failures, becomes more concerned about his speech, and eventually begins to include *stutterer* as a major component of his self-identity. As severity increases, we may see facial grimaces, and the stutterer may seem to have difficulty regulating his breathing during speech, and he struggles to make his articulators move when he wants them to move.

Most experts believe that the prognosis for the adult stutterer is not good. He may learn how to control his speech to the extent that he can dramatically improve his ability to communicate, but it is not likely he will ever again be a *normal speaker.* On those rare occasions when an adult stutterer is completely liberated from his disorder, the liberation is typically the product of a life-altering experience.

The treatment of stuttering is much too complex to discuss here. Some cynics suggest that it is ludicrous to suggest that a disorder about which so little is known with certainty can be treated at all. We would remind you that there are many human problems, as faintly understood as stuttering, that we treat and should treat. Physicians treat the various cancers that afflict human beings, and they treat heart disease, arthritis, multiple sclerosis, muscular dystrophy, cystic fibrosis, Alzheimer's disease, and many other illnesses even though there is much we do not understand about the causes of these conditions and about why some people are more vulnerable to these conditions than others. Physicians treat based on what they do know, and they treat based on their best hypotheses about what are the most reasonable intervention strategies. Some of these treatments work, and some fail. Some work for some people but not for others. Medical scientists learn from the successes and the failures, and their knowledge advances; as their knowledge advances, their treatments become more viable and effective. They also suggest things people can do to prevent the occurrence of these conditions. These suggestions are not always, or even usually, based on irrefutable facts. They are grounded in best guesses based on what they do know or think they know.

Speech–language pathologists treat stuttering, and other communication disorders, from this same perspective. Any viable treatment is a hypothesis, based on the information we have gathered about the disorder and the person who owns it. Whatever therapy we employ in the treatment of stuttering will not work for every client because the disorder is not the same for every person who stutters and because not all people who stutter are the same. We do know that if stuttering is addressed early, the prognosis is excellent. Might some of these clients have spontaneously recovered without the treatment? They probably would have, but that does not obviate the decision to treat because we cannot know who will spontaneously recover and who will not. When there is any doubt about whether a child is stuttering or producing normal nonfluencies, an evaluation is in order. If the evaluation indicates that a problem may exist, the problem should be addressed. In the case of stuttering, the old adage that an ounce of prevention is worth a pound of cure holds very true. If we can prevent early stuttering from progressing to established stuttering, the outcome has a good chance of being favorable.

As noted at the beginning of this section, the term *stuttering* is often applied to disorders that do not fit the profile of developmental stuttering. Some individuals have fluency problems that are clearly and directly connected to neuropathologies. Although these individuals may produce some behaviors that are produced by developmental stutterers, there are differences between developmental stuttering and *neurogenic stuttering*. Other people may have a fluency disorder that is the product of a psychological problem, a disorder called *psychogenic stuttering* or *hysterical stuttering*. Again, some common ground is shared by developmental stuttering and psychogenic stuttering, but important differences are evident as well. Finally, a disorder called *cluttering* differs from stuttering in many respects even though both are fluency disorders.

Neurogenic Stuttering

Stuttering that begins after an individual suffers damage to the central nervous system (CNS) has been described by many authors, including Davis (1993), Hertrich and Ackermann (1994), Mavlov (1994), and Nagafuchi (1994). In most cases described by these and other writers, the individuals had no history of stuttering prior to the CNS damage. The onset of stuttering was sudden and associated with a specific, documented CNS injury. In some cases, the individual had a history of stuttering that either reappeared or noticeably worsened after the neurological damage. Damage to the CNS can be caused by a cerebral vascular accident (stroke), a blow to the head, the development of a tumor, a reaction to drugs, dementia, or a number of diseases that affect the nervous system.

As his disorder becomes more severe, the developmental stutterer adds what are called *secondary symptoms* to his repertoire of behaviors. These include facial grimaces, head jerks, and extraneous movements in the limbs that reflect his struggle to fight through moments of stuttering. The neurogenic stutterer is less likely to acquire these secondary symptoms.

Psychogenic Stuttering

Cases of psychogenic stuttering were widely reported in the older stuttering literature (Bluemel, 1935; Breuer & Freud, 1936; Preacher & Harris, 1946), but even at the end of the twentieth century, cases of individuals who stutter as the result of a psychological problem have been identified (Attanasio, 1987; Mahr & Leith, 1992; Roth et al., 1989). As with neurogenic stuttering, the onset in psychogenic stuttering tends to be sudden and appears to be associated with a specific, identifiable psychological trauma. In some cases, the trauma is the result of violence the individual has experienced or observed. In other cases, the trauma is associated with a powerful and aversive life-altering experience, such as the sudden, unexpected death of a loved one or an unusually acrimonious divorce. Unlike the developmental stutterer who stutters in response to certain situational and linguistic cues, the psychogenic stutterer tends to stutter in all communicative situations. She does not develop secondary behaviors such as facial grimaces and head jerks. She does not avoid words or speaking situations, and she tends to be so completely unconcerned about her stuttering that she is essentially detached from it (Freund, 1966).

Cluttering

Cluttering is as misunderstood a communication disorder as stuttering, and it has received far less attention from U.S. authors than European authors (St. Louis & Rustin, 1992). Cluttering is as difficult to define as stuttering. The most commonly referenced definition belongs to Weiss (1964):

> Cluttering is a speech disorder characterized by the clutterer's unawareness of his disorder, by a short attention span, by disturbances in perception, articulation and formulation of speech, and often by excessive speed of delivery. It is a disorder of thought processes preparatory to speech and based on a hereditary disposition. Cluttering is a verbal manifestation of Central Language Imbalance, which affects all channels of communication. (p. 1)

The "problem" then, according to Weiss, is a language problem. Cluttering is just one symptom of that problem. Others include delayed speech, developmental phonological disorders, reading and writing disorders, disorders of rhythm and musicality, and even general behavioral problems such as restlessness and disorderliness. Daly (1993) provides more specific details about the speech and language behaviors of clutterers in his definition:

> Cluttering is a disorder of both speech and language processing that frequently results in rapid, disrhythmic, sporadic, unorganized, and often unintelligible speech. . . . Those who clutter confuse their listeners with incomplete and awkward

sentences, false starts, sound sequencing errors, and word-retrieval problems. Their garbled speech is confounded by a lack of clarity of inner language formulation. (p. 7)

Final Thoughts

We have come to the end of our story. As you have progressed through the pages of this book, we hope you have developed a new appreciation for the miracle of speech and language. We may never fully understand how human beings can think, edit thoughts, pull language from their memory banks, transform language into speech, and combine speech with all the critical aspects of nonverbal communication. We should, however, appreciate that this communicative ability is one of the great gifts humans pass from generation to generation.

Although there is a powerful innate drive to acquire language and to speak in all human children, parents should do all they can to encourage their children during the acquisition period. Parents and teachers are usually the first to notice when a child is having difficulty with speech and language. It is their responsibility to seek professional help from speech–language pathologists who are qualified to diagnose and treat communication problems. If there is any doubt about whether a child has a communication disorder, the child should be evaluated and treated, if necessary. It is far easier to treat communication disorders in their early stages than after inappropriate habits have become established. The child who can talk has one of the most important tools she needs to explore and understand the exciting world awaiting her.

Review Questions

1. Why is it difficult to determine what constitutes a communication defect?

2. In your own words, and taking into account our discussion of the inherent problems in differentiating between "normal" and "abnormal" speech and language, define *communication defect*.

3. How do categories of communication disorders differ when we classify them by symptoms as opposed to classifying them by causes?

4. What does the term *functional* mean, and why is it inappropriate to think of *functional* as a synonym for *nonorganic*?

5. What is the difference between *phonology* and *articulation*? What is the difference between a *phonological disorder* and an *articulation disorder*?

6. Discuss the problems associated with terms such as *language disorder* and *language delay*. Why is *language impairment* a better term?

7. Why should we avoid using terms such as *autistic language* or *mentally retarded language*?

8. What is meant by *specific language impairment*? How do the language behaviors of SLI children compare to the language behaviors of normally developing children?

9. How do the language behaviors of mentally retarded children compare to the language behaviors of normally developing children?

10. What is *autism?* Identify some of the behaviors and problems commonly associated with autism.
11. Describe the language behaviors commonly associated with autism and explain how these behaviors are related to other problems typically experienced by autistic children.
12. What is a *traumatic brain injury?* What are some of the common ef-

fects of TBI on a child's behavior in general and on language behavior specifically?
13. In what major ways can the voice be disordered?
14. Why is stuttering such a difficult disorder to define?
15. Compare and contrast the following types of stuttering: *developmental, neurogenic,* and *psychogenic.*

References and Suggested Readings

Ad Hoc Committee on Service Delivery in the Schools, ASHA. (1993). Definitions of communication disorders and variations. *ASHA, 35*(3) (Suppl. 10), 40–41.

Ainsworth, S., & Fraser, J. (Eds.). (1988). *If your child stutters: A guide for parents* (3rd ed.). Memphis, TN: Speech Foundation of America.

Aram, D. (1991). Comments on specific language impairment as a clinical category. *Language, Speech, and Hearing Services in Schools, 22,* 84–87.

Aronson, A. (1985). *Clinical voice disorders* (2nd ed.). New York: Thieme-Stratton.

Attanasio, J. (1987). A case of late-onset or acquired stuttering in adult life. *Journal of Fluency Disorders, 12,* 287–290.

Bartolucci, G., Pierce, S., Streiner, D., & Eppel, P. (1976). Phonological investigation of verbal autistic and mentally retarded subjects. *Journal of Autism and Childhood Schizophrenia, 6,* 303–316.

Bernthal, J., & Bankson, N. (2004). *Articulation and phonological disorders* (5th ed.). Boston: Allyn & Bacon.

Bishop, D., & Adams, C. (1992). Comprehension problems in children with specific language impairment:

Literal and inferential meaning. *Journal of Speech and Hearing Research, 35,* 119–129.

Bleumel, C. (1935). *Stammering and allied disorders.* New York: Macmillan.

Bloodstein, O. (1979). *Speech pathology, an introduction.* Boston: Houghton Mifflin.

Bloodstein, O. (1990). On pluttering, skivering, and floggering: A commentary. *Journal of Speech and Hearing Disorders, 55,* 392–393.

Bloodstein, O. (1993). *Stuttering: The search for a cause and cure.* Boston: Allyn & Bacon.

Bloodstein O. (1995). *A handbook on stuttering* (5th ed.). San Diego, CA: Singular.

Boone, D., McFarlane, S., & Von Berg, S. (2005). *The voice and voice therapy* (7th ed.). Boston: Allyn & Bacon.

Breuer, J., & Freud, S. (1936). *Studies in hysteria* (Nervous and Mental Disease Monograph Series No. 61). New York: Nervous and Mental Disease Publishing.

Brutten, G., & Shoemaker, D. (1967). *The modification of stuttering.* Upper Saddle River, NJ: Prentice Hall.

Canter, G. (1971). Observations on neurogenic stuttering: A contribution to differential diagnosis. *British Journal of Disorders of Communication, 6,* 139–143.

Coggins, T. (1979). Relational meaning encoded in two-word utterances of Stage I Down's syndrome children. *Journal of Speech and Hearing Research, 22,* 166–178.

Conture, E. (1990). *Stuttering* (2nd ed.). Upper Saddle River, NJ: Prentice Hall.

Conture, E. (2001). *Stuttering, its nature, diagnosis, and treatment.* Boston: Allyn & Bacon.

Conture, E., & Kelly, E. (1991). Young stutterers' nonspeech behaviors during stuttering. *Journal of Speech and Hearing Research, 34,* 1041–1056.

Coriat, I. (1933). Psychoanalytic concept of stammering. *Nervous Child, 2,* 167–171.

Craig, H. (1993). Social skills of children with specific language impairment: Peer relationships. *Language, Speech, and Hearing Services in Schools, 24,* 206–215.

Creaghead, N., Newman, P., & Secord, W. (Eds.) (1989). *Assessment and remediation of articulatory and phonological disorders* (2nd ed.). Upper Saddle River, NJ: Merrill/Prentice Hall.

Crowe Hall, B. (1991). Attitudes of fourth and sixth graders toward peers with mild articulation disorders. *Language, Speech, Hearing Services in Schools, 22,* 334–340.

Curlee, R., & Perkins, W. (Eds.). (1984). *Nature and treatment of stuttering: New directions.* San Diego, CA: College-Hill.

Curlee, R., & Siegel, G. (Eds.). (1997). *Nature and treatment of stuttering: New directions.* Boston: Allyn & Bacon.

Curtis, S., Katz, W., & Tallal, P. (1992). Delay versus deviance in the language acquisition of language-impaired children. *Journal of Speech and Hearing Research, 35,* 373–383.

Daly, D. (1993). Cluttering: The orphan of speech–language pathology. *ASHA, 2,* 6–8.

Davis, G. (1993). *A survey of adult aphasia* (2nd ed.). Upper Saddle River, NJ: Prentice Hall.

Donnellan, A., & Kilman, B. (1986). Behavioral approaches to social skill development in autism. In E. Schopler & G. Mesibov (Eds.), *Social Behavior in Autism.* New York: Plenum.

Egland, G. (1970). *Speech and language problems: A guide for the classroom teacher.* Upper Saddle River, NJ: Prentice Hall.

Ewing-Cobbs, L., Fletcher, J., & Leven, H. (1985). In M. Ylvisaker (Ed.), *Head Injury Rehabilitation: Children and Adolescents.* Austin, TX: PRO-ED.

Fay, W., & Schuler, A. (1980). *Emerging language in autistic children.* Baltimore: University Park Press.

Fein, D. (1983). The prevalence of speech and language impairments. *ASHA, 25,* 37.

Fey, M. (1992). Articulation and phonology: Inextricable constructs in speech pathology. *Language, Speech, and Hearing Services in Schools, 23,* 225–232.

Freund, H. (1966). *Psychopathology and the problems of stuttering.* Springfield, IL: Thomas.

Goehl, H., & Kaufman, P. (1984). Do the effects of adventitious deafness include disordered speech? *Journal of Speech and Hearing Disorders, 49,* 58–64.

Grossman, I. (1983). *Classification in mental retardation.* Washington, D.C.: American Association on Mental Deficiency.

Guitar, B. (1998). *Stuttering: An integrated approach to its nature and treatment* (2nd ed.). Baltimore: Williams & Wilkins.

Ham, R. (1990). *Therapy of stuttering, preschool through adolescence.* Upper Saddle River, NJ: Prentice Hall.

Hegde, M. (2004). *Introduction to communicative disorders* (3rd ed.). Austin, TX: PRO-ED.

Hertrich, I., & Ackermann, H. (1994). Acquired stuttering in Parkinson syndrome. *Journal of Fluency Disorders, 19,* 179.

Hobbs, J. (Ed.) (1987). *Cleft lip and cleft palate from birth to three years.* Pittsburgh: American Cleft Palate Educational Foundation.

Hobbs, J. (Ed.) (1987). *Cleft lip and cleft palate: The child from three to twelve years.* Pittsburgh: American Cleft Palate Educational Foundation.

Hulit, L. (1989). A stutterer like me. *Journal of Fluency Disorders, 14,* 209–214.

Hulit, L. (2004). *Straight talk on stuttering* (2nd ed.). Springfield, IL: Thomas.

Hulit, L., & Wirtz, L. (1994). The association of attitudes toward stuttering with selected variables. *Journal of Fluency Disorders, 19,* 247–267.

Ingram, D. (1991). *Phonological disability in children* (2nd ed.). San Diego, CA: Singular.

Johnson, B. (1996). *Language disorders in children: An introductory clinical perspective.* Albany, NY: Delmar.

Johnson, W. (1946). *People in quandaries.* New York: Harper.

Johnson, W., et al. (1967). *Speech-handicapped school children* (3rd ed.). New York: Harper & Row.

Kamhi, A. (1981). Developmental vs. difference theories of mental retardation: A new look. *American Journal of Mental Deficiency, 86,* 1–7.

Larkins, P. (1985). *Speech-language pathology update.* Rockville, MD: American Speech–Language–Hearing Association.

Lass, N., Ruscello, D., Schmitt, J., Pannbacker, M., Orlando, M., Dean, K., Ruziska, J., & Bradshaw, K. (1992). Teachers perceptions of stutterers. *Language, Speech, Hearing Services in Schools, 23,* 78–81.

Lebrun, Y., Leleux, C., Rousseau, J., & Devreux, F. (1983). Acquired stuttering. *Journal of Fluency Disorders, 8,* 323–330.

Leonard, L. (1987). Is specific language impairment a useful construct? In S. Rosenberg (Ed.), *Advances in applied psycholinguistics* (Vol. 1). Cambridge: Cambridge University Press.

Leske, M. (1981a). Prevalence estimates of communicative disorders in the U.S.: Language, hearing and vestibular disorders. *ASHA, 23,* 229–237.

Leske, M. (1981b). Prevalence estimates of communicative disorders in the U.S.: Speech disorders. *ASHA, 23,* 217–225.

Mahr, G., & Leith, W. (1992). Psychogenic stuttering of adult onset. *Journal of Speech and Hearing Research, 35,* 283–286.

Martin, H., McConkey, R., & Martin, S. (1984). From acquisition theories to intervention strategies: An experiment with mentally handicapped children. *British Journal of Disorders of Communication, 19,* 3–14.

Mavlov, L. (1994). Mechanisms of fluency disorders in neocerebellar dysarthria and premotor articulatory apraxia. *Journal of Fluency Disorders, 19,* 192–193.

McTear, M., & Conti-Ramsden, G. (1991). *Pragmatic disability in children.* San Diego, CA: Singular.

Miller, S., & Madison, C. (1984). Public school voice clinics. I: A working model. *Language, Speech and Hearing Services in Schools, 15,* 51–57.

Mirenda, P., & Donnellan, A. (1986). Effects of adult interaction style on conversational behavior in students with severe communication problems. *Language, Speech, and Hearing Services in Schools, 17,* 126–141.

Mowrer, D. (1990). *Methods of modifying speech behaviors* (2nd ed.). Prospect Heights, IL: Waveland.

Nagafuchi, M. (1994). Acquired stuttering due to damage to the left premotor area. *Journal of Fluency Disorders, 19,* 195.

Nelson, N. (1993). *Childhood language disorders in context: Infancy through adolescence.* New York: Macmillan.

Nippold, M. (1990). Concomitant speech and language disorders in stuttering children: A critique of the literature. *Journal of Speech and Hearing Disorders, 55,* 51–60.

Owens, R. (2004). *Language disorders: A functional approach to assessment and intervention* (4th ed.). Boston: Allyn & Bacon.

Pannbacker, M. (1992). Some common myths about voice therapy. *Language, Speech, Hearing Services in Schools, 23,* 12–19.

Paul, R. (1987). Communication in autism. In D. J. Cohen & A. M. Donnellan (Eds.), *Handbook of autism and pervasive developmental disorders.* New York: Wiley.

Perkins, W. (1978). *Human perspectives in speech and language disorders.* St. Louis: Mosby.

Perkins, W. (1990). What is stuttering? *Journal of Speech and Hearing Disorders, 55,* 370–382.

Preacher, W., & Harris, W. (1946). Speech disorders in World War II: VIII. Stuttering. *Journal of Speech Disorders, 11,* 303–308.

Ritvo, E., & Freeman, B. (1978). National Society for Autistic Children definition of the syndrome of autism. *Journal of Autism and Childhood Schizophrenia, 8,* 162–167.

Roth, C., Aronson, A., & Davis, L. (1989). Clinical studies in psychogenic stuttering of adult onset. *Journal of Speech and Hearing Disorders, 54,* 634–646.

Ruscello, D., St. Louis, K., & Mason, N. (1991). School-aged children with phonologic disorders: Coexistence with other speech/language disorders. *Journal of Speech and Hearing Research, 34,* 236–242.

Scheerenberger, R. (1987). *A history of mental retardation.* Baltimore: Brookes.

Shames, G., & Rubin, H. (Eds.). (1986). *Stuttering: Then and now.* Upper Saddle River, NJ: Merrill/Prentice Hall.

Shewan, C. (1988). *ASHA work force study: Final report.* Rockville, MD: American Speech–Language–Hearing Association.

Shewan, C., & Malm, K. (1990). The prevalence of speech and language impairments. *ASHA, 32,* 108.

Silverman, E., & Zimmer, C. (1975). Incidence of chronic hoarseness among school-age children. *Journal of Speech and Hearing Disorders, 40,* 211–215.

Silverman, F. (1996). *Stuttering and other fluency disorders* (2nd ed.). Boston: Allyn & Bacon.

Skinner, P., & Shelton, R. (Eds.). (1985). *Speech, language and hearing.* New York: Wiley.

Stark, R., & Tallal, P. (1988). *Language, Speech, and Reading Disorders in Chil-*

dren: Neuropsychological Studies. San Diego, CA: College-Hill.

Starkweather, C. (1987). *Fluency and stuttering.* Upper Saddle River, NJ: Prentice Hall.

Starkweather, C., & Givens-Ackerman, J. (1997). *Stuttering.* Austin, TX: PRO-ED.

St. Louis, K., & Rustin, L. (1992). Professional awareness of cluttering. In F. Myers & K. St. Louis (Eds.), *Cluttering: A clinical perspective,* (pp. 23–35). Leicester, England: Far Communications.

Stoel-Gammon, C. (1990). Down syndrome: Effects on language development. *ASHA, 32,* 42–44.

Swisher, L., & Demetras, M. (1985). The expressive language characteristics of autistic children compared with mentally retarded or specific language-impaired children. In E. Schopler & G. B. Mesibov (Eds.), *Communication problems in autism.* New York: Plenum.

Tager-Flusberg, H. (1985). The conceptual basis for referential word meaning in children with autism. *Child Development, 56,* 1167–1178.

Van Riper, C. (1973). *The treatment of stuttering.* Upper Saddle River, NJ: Prentice Hall.

Van Riper, C. (1992). *The Nature of Stuttering,* 2nd ed. Prospect Heights, IL: Waveland.

Van Riper, C., & Erickson, R. (1996). *Speech correction: An introduction to speech pathology and audiology* (9th ed.). Boston: Allyn & Bacon.

Wall, M., & Meyers, F. (1984). *Clinical management of childhood stuttering.* Baltimore: University Park Press.

Weiss, C., Gordon, M., & Lillywhite, H. (1987). *Clinical management of articulatory and phonologic disorders* (2nd ed.). Baltimore: Williams & Wilkins.

Weiss, D. (1964). *Cluttering.* Upper Saddle River, NJ: Prentice Hall.

Weiss, D. (1967). Similarities and differences between cluttering and stuttering. *Folia Phoniatrica, 19,* 98–104.

Wetherby, A. (1986). Ontogeny of communicative functions in autism. *Journal of Autism and Developmental Disorders, 16,* 295–316.

Wilson, D. (1979). *Voice problems in children* (2nd ed.). Baltimore: Williams & Wilkins.

Wingate, M. (1997). *Stuttering: A short history of a curious disorder.* Westport, CT: Bergin & Garvey.

Winitz, H. (1988). *Human communication and its disorders: A review.* Norwood, NJ: Ablex.

Yairi, E. & Grinager Ambrose, N. (2004). *Early childhood stuttering.* Austin, TX: Pro-Ed.

Appendix

The Anatomical
and Physiological Bases
of Speech, Language,
and Hearing

Some of you will have a more thorough understanding of the anatomy and physiology of speech and hearing than others. Some will have no background in this area. All students of human communication development, regardless of knowledge level,

need to be reminded that the speech portion of human communication is a physiological process. To understand fully how speech and language development occurs, therefore, one must have some appreciation for the anatomical equipment that makes the human communication system work. This chapter introduces the novice to basic information about the anatomy and physiology of speech and hearing and provides an adequate review if you already have a background. Specifically, this chapter is designed to facilitate understanding of the following topics:

- The integration of respiration, phonation, articulation, and resonation in the production of speech
- *Respiration:* the power source for speech

- *Phonation:* using the larynx to generate voice
- *Resonation:* shaping the cavities of the speech mechanism to modify the tones of speech
- *Articulation:* using the structures of the mouth to produce the sounds of speech
- The *human nervous system:* linking the brain to the muscles of speech
- The *ear:* moving sound waves from the pinna to the brain

It is impossible really to understand human speech without examining the anatomic structures and physiological processes that produce speech. Speech is, after all, the direct result of muscle contractions innervated by the nervous system which move structures in ways that force air out of the lungs, vibrate that air, resonate it, and break it up into speech sounds. In this chapter, we look at the structures which together make up what we call the speech machine. We also examine the hearing mechanism, which is important to speech in two ways. First, we receive the speech of others through the hearing mechanism. Unless there are ears to hear what is said, we cannot complete the **vocal-auditory channel,** one of the design-features of speech (Hockett, 1960). Second, the speaker depends on the ability to hear himself so that he can monitor the content of his speech as well as things like rate, pitch, stress, rhythm, and articulatory accuracy.

Speech as the Product of Borrowed Structures

All of the structures involved in producing speech are designed for other, more basic, biological purposes. Breathing, for example, is important for speech, but the primary reason a person breathes is to absorb oxygen into the bloodstream and to release waste in the form of carbon dioxide. The *larynx,* commonly called the *voice box,* is a valve in the throat that prevents the ingestion of foreign substances into the lungs. The tongue, which plays a major role in the production of speech sounds, exists primarily to facilitate eating. Every structure that is a part of the speech machine is, in a sense, borrowed from the body's life maintenance systems. Human beings have adapted certain bodily structures for the purpose of producing speech.

You should not interpret this to mean that speech is the product of an anatomy ill-suited for this purpose. On the contrary, every part of the body that plays a role in speech is ideally designed in structure and function for speech, but we should never forget that speech is an activity that is overlaid on biological functions that are more basic to our physical survival than is speech. This is one of the wonders of human oral communication—that we have been able to use structures intended for other purposes to create a communication system that is convenient and efficient and unmatched in power and sophistication by any other communication system in the animal kingdom. Other primates, for example, have anatomies remarkably similar to ours, but they have not been able to adapt their structures to produce oral communication systems even remotely comparable to speech. The structures themselves, while similar, are not capable of the intricate, controlled adjustments required for speech. The larynx of a chimpanzee, for example, resembles the human larynx, but the vocal folds in the chimpanzee's larynx do not allow the same range of length and tension adjustments as are possible in human vocal folds. Although it is true, therefore, that the structures humans use to produce speech have more fundamental vegetative responsibilities, they work so well for speech that they could have been specifically designed for that purpose.

The Four Processes of Speech

Speech can be most easily understood as the product of four separate but inextricably related processes: respiration, phonation, resonation, and articulation. As indicated in Figure A.1, each process makes a specific contribution to the end product. **Respiration** or breathing provides the power for speech. The speaker inhales to capture air in the lungs and then, in a controlled manner, exhales to force a column of air into the larynx. **Phonation** occurs when the vocal folds of the larynx are drawn together by contraction of specific muscles, and the exhaled air causes the folds to vibrate in a manner that disturbs or vibrates the air column. As the vibrating air column passes through the throat, mouth, and sometimes the nasal cavities, it is **resonated,** which means that the tone of the noise from the vocal folds is modified according to the size and shape of the resonating cavities. As the vibrating and resonated air column passes through the mouth, the tongue, teeth, and other structures in the mouth break up the airstream into the sounds of speech, a process called **articulation.**

As described here and depicted in Figure A.1, the reader might get the impression that there is a discrete order from one process to the next, beginning with respiration. It is more accurate to understand speech as the product of the successive and simultaneous interactions of these four processes. In other words, it is true that speech must begin with exhalation, and the air stream must be phonated before it can be resonated, and it is articulated as it passes out of the mouth, but in continuous speech, all four of these processes are occurring in a precisely integrated and synchronized manner. While one part of the vibrating air column is being articulated, another part of the air column is just beginning the journey from the lungs into the larynx.

For the sake of convenience, we will look at each process as a separate entity, but you should remember that, like any machine, each part of the speech machine depends on every other part, and the machine functions only as the parts work

Figure A.1 The Processes of Speech

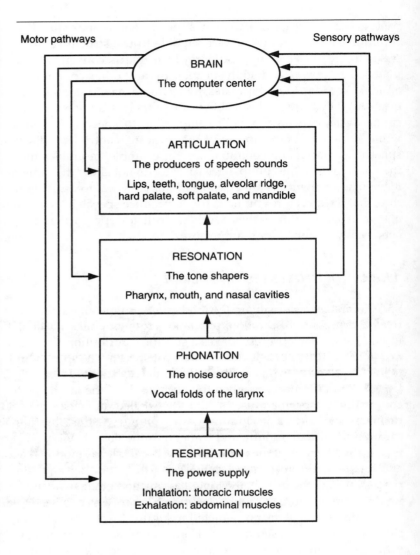

Motor pathways

Sensory pathways

BRAIN

The computer center

ARTICULATION

The producers of speech sounds

Lips, teeth, tongue, alveolar ridge, hard palate, soft palate, and mandible

RESONATION

The tone shapers

Pharynx, mouth, and nasal cavities

PHONATION

The noise source

Vocal folds of the larynx

RESPIRATION

The power supply

Inhalation: thoracic muscles
Exhalation: abdominal muscles

together. Many man-made machines have become so complicated in their structures and functions that they must be managed by internal computers. The human speech machine is also incredibly complex and also requires an internal computer to make sure all the parts function in proper synchrony. The speech machine's computer is the brain. It is the brain that coordinates the activities of all the processes of speech and ensures that the product is speech, not gibberish. As indicated in Figure A.1, the brain sends out instructions along motor pathways to the structures involved in each process and constantly monitors how these structures are responding by analyzing the data sent back by the sensory pathways. Normal speech is maintained only if correct instructions are sent to the speech structures and reliable feedback is received from them.

Respiration

As has already been noted, the primary biological function of respiration is the exchange of life-sustaining oxygen for carbon dioxide. Breathing for life is involuntary and rhythmic. About 50 percent of each breathing cycle is spent on inhalation and about 50 percent on exhalation. Breathing for speech is very different. The speaker exercises voluntary control over the breathing cycle, especially exhalation, which forces air through the vocal tract. During speech, about 15 percent of the breathing cycle is devoted to inhalation and 85 percent to exhalation.

The Structures of Breathing

The primary muscle involved in inhalation is the **diaphragm,** which separates the trunk of the body into two sections. The section above the diaphragm is called the **thorax,** the cavity that houses the lungs, and the section below the diaphragm is called the **abdomen,** the cavity that houses internal organs including the kidneys, liver, and intestines.

The bony framework of the thorax (Figure A.2) is composed of twelve **thoracic vertebrae** posteriorly, the **sternum** (breastbone) anteriorly, and twelve pairs of **ribs** laterally. The **lungs,** located inside the thorax, are the structures that exchange carbon dioxide and oxygen. The bases of the lungs rest on top of the diaphragm. Two moist membranes called **pleurae** surround the lungs. The lungs themselves consist of spongy tissue that is highly elastic, but there are very few muscle fibers in the lungs, which means they are passive structures. They receive air. They do not suck in air, as some people think. The lungs receive air during inhalation when the thorax expands, creating a difference in air pressure in the lungs compared to the air pressure outside the body. Breathing depends on a very basic principle of physics known as Boyle's law.

The Application of Basic Physics to Breathing

According to Boyle's law, "If a gas is kept at a constant temperature, pressure and volume are inversely proportional to one another and have a constant product" (Zemlin, 1988, p. 33). This means that if we have a given number of gas molecules at a constant temperature, we can change the pressure exerted by those molecules by changing the volume of the container. If we double the volume of the container, the pressure is reduced by one-half. If we triple the volume of the container, the pressure

Figure A.2 The Thorax: Front and Rear Views

Sternum

Front view

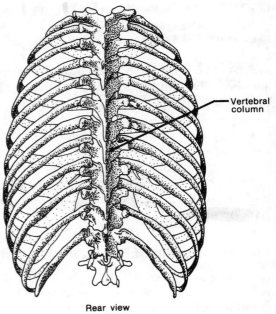

Vertebral column

Rear view

is reduced to one-third of the original pressure, and so on. However, if we cut the volume of the container in half, the pressure exerted by the gas molecules doubles, and if we reduce the volume to one-third of the original volume, the pressure triples, and so on.

Consider how this law is applied to breathing. The lungs are housed inside the thorax, an airtight cavity connected to the outside air through the **trachea** or windpipe and the mouth and nose. If the volume of the thorax is increased, the air pressure inside the lungs decreases proportionately, and what will happen if the pressure inside is less than the pressure outside when there is a direct connection between the lungs and the outside air? Air will rush into the lungs to make the pressures equal, of course. Therefore, **inhalation** occurs when the volume of the thorax is increased, creating pressure in the lungs that is less than the outside pressure. In **exhalation,** the volume of the thorax is reduced, creating pressure inside the lungs that is greater than the outside pressure, and what happens? Air rushes out of the lungs until the pressures are equal again. Breathing then depends on the very practical application of Boyle's law and the simple principle of equilibrium. What remains to be understood is how the volume of the thorax is increased in inhalation and decreased in exhalation.

Inhalation and Exhalation during Quiet Breathing

During normal quiet breathing, the amount of oxygen inhaled is approximately equal to the volume of carbon dioxide exhaled, and a complete inhalation-exhalation cycle occurs about twelve to fifteen times per minute.

The diaphragm is dome-shaped in its resting configuration. Inhalation begins when the diaphragm contracts or flattens, resulting in an increase in the vertical dimension of the thorax (Figure A.3). At the same time, muscles attached to the ribs contract, lifting the ribs and swinging them upward and outward in much the same way the handle on a bucket moves away from the side of a bucket when it is lifted (Figure A.4). This action also causes the sternum to be moved up and out. The muscles of inhalation, therefore, cause the thorax to be increased from side to side, front to back, and in the vertical dimension. The lungs, which are effectively attached to the sides of the thorax by the pleurae that surround them, expand when the thorax expands. This action creates reduced air pressure in the lungs relative to the outside air pressure, and air rushes into the lungs until the pressures are equal, completing the inhalation portion of the respiratory cycle.

Exhalation in quiet breathing is a passive process, not involving muscle activity. After the lungs fill with air, the muscles of inhalation relax, reducing the volume of the thorax and creating another imbalance of inside and outside pressures. Air now flows out of the lungs until the pressures are equal again. This completes exhalation and one complete cycle of respiration. We do this automatically and rhythmically about twelve to fifteen times per minute, whether asleep or awake (Zemlin, 1988, p. 94). There are obviously more cycles per minute when we are active than when we are relaxed, and when we sleep soundly, the number of cycles per minute is further reduced.

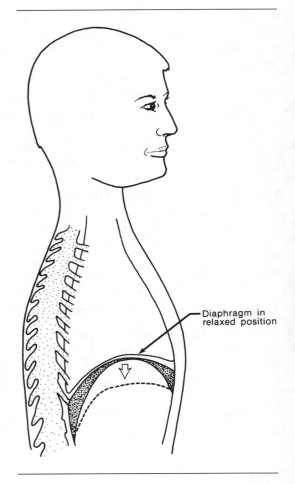

Figure A.3 Vertical Increase in Thoracic Volume as Diaphragm Contracts

Diaphragm in relaxed position

Breathing for Speech

Breathing for speech differs radically from breathing for life. As mentioned earlier, speech is a muscular activity requiring the precise synchronization of all four processes of speech, including respiration. Breathing for speech necessitates delicate control of each respiratory cycle and particularly the exhalation portion of the cycle. When we breathe for speech, we extend and control exhalation for up to fifteen seconds. If we were unable to do this, talking time would be restricted to 2.5-second spurts, the average duration of exhalation during quiet breathing (Zemlin, 1990, p. 80). We would be able to produce only a few words at a time instead of the lengthy sentences that characterize normal speech.

Figure A.4 Lateral and Anteroposterior Expansions of the Thorax

Air is drawn in

Sternum moves forward

Ribs are lifted

Contracted diaphragm

Side-to-side and front-to-back expansion

Resemblance between lifted bucket handle and lifted ribs

Relaxed diaphragm

Thorax at rest

In addition to changing the nature of the respiratory cycle, speech affects breathing by introducing varying degrees of airflow resistance at a number of places in the speech mechanism. If the vocal folds are brought together, for example, and the lips or the tongue are positioned for the production of certain sounds, the power of exhalation must be great enough to force air through the constriction points. Instead of just relaxing the muscles of inhalation as we do during quiet breathing, we must partially contract these muscles and actively contract muscles of exhalation to maintain sufficient airflow force and control for speech production. Breathing for speech, therefore, requires a complex balance of the muscle activities involved in inhalation and exhalation, a balance that allows us to sustain exhalation for periods up to six times longer than exhalation during quiet breathing. The air we exhale for speech moves into the larynx, the tone-producing structure in the speech machine.

Phonation

The **larynx** is a structure in the anterior neck commonly known as the *voice box*. The **vocal folds** are the components in the larynx responsible for generating the noise upon which speech is superimposed. The larynx sits on top of the trachea and is suspended by means of muscles and ligaments from a U-shaped bone called the **hyoid**. Although the hyoid is not part of the larynx, it is important to laryngeal function because a number of laryngeal muscles are attached to it.

As mentioned earlier, the larynx acts as a valve to prevent foreign materials from entering the trachea and lungs. If something threatens to enter, the vocal folds close while exhalation continues until the force of the air below the folds literally blows them open. You may recognize this action as the cough.

The secondary function of the larynx is sound production, a purpose for which it is ideally constructed. The vocal folds are relatively long and are capable of the wide range of adjustments in length and tension that are essential for voice production. During normal quiet breathing, the vocal folds are relatively wide open, but during speech, they are drawn together to obstruct the flow of air from the lungs, setting up the conditions necessary for vocal fold vibration. We will take a closer look at the mechanics of voice production after we examine the structure of the larynx.

The Parts of the Voice Generator

The larynx is composed of nine cartilages (Figure A.5) bound together by a complex network of membranes. The inside of the larynx is lined with a membrane that is continuous with the membrane lining the trachea below and the pharynx above. There are three single cartilages in the larynx and three pairs of smaller cartilages. We are concerned with only the most important of these cartilages: thyroid, cricoid, epiglottis, and the arytenoids.

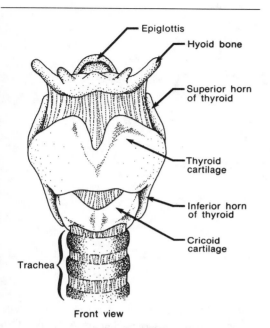

Epiglottis

Hyoid bone

Superior horn
of thyroid

Thyroid
cartilage

Inferior horn
of thyroid

Cricoid
cartilage

Trachea

Front view

Figure A.5 The Cartilages of the
Larynx: Front and Rear
Views

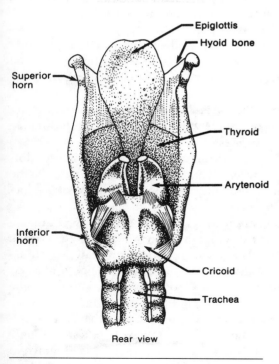

Epiglottis

Hyoid bone

Superior
horn

Thyroid

Arytenoid

Inferior
horn

Cricoid

Trachea

Rear view

Figure A.6 The Arytenoid Cartilages and Related Structures

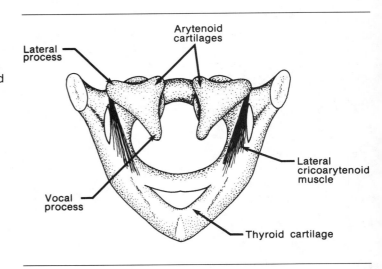

The **thyroid** is the largest of the laryngeal cartilages. It is the part of the larynx that tends to protrude in the neck and is often referred to as the Adam's apple. This unpaired cartilage is made up of two plates joined in front in a V shape whose open portion faces toward the back. Each plate has two projections called **horns.** The **superior horn** extends upward toward the hyoid bone, and the **inferior horn** extends downward to connect with the cricoid cartilage. This pivotal connection allows the thyroid cartilage to be tilted downward and forward, an action that lengthens the vocal folds.

The lowermost portion of the larynx is the **cricoid** cartilage, which sits on the top of the trachea. The cricoid is in the shape of a ring, with a plate on the posterior side and a narrower band forming the front and sides.

Attached to the angle of the thyroid is the third single cartilage called the **epiglottis,** which is shaped something like a narrow leaf. It is attached at its top margin to the hyoid bone by a ligament. Even though the epiglottis is an interesting-looking structure, it makes little, if any, contribution to speech.

The only paired cartilages that are important to laryngeal function are the roughly pyramid-shaped **arytenoids** (Figure A.6), which are situated on top of the posterior plate of the cricoid. Each arytenoid has a **vocal process** and a **lateral** or **muscular** process. The vocal processes extend anteriorly and have the vocal folds attached to them. The lateral processes have muscles attached to them that act to move the vocal folds together or apart.

As has already been mentioned, the vocal folds (Figure A.7) are the vibrating elements of the larynx and consist of muscles and ligaments. They originate at the angle of the thyroid, extend posteriorly along the inner sides of the thyroid, and attach to the vocal processes of the arytenoids. As indicated in Figure A.7, each vocal fold ex-

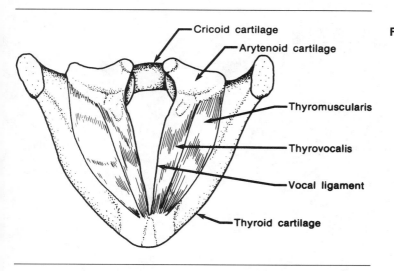

Figure A.7 The Vocal Folds

Labels: Cricoid cartilage, Arytenoid cartilage, Thyromuscularis, Thyrovocalis, Vocal ligament, Thyroid cartilage

tends into the opening of the larynx like a shelf. The space between the folds is called the **glottis.** The glottis varies in width, depending on which laryngeal muscles contract and how much they contract. During normal breathing, the glottis is relatively wide open. When the speaker whispers, the front part of the glottis closes, but the posterior portion remains open. During full voice, the folds are closed along their entire length, and the glottis disappears.

Making the Voice Generator Work

Muscles in the larynx allow the speaker to open and close the vocal folds, and the muscles making up the vocal folds allow the speaker to make the folds tense or lax. These adjustments are basic to producing the voice. Muscles that have both of their attachments within the larynx itself are **intrinsic muscles** of the larynx. These are the muscles primarily responsible for the adjustments necessary for voice production. The extrinsic muscles, with one attachment in the larynx and the other attachment outside the larynx, move the entire structure up and down, but these adjustments have little to do with generating voice. This section, therefore, focuses on those intrinsic muscles most directly involved in opening and closing the vocal folds.

The muscles whose primary responsibility is to open the vocal folds are called **abductors.** To **abduct** means to move or pull away from the middle. In the case of laryngeal function, the abductors pull the vocal folds away from one another, opening the glottis between them. Those muscles primarily responsible for closing the vocal folds are called **adductors,** which means that they move the vocal folds toward the middle, effectively closing the glottis.

Figure A.8 The Action of the Posterior
Cricoarytenoid Muscles:
Abduction

Posterior view

Top view

The muscles of abduction are the **posterior cricoarytenoid** muscles (Figure A.8). As is true of most muscles of the body, the name itself identifies the points of attachment. These muscles originate on both sides of the posterior plate of the cricoid cartilage and attach to the lateral or muscular processes of the arytenoid cartilages. When these muscles contract, they pull the arytenoids in a manner that causes them to rotate, opening the folds attached to their vocal processes.

Adduction of the vocal folds is accomplished by contraction of the paired **lateral cricoarytenoid** muscles and the **interarytenoid** muscles (Figure A.9). The lateral cricoarytenoid muscles originate on the sides of the cricoid cartilage and insert into the lateral processes of the arytenoids. When they contract, they pull the vocal processes and the attached vocal folds toward the middle, partially closing the glottis. To achieve complete closure of the vocal folds, the interarytenoids must also be in-

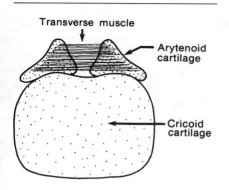

Transverse muscle

Arytenoid cartilage

Cricoid cartilage

Figure A.9 The Interarytenoid Muscles: Transverse and Oblique (Rear View)

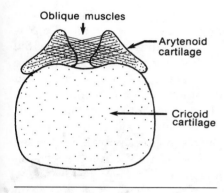

Oblique muscles

Arytenoid cartilage

Cricoid cartilage

volved. Actually several interarytenoid muscles, as the name implies, run between the arytenoid cartilages. The **transverse interarytenoid,** an unpaired muscle, courses from the outside edge of one arytenoid to the outside edge of the other. Each of the two **oblique interarytenoid** muscles originates on the lower outside edge of one arytenoid and attaches to the top or apex of the other. When the interarytenoid muscles contract, they pull the arytenoid cartilages and the vocal folds together, and when they work together with the lateral cricoarytenoid muscles, they completely close the vocal folds.

We have now examined all of the laryngeal parts that are active in generating the tone upon which speech is produced. The laryngeal tone is the result of very rapid vocal fold vibrations. Consider what happens in a single cycle of vibration: (1) The vocal folds are adducted to restrict the flow of air from the lungs. (2) At the same time as the folds are being adducted, exhalation is producing increased air pressure beneath the folds. (3) When this pressure is sufficient, the folds are blown apart, releasing a small puff of air into the trachea above. (4) This release results in reduced pressure beneath the folds. (5) The reduction of air pressure combined with the elasticity of the folds forces the folds to snap back together, ready to be blown apart again when the pressure builds up. This five-step sequence is repeated 120 to 145 times per second in adult males and 200 to 260 times per second in adult females (Zemlin, 1990, p. 93).

Pitch changes are accomplished by varying the length and mass of the folds. In general, pitch rises when there is an increase in length and a decrease in mass, adjustments that result in more rapid vocal fold vibrations. The tone produced by the larynx is most often called the **glottal** or **laryngeal tone.** It sounds like the combination of a hum and a buzz until it is shaped by the resonating cavities of the neck and head and eventually broken up by the articulators into the speech sounds we combine into words and sentences.

Resonation

The next speech process is **resonation.** Have you ever blown over the top of a partially filled bottle of pop? The sound you hear results from the size and shape of the resonating cavity, in this case the space in the bottle above the pop. If you drink more of the pop and blow over the top again, the tone will change. The change is the result of a larger and, depending on bottle shape and the amount of pop remaining, differently shaped resonating cavity. In other words, if the tone fed into the bottle remains constant, but the size and shape of the resonating cavity within the bottle changes, the resulting tones will change. In general, the larger the resonating cavity, the lower the perceived pitch of the tone, because the larger cavity will reinforce the lower frequencies in the original tone. Resonance in speech, therefore, is the process whereby certain frequencies in the laryngeal tone are reinforced or emphasized depending on the size and shape of the speech resonators, including the pharynx, mouth, and nasal cavities (Figure A.10). Although a bottle's resonating cavity has a fairly limited range of adjustments, the resonating cavities for speech are capable of seemingly limitless adjustments.

Although resonation is important for shaping all speech sounds, it is particularly important for vowels. The primary characteristic differentiating vowels from consonants is that they are open sounds, produced with a relatively free flow of air. There is very little constriction anywhere in the vocal tract when a vowel is produced. Say the following sounds aloud: "p," "t," "k." Notice that the airflow is actually stopped and released on these sounds. Now say "s," "f," and "th." Notice that the flow of air continues, but it is constricted. Now produce a few vowels aloud such as "a," "o," and "e." There is little restriction of air flow in the mouth. Now try producing a constant laryngeal tone and simply change the size and shape of your mouth by opening it wide and narrowing the opening, by lifting the tongue and lowering it without touching anything, and by moving the tongue forward and pulling it back. These are the kinds of adjustments we make to produce different vowels. When we produce a vowel like the "ee" in *feet,* we create a narrow, high, front-of-the-

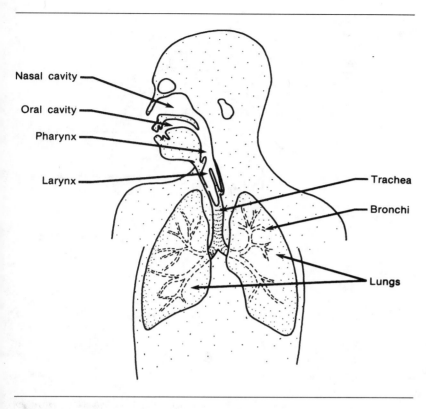

Figure A.10 The Resonating Cavities

mouth resonating cavity. When we produce a vowel like the "a" in *father*, we shape a wide, low, back-of-the-mouth cavity. Notice that the "ee" sounds higher in pitch than the "a," even though the laryngeal tone remains the same. Keep in mind that we have considered changes only in the mouth. The pharynx, which connects the trachea and the mouth, is a muscular structure capable of many adjustments, and it is constantly changing its shape during speech, adding subtle resonated qualities to the laryngeal tone.

It is generally understood that the nasal cavities are opened for resonation only for the production of the consonants *m, n,* and *ng.* We actually experience some nasal resonation on vowels in words containing these consonants because we cannot close off the nasal cavities quickly enough to eliminate the nasal quality. You may also have noticed that there is a nasal quality in some dialects of American English, particularly in the southern and southwestern parts of the country.

Figure A.11 The Articulators

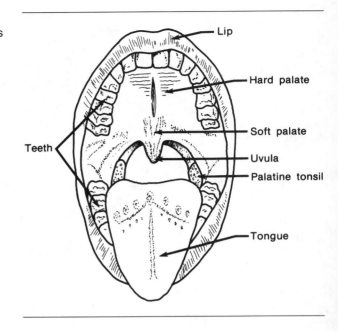

Lip

Hard palate

Soft palate

Uvula

Palatine tonsil

Teeth

Tongue

Articulation

We now come to the final process of speech, **articulation,** which is most simply understood as the breaking up of the air stream into the sounds of speech by the structures of the mouth. It should be clear at this point, however, that it is not possible to separate articulation from the other processes of speech, particularly resonation, with which it is closely integrated. Although it is true, for example, that vowels are primarily the products of resonation, they are also the products of articulatory adjustments, especially varying jaw openings and tongue manipulations. We most commonly associate articulation with consonants, but as has already been noted, the consonants *m, n,* and *ng* are very much the products of nasal resonance. Whatever separation we make between resonation and articulation, therefore, is somewhat arbitrary and must be understood as an effort to emphasize and clarify the most important function of each process. With that purpose in mind, it is reasonable and accurate to note that resonation is primarily concerned with vowel production, and articulation is primarily concerned with consonant production, although each process is involved in the production of all speech sounds.

The articulators include the teeth, tongue, lips, alveolar ridge, hard palate, soft palate (velum), and the jaw (Figure A.11). Notice that some of these structures can move and others are fixed. The tongue, lips, soft palate, and the jaw can move, but not at the same speeds. The tongue is capable of relatively rapid movements, but the soft palate moves very slowly. The soft palate is the muscular tissue at the posterior end of the roof of the mouth. For all of the sounds of speech, except "m," "n," and "ng," it lifts up and back to close off the opening between the mouth and the nasal cavities. The alveolar ridge is the bony shelf into which the upper teeth are set. The hard palate is the bony portion of the roof of the mouth. These structures and the teeth do not move. Another way to understand articulation, therefore, is that the mobile articulators move toward and away from, and sometimes make contact with, the fixed articulators. These adjustments account for how most, but not all, speech sounds are articulated, since the sounds "k," "g," and "ng" involve contacts between the back of the tongue and the soft palate, two mobile articulators.

The Four Processes in Review

Now that we have examined each process as a separate part of the anatomy and physiology of speech, we will consider how they work together in the simple production of the word *be.*

The speaker inhales by contracting the diaphragm and the muscles of the thorax, which has the effect of increasing the volume of the thorax in the vertical, side-to-side, and front-to-back dimensions. This increase in volume creates reduced pressure in the lungs, which expand along with the expanding thorax. Air comes into the lungs until the pressure in the lungs equals the pressure outside the body. The speaker then exhales by relaxing most of the muscles of inhalation and contracting the muscles of exhalation in a prolonged and controlled manner. These actions push a column of air out of the lungs, through the trachea, and into the larynx.

Since both sounds in the word *be* require vocal fold vibration, the speaker contracts the adductor muscles to bring the vocal folds together. As the column of air is pushed through the folds by the forces of exhalation, the folds vibrate, creating a disturbance in the particles of air we refer to as the *glottal* or *laryngeal tone.* The now-vibrating column of air passes out of the larynx into the pharynx.

The speaker adjusts the *resonators,* including the pharynx, mouth, and nasal cavities, to shape the laryngeal tone according to the characteristics of the sounds being produced. In producing *"be,"* for example, the speaker will lift the soft palate to close off the nasal cavities because the sounds in the word do not receive nasal resonance. The speaker closes the lips to stop the flow of air and then quickly releases this closure to *articulate* the "b" sound and, at the same time, raises the tongue toward the front part of the hard palate to create the high, narrow resonating chamber for the "e." The vocal folds vibrate throughout the entire production.

You should once again be impressed with the complexity of these adjustments and the speed at which they occur. The human anatomy has been ideally developed for the production of speech, and the physiology involved occurs so naturally and effortlessly that we make these rapid, intricate adjustments thousands upon thousands of times every day without giving them a conscious thought.

The Brain: The Computer Center for Speech and Language

The reason speech is produced with so little conscious effort is that the speech machine is directed by a central nervous system unmatched in any other animal on earth. Some physiological functions in humans and all animals are automatic, of course. Our hearts beat and we breathe without any conscious efforts on our parts, whether we are awake or asleep.

The behaviors of speech and language are voluntary and require more conscious control than breathing, but they require far less direct attention than, for example, putting thread through the eye of a needle. Remember, too, that people sometimes talk while they are asleep, so the behaviors of speech and language are voluntary, but they are so natural and instinctive and require so little effort that we can sometimes talk in our sleep. This would not be possible without the complex and highly reliable nervous system that serves as a kind of computer center for speech and language.

A detailed description of neuroanatomy and neurophysiology is beyond the scope of this book, but if you want to learn more about these subjects, see the list of readings at the end of this appendix. For our purposes, we will focus on the major features of the human nervous system, and especially on those parts that are most directly related to speech, language, and hearing.

The nervous system can be arbitrarily divided into two major divisions: (1) central nervous system and (2) peripheral nervous system. The **central nervous system** (Figure A.12) includes the brain and the spinal cord. The brain is divided into halves called the right and left **cerebral hemispheres,** the **brain stem,** and the **cerebellum.** The brain is encased in the skull, and the spinal cord is surrounded by the bony **vertebral column,** sometimes called the **spinal column.**

The peripheral nervous system consists of all the cranial and spinal nerves that carry information to the brain in the form of sensations such as hearing, pain, or temperature, and information from the brain in the form of motor commands to the muscles of the body.

The most basic anatomic unit of the nervous system is the **neuron.** There are millions of neurons in the body, which are organized into complex networks or circuits. Any message carried anywhere in the nervous system is carried by the tiny neuron.

Speech and Language Functions of the Brain

Even though the speech and language functions of the brain are not fully understood, we have been able to identify certain areas of the cerebral hemispheres that have primary responsibilities for this uniquely human range of behaviors. What follows is a brief overview of the information researchers have gathered over the years about those structures they believe are most closely associated with speech and language functions. Be forewarned: Because this is only an overview and intentionally introductory in nature, we will focus only on the most obvious relevant structures. If you are interested in a more detailed description of all neural structures believed to be rel-

Figure A.12 The Central Nervous System

evant to speech and language functions, consult the references and suggested readings included at the end of this appendix.

The Cerebrum: Left and Right Cerebral Hemispheres

The **cerebrum,** the largest portion of the brain, is incompletely divided into two hemispheres. The two halves of the cerebrum are connected by a large band of neural fibers known as the **corpus callosum,** a structure that serves as a major communication pathway between the two hemispheres. Although we cannot generalize left and right hemispheric functions for all people, it is appropriate to indicate that in most people the left hemisphere has greater responsibilities for speech and language activities than the right. Three areas of the left hemisphere and a bundle of neural fibers (Figure A.13) are of particular interest: **Wernicke's area, Broca's area,** the **motor cortex,** and the **arcuate fasciculus.** Wernicke's area is primarily concerned with the comprehension and formulation of language. Language information is transmitted to Broca's area from Wernicke's area via a bundle of neural fibers called the arcuate fasciculus. The term *fasciculus* refers to a bundle of nerve fibers that share a common origin, termination, and function. In Broca's area, language information is organized into the appropriate articulatory motor sequences for speech. These motor commands are then transmitted to the motor cortex. The neural messages carrying speech and language information are eventually sent to the speech musculature along special pathways that will be described in the next section.

The right hemisphere is less involved with speech and language than the left, but it does contribute to the processing of emotional content that often underlies speech and language. There is also evidence that the melodic patterns we superimpose on speech when we sing are associated with right hemispheric functions (Blumstein & Cooper, 1974; Knox & Kimura, 1970).

The suggestion here is that functions of the hemispheres are highly specialized, and although areas in each hemisphere do seem to have specific functions, it is important to understand that there is significant integration of the functions of the cerebrum. For example, we have noted that emotional processing is associated with the right hemisphere, and language and speech functions are associated with the left hemisphere. It should be immediately clear, however, that we can communicate emotional messages through speech and language only if the two hemispheres interact with one another in a manner that allows us to integrate emotional messages into language form, which are then expressed in meaningful speech.

Motor Speech Control

How do we get our speech and language messages from the cerebrum to the muscles of speech? Once thoughts are formulated and put into language form, the cerebrum sends the motor messages of speech along a complex neural network of special pathways within the central nervous system. The information contained in these pathways ultimately reaches the various motor portions of the cranial and spinal nerves that constitute the peripheral nervous system. The peripheral nerves are connected to the muscles of the body and are the final pathways over which the messages will be delivered.

It may help to think of this process of getting motor commands from the cerebrum to the structures of speech as being analogous to a relay race. The "runners" who will be the initial carriers of information in this complicated delivery system are the many neurons that make up specialized pathways in the central nervous system. Positioned at strategic locations within the nervous system are the other runners or neurons that make up the cranial and spinal nerves of the peripheral nervous system. Once the communication plan is developed, the runners of the central nervous system are given complex messages, which they carry to the runners of the peripheral nervous system by way of the special pathways. Upon reaching the stations where

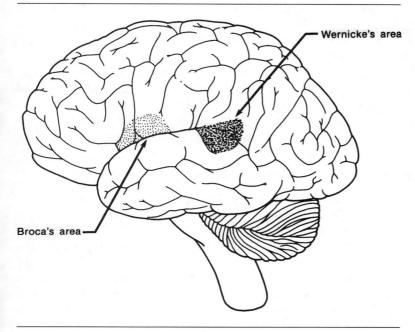

Figure A.13 Left Cerebral Hemisphere

Wernicke's area

Broca's area

the peripheral nervous system runners are waiting, the messages are passed on and carried by those runners to the muscles of the body that must be activated to produce the message in its final form—speech.

Central Nervous System Pathways: The Beginning of the Race

One of the special pathways of the central nervous system is called **pyramidal** because the tiny neurons that give rise to this system have cell bodies shaped like pyramids. This part of the system has **direct** input into the motor cranial and spinal nerves that represent the second leg in the relay race to the structures of speech. The pyramidal pathway controls refined, intricate movements in structures such as the lips and tongue. This kind of control is crucial to an activity like speech, which is the product of complex, precise, and delicately integrated motor adjustments.

The **extrapyramidal** system has a more **indirect** connection to the motor cranial and spinal nerves than the pyramidal, and it is responsible for providing commands for more gross and unskilled motor activities such as those involved in postural adjustment. We might refer to the act of writing to provide a simple example of the difference between pyramidal and extrapyramidal responsibilities. When you write, the extrapyramidal tract gets your hand to the paper, and the pyramidal tract controls the fine-motor skills necessary for you to write on that paper. In the context of our relay race analogy, the runners in the extrapyramidal system stop at a number of locations within the central nervous system to gather additional information in order to make the necessary adjustments to provide a background against which the pyramidal system makes its more precise, finely tuned movements.

The cerebellum coordinates the activities controlled by the pyramidal and extrapyramidal systems. It is constantly receiving sensory information about the status of the muscles and limbs of the body and monitors the motor commands being sent along the pyramidal and extrapyramidal pathways. Using this steady flow of information to and from the central nervous system, the cerebellum makes crucial adjustments in commands to ensure that the final motor products are performed as accurately as possible.

Peripheral Nervous System Pathways: The Relay Race Continues

The commands that have been formulated in the cerebral hemispheres, carried through the central nervous system along the pyramidal and extrapyramidal pathways, and fine-tuned by the cerebellum are now passed to the message carrier who will run along the pathways of the cranial and spinal nerves that comprise the peripheral nervous system.

There are twelve pairs of **cranial nerves.** Some of these nerves carry only sensory information, some only motor, and others are mixed and carry both sensory and motor information. Only six of the cranial nerves are concerned with motor speech (Figure A.14).

There are thirty-one pairs of **spinal nerves,** and they are all mixed; that is, they carry both sensory and motor information. More than half of these nerves control the muscles of respiration. Since, as we observed earlier in this chapter, controlled and prolonged exhalation is crucial to speech production, these nerves make important contributions to the speech machine.

The Relay Race in Review: Instant Replay

There is much that is not understood about the nervous system in general and much not known about those functions related to speech and language. We do know, however, that the nervous system is organized in a hierarchical manner. That is, at some levels in the system information is developed, refined, and integrated as it works its way to the speech musculature.

Using the relay race analogy, we can now summarize the process. At the highest level in the system, the cerebrum, thoughts are developed, and language to express those thoughts is formulated. The message is carried by runners along the pyramidal and extrapyramidal pathways of the central nervous system. These runners carry the message through the cerebellum, which fine-tunes the motor commands, before they hand off the message to other runners who carry the message along the pathways of the cranial and spinal nerves involved in speech. The race ends when the commands reach the muscles of the speech structures, which contract in patterns producing strings of sounds that are a direct translation of the original thought.

In continuous speech, of course, the relay race is infinitely more complicated than this summary indicates because new thoughts, new language forms, and new motor

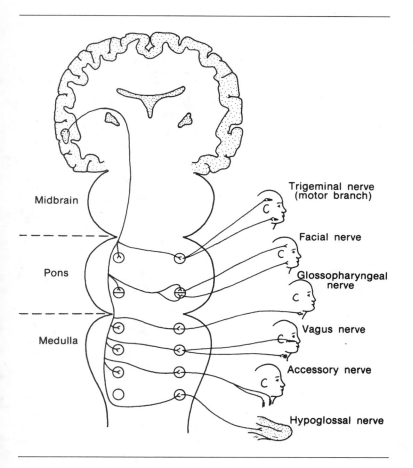

Figure A.14 Pyramidal Fibers Serving Motor Cranial Nerves of Speech

messages are being sent and monitored and fine-tuned constantly. The nervous system carries so much information so quickly with such tremendous efficiency that it makes the most sophisticated telephone systems invented by humans and hyped by Madison Avenue look like tin cans connected by kite string.

The Ear: An Energy Transformer

It is impossible to understand speech as a physiological process without considering the hearing mechanism that allows us to receive speech and monitor our own speech productions. You will quickly appreciate the importance of hearing if you consider how the child learns to talk. She does not buy a "How to Talk" manual, and she does not enroll in Human Speech 101 at the local university. She learns to talk by *listening* to the speech around her. If a child has any significant deficit in hearing, it is highly

Figure A.15 The Outer Ear

Pinna

External
auditory
meatus

likely that the acquisition of speech will be impaired. At the other end of the age spectrum, a normally speaking adult who loses hearing later in life will not lose language but may experience some deterioration in speech because he cannot hear his own productions. Articulation may not be as precise as it once was, for example, and there may be some nasality on speech sounds that are not supposed to have nasal resonance. The point is simple but important. Hearing is as crucial to normal speech as any other part of the complete anatomical and physiological speech package.

The human hearing mechanism is an extraordinary energy transformer, and tracing the changes in energy forms is one of the best ways to understand the parts of the hearing system and how they are related to one another. For the sake of convenience, we will consider the three traditional anatomic divisions of the ear—*outer, middle,* and *inner*—but it is important to note that the outer and middle ears function together to transform acoustic energy into mechanical energy.

The Outer Ear

Sound travels to the outer ear (see Figure A.15) in the form of sound waves that, as we noted in the first chapter, are disturbances of air particles characterized by compressions and rarefactions. These waves are caught by the *pinna,* the visible fleshy part of the ear attached to the side of the head. The pinna contributes minimally to our abil-

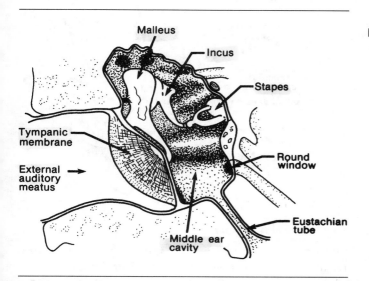

Figure A.16 The Middle Ear

ity to hear, but it does serve to direct sound waves into the **external auditory meatus** or ear canal. This canal is slightly curved, about an inch long and a quarter of an inch across, dimensions that make it a resonator specifically tuned to the frequencies of speech sounds. At the end of the canal is the **tympanic membrane** or eardrum, which serves as the boundary between the outer and middle ears.

The Middle Ear

In the middle ear (see Figure A.16), the tympanic membrane is semitransparent and is usually pearl gray when it is healthy. The center of the membrane is pulled in because it is attached to one of the tiny bones in the middle ear. The tympanic membrane absorbs the acoustic energy of sound waves and transforms it into mechanical energy, which is the vibration of a solid material.

The tiny bones in the middle ear, called the **ossicles,** are the **malleus** (hammer), **incus** (anvil), and **stapes** (stirrup). The malleus is the largest ossicle, and its "handle" is attached to the center of the tympanic membrane. The middle ossicle is the incus, which is attached to the innermost ossicle, the stapes. The bottom part of the stapes, known as the footplate because of its similarity to the footplate of the stirrup of a saddle, fits into an oval-shaped hole in the bony wall of the inner ear called the **oval window.**

The ossicles operate together in transferring energy from the tympanic membrane to the oval window and, for this reason, are often referred to as the *ossicular chain.* This chain is suspended in the air-filled cavity of the middle ear by ligaments and muscles and spans the cavity like a bridge.

Figure A.17 The Inner Ear in Relation to Middle Ear Structures

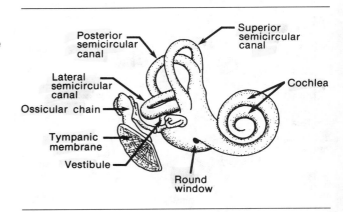

The physics involved in how the ossicular chain and the eardrum function to transfer energy from the outer to inner ears is beyond the scope of this discussion. It is enough to consider that the ossicles take all the energy captured on the surface of the tympanic membrane and focus this energy onto the much smaller surface of the oval window. The surface area difference between the eardrum and the oval window, when coupled with a lever action of the ossicles, causes an increased concentration of energy at the oval window. Perkins and Kent (1986, p. 251) have likened this to a woman wearing spike heels trying to walk across a wet lawn. Regardless of how petite she is, her total body weight will be focused on the small heels, causing them to sink into the ground. In the same way, all of the sound energy captured on the tympanic membrane is focused onto the much smaller footplate of the stapes. The increased concentration of energy achieved by the tympanic membrane and the ossicular chain is necessary to set the dense fluids of the inner ear into motion.

The Inner Ear

Although the inner ear is very small, its anatomy is complex and its functions not fully understood. Before we continue to trace hearing through the inner ear, we need to examine its anatomy. The inner ear (Figure A.17) actually serves two functions. It contains structures important to hearing, of course, but it also contains a system we use to maintain balance or equilibrium. The structures of equilibrium are called the **semicircular canals.** Even though the inner ear has two functions, the divisions are connected and share the same fluid system.

The inner ear is encased in the temporal bone of the skull. The division containing the organs of hearing is called the *cochlea,* a structure that coils about two and a half times around a cone-shaped bone called the **modiolus.** The nerve pathways from the cochlea feed into the modiolus where they merge into the **auditory nerve,** which carries hearing messages to the brain.

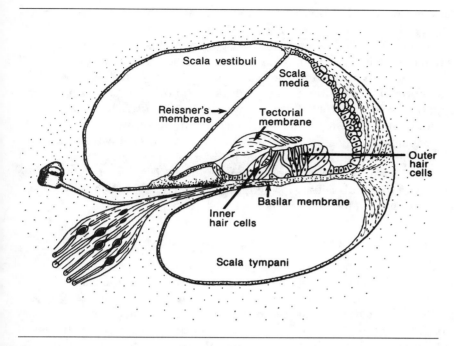

Figure A.18 Cross Section of the Cochlea

Figure A.18 shows a cross section of the cochlea. Imagine that we have uncoiled the cochlea, laid it lengthwise, and cut it. This figure shows what you would see if you looked through the cochlea as you might look through a pipe. Remember that everything you see here continues along the length of the structure. The cochlea is actually a bony tube containing two membranes that divide the tube into three sections: the **scala vestibule, scala media,** and **scala tympani.** The scala vestibule and scala media are separated by **Reissner's membrane,** and the scala media and scala tympani are separated by the **basilar membrane.** All three of these divisions are filled with fluid. The scala vestibule and scala tympani, which are connected at the top of the cochlea through a small opening called the **helicotrema,** are filled with fluid called **peri-lymph.** The fluid in the scala media is called **endolymph.**

The **organ of Corti,** sometimes called the essential or end organ of hearing, is situated along the length of basilar membrane. It consists of thousands of tiny auditory nerve receptors with **hair cells** that are the delicate final endings of the auditory nerve. These receptors and their hair cells are arranged into one inner row and three outer rows along the basilar membrane. A jellylike structure called the **tectorial membrane** hangs suspended over the tops of these highly sensitive hair cells. The tectorial membrane is a relatively free-floating membrane that responds to movements in the fluid of the scala media.

The oval window, which is occupied by the footplate of the stapes, serves as the communicating link between the middle ear and the scala vestibuli of the inner ear. The **round window** is located below the oval window and is adjacent to the scala tympani section of the inner ear. Sound vibrations enter the cochlea through the oval window. When the stapes pushes into the oval window, the mechanical energy of the ossicles is transformed into hydraulic energy in the form of fluid motion. The pressure of this motion is relieved by the round window, which moves toward the middle ear as the footplate of the stapes moves inward toward the inner ear.

There is some uncertainty about what happens next. We do know that motion of the fluids in the inner ear causes the tectorial membrane to move in a manner that somehow excites the hair cells, triggering neural impulses. The net result is that the hydraulic energy of the fluids is transformed into neural energy, which is carried by the peripheral pathways of the auditory nerve to the brain.

Tracing the Pathway of Hearing: A Brief Summary

By way of summarizing the hearing mechanism, we will follow a sound wave through the system and note the major structures of hearing along the way.

The sound wave is captured by the pinna, directed into the external auditory meatus, and strikes the surface of the tympanic membrane, setting it into vibration. This vibration is carried by the ossicles across the middle ear cavity and is focused onto the footplate of the stapes in the oval window. The inward movement of the stapes sets the perilymph of the scala vestibuli into motion, which causes Reissner's membrane to move, which then causes motion in the endolymph of the scala media. The motion of the endolymph causes movement of the tectorial membrane and movement along the basilar membrane. The motion finally makes its way along the scala tympani to the round window, which bulges slightly into the middle ear cavity. The motion of the tectorial membrane triggers neural responses in the hair cells, which are connected to the peripheral pathways of the auditory nerve. The auditory nerve carries the hearing information to the brain where it is processed.

Finally, notice the transformations of energy accomplished by the hearing mechanism. The acoustic energy of the sound wave is transformed into mechanical energy by the tympanic membrane and the ossicles. This mechanical energy is transformed into hydraulic energy by the fluids of the inner ear. The hydraulic energy is eventually transformed into neural energy by the action of the tectorial membrane and the hair cells.

The Complete Speech and Language Machine

We have now examined the anatomy and physiology, albeit briefly and superficially, of the structures that make up the speech machine. It is a complex system of systems, each part precisely and efficiently integrated with every other part and directed by a reliable and constantly adapting central nervous system. Humans are born with all this equipment, and we quickly and easily adapt it for expressing language through speech.

Review Questions

1. Identify and define the four processes of speech. How are they integrated to produce speech?
2. How does quiet breathing differ from breathing for speech?
3. What happens in a single cycle of vocal fold vibration?
4. Describe the role of resonation in speech production.
5. What are the articulators? Which are mobile and which are fixed?
6. Trace the neurological relay race from the cerebrum to the muscles of speech.
7. Trace the journey of a sound wave from the pinna to the brain.

References and Suggested Readings

Abbs, J., Gracco, V., & Cole, K. (1984). Control of multimovement coordination: Sensorimotor mechanisms in speech motor programming. *Journal of Motor Behaviors, 16,* 195.

Barlow, S., & Abbs, J. (1978, November). *Some evidence of auditory feedback contributing to the ongoing control of speech production.* Paper presented at American Speech and Hearing Association Convention, San Francisco.

Bateman, H., & Mason, R. (1984). *Applied anatomy and physiology of the speech and hearing mechanism.* Springfield, IL: Thomas.

Bell-Berti, F. (1975). Control of pharyngeal cavity size for English voiced and voiceless stops. *Journal of the Acoustical Society of America, 57,* 456–461.

Berti, F., & Hirose, H. (1975). Palatal activity in voicing distinctions: A simultaneous fiberoptic and electromyographic study. *Journal of Phonetics, 3,* 69–74.

Bless, D., & Miller, J. (1972, November). *Influence of mechanical and linguistic factors on lung volume events during speech.* Paper presented at American Speech and Hearing Association Convention, San Francisco.

Blumstein, S., & Cooper, W. (1974). Hemispheric processing of intonational contours. *Cortex, 10,* 146–158.

Borden, G. (1980). Use of feedback in established and developing speech. In N. Lass, (Ed.), *Speech and language advances in basic research and practice* (Vol. 3). New York: Academic Press.

Borden, G., & Harris, K. (1984). *Speech science primer* (2nd ed.). Baltimore: Williams & Wilkins.

Brown, J. (1975). On the neural organization of language: Thalamic and cortical relationships. *Brain and Language, 2,* 18–30.

Calvin, W., & Ojemann, G. (1980). *Inside the brain.* New York: New American Library.

Darley, F., Aronson, A., & Brown, J. (1975). *Motor speech disorders.* Philadelphia: Saunders.

Denes, P., & Pinson, E. (1993). *The speech chain* (2nd ed.). New York: Freeman.

Dimond, S., & Beaumont, J. (1974). Experimental studies of hemispheric function in the human brain. In S.

Dimond & J. Beaumont (Eds.), *Hemispheric function in the human brain.* New York: Wiley.

Fritzel, B. (1969). The velopharyngeal muscles in speech: An electromyographic and cinefluorographic study. *Acta Otolaryngology* (Stockholm), Suppl. 250.

Galaburda, A., & Sanides, F. (1980). Cytoarchitectonic organization of the human auditory cortex. *Journal of Comparative Neurology, 190,* 597–610.

Hixon, T. (1987). Respiratory function in speech. In T. Hixon (Ed.), *Respiratory function in speech and song.* Boston: College-Hill.

Hockett, C. (1960). The origins of speech. *Scientific American, 203,* 89–97.

Hoit, J., Hixon, T., Watson, P., & Morgan, W. (1990). Speech breathing in children and adolescents. *Journal of Speech and Hearing Research, 33,* 51–69.

Hollien, H. (1960a). Some laryngeal correlates of vocal pitch. *Journal of Speech and Hearing Research, 3,* 52–58.

Hollien, H. (1960b). Vocal pitch variations related to changes in vocal fold length. *Journal of Speech and Hearing Research, 3,* 150–156.

Hutchinson, J., & Putnam, A. (1974). Aerodynamic aspects of sensory deprived speech. *Journal of the Acoustical Society of America, 56,* 1612–1617.

Isshiki, N. (1959). Regulatory mechanism of the pitch and volume of voice. *Otorhinolaryngology Clinic* (Kyoto), *52,* 1065.

Isshiki, N. (1964). Regulatory mechanisms of voice intensity variation. *Journal of Speech and Hearing Research, 7,* 17–29.

Isshiki, N., & Ringel, R. (1964). Air flow during the production of selected consonants. *Journal of Speech and Hearing Research, 7,* 233–244.

Kahane, J., & Folkins, J. (1984). *Atlas of speech and hearing anatomy.* Upper Saddle River, NJ: Prentice Hall.

Kelso, J., Tuller, B., & Harris, K. (1983). A dynamic pattern perspective on the control and coordination of movement. In P. MacNeilage (Ed.), *The production of speech.* New York: Springer.

Kent, R. (1984). Brain mechanisms of speech and language with special reference to emotional interactions. In R. Naremore (Ed.), *Language science: Recent advances.* San Diego, CA: College-Hill.

Knox, C., & Kimura, D. (1970). Cerebral processing of nonverbal sounds in boys and girls. *Neuropsychologia, 8,* 227–237.

Kuehn, D., Lemme, M., & Baumgartner, J. (eds.). (1989). *Neural bases of speech, hearing, and language.* Boston: College-Hill.

Lieberman, P. (1975). *On the origins of language: An introduction to the evolution of human speech.* Series in Physical Anthropology. New York: Macmillan.

Liebman, M. (1991). *Neuroanatomy made easy and understandable* (4th ed.). Rockville, MD: Aspen.

Lubker, J. (1968). An electromyographic-cinefluorographic investigation of velar function during normal speech production. *Cleft Palate Journal, 5,* 1–18.

Marin, O., Schwartz, M., & Saffran, E. (1979). Origins and distribution of language. In M. Gazzaniga (Ed.), *Handbook of behavioral neurobiology.* New York: Plenum.

MacNeilage, P. (1970). Motor control of serial ordering of speech. *Psychological Review, 77,* 182–196.

McKeough, D. (1982). *The coloring review of neuroscience.* Boston: Little, Brown.

Millikan, C., & Darley, F. (1967). *Brain mechanisms underlying speech and language.* New York: Grune & Stratton.

Moll, K., & Daniloff, R. (1971). Investigation of the timing of velar movements during speech. *Journal of the Acoustical Society of America, 50,* 678–684.

Netsell, R., Kent, R., & Abbs, J. (1980). The organization and reorganization of speech movement. *Society of Neuroscience Abstracts, 6,* 462.

Negus, V. (1962). *The comparative anatomy and physiology of the larynx.* New York: Hafner.

Ornstein, R., & Thompson, R. (1984). *The amazing brain.* Boston: Houghton Mifflin.

Perkins, W., & Kent, R. (1986). *Functional anatomy of speech, language, and hearing: A primer.* Boston: College-Hill.

Putnam, A., & Ringel, R. (1979). Oral sensation and perception. In W. Williams & D. Goulding (Eds.), *Articulation and learning.* Springfield, IL: Thomas.

Scott, C., & Ringel, R. L. (1971). Articulation without oral sensory control. *Journal of Speech and Hearing Research, 14,* 804–818.

Subtelny, J., Oya, N., & Subtelny, J. (1972). Cineradiographic study of sibilants. *Folia Phoniatrics* (Basel), *24,* 30–50.

Sussman, H. (1979). Evidence for left hemisphere superiority in processing movement-related tonal signals. *Journal of Speech and Hearing Research, 22,* 224–235.

Tucker, D. (1981). Lateral brain function, emotion and conceptualization. *Psychological Review, 89,* 19–46.

Zemlin, W. (1988). *Speech and hearing science, anatomy and physiology* (3rd ed.). Upper Saddle River, NJ: Prentice Hall.

Zemlin, W. (1990). Anatomy and physiology of speech. In G. Shames & E. Wiig (Eds.), *Human communication disorders* (3rd ed.). Upper Saddle River, NJ: Merrill/Prentice Hall.

Name Index

Subject Index

Photo Credits